Studies in the Psychosocial

Studies in the Psychosocial seeks to investigate the ways in which psychic and social processes demand to be understood as always implicated in each other, as mutually constitutive, co-produced, or abstracted levels of a single dialectical process. As such it can be understood as an interdisciplinary field in search of transdisciplinary objects of knowledge. Studies in the Psychosocial is also distinguished by its emphasis on affect, the irrational and unconscious processes, often, but not necessarily, understood psychoanalytically. Studies in the Psychosocial aims to foster the development of this field by publishing high quality and innovative monographs and edited collections. The series welcomes submissions from a range of theoretical perspectives and disciplinary orientations, including sociology, social and critical psychology, political science, postcolonial studies, feminist studies, queer studies, management and organization studies, cultural and media studies and psychoanalysis. However, in keeping with the inter- or transdisciplinary character of psychosocial analysis, books in the series will generally pass beyond their points of origin to generate concepts, understandings and forms of investigation that are distinctively psychosocial in character.

More information about this series at
http://www.palgrave.com/gp/series/14464

Kjetil Moen

Death at Work

Existential and Psychosocial Perspectives on End-of-Life Care

palgrave
macmillan

Kjetil Moen
University of Stavanger
Stavanger, Norway

Studies in the Psychosocial
ISBN 978-3-030-07991-8 ISBN 978-3-319-90326-2 (eBook)
https://doi.org/10.1007/978-3-319-90326-2

Cover credit: Artepics/Alamy Stock Photo

Printed on acid-free paper

This Palgrave Macmillan imprint is published by the registered company Springer International Publishing AG part of Springer Nature
The registered company address is: Gewerbestrasse 11, 6330 Cham, Switzerland

To all those encountering Death at Work

—

To Daniel August, Maria Thalia and Markus Aleksander

Beautiful expressions of Life at Work

Preface

Although this book builds on a thesis and is mainly aimed at academics and students, my hope is that practitioners in various relation-intense fields will find it both accessible and rewarding. Hence, the intention has been to transform the thesis into a reader-friendly book without losing its academic qualities.

Despite being shorter than the original thesis from which it developed, the book is nonetheless long and detailed. By allowing detailed insight into the deliberations underpinning the choices made, space is offered in which the dynamics between the interviewer and interviewee, as well as between the researcher and his subject, can be explored by the reader. Though there is a rationale for the length and sequence of the chapters, there are many ways to get through the book, and the reader is of course free to find his or her own. If the philosophical underpinnings elaborated in Chapters 2 and 3 are of no value to a reader, he or she will feel free to move on to the narrative accounts in Chapters 4 through 8.

It has been noted that a problem with some qualitative studies is the absence of a clear statement linking the method used and the philosophical underpinnings that should guide it (Stubblefield & Murray, 2002). The point has also been made that qualitative studies too often fail to sufficiently describe "the narratives of the participants, the presuppositions of the researcher and the processes by which these viewpoints are merged" (Draucker, 1999, 361), thus leaving the reader without an explanation of how formulations were arrived at from the data. Even though theoretical and methodological considerations might be regarded as of interest to the few, even though a *sine qua non* for a thesis, the above considerations have prompted me to also include them in the book (Chapters 2 and 3).

Death at Work is a narrative study that takes care to linger sufficiently on how the individual makes sense of his/her world before concluding how the professionals (in the plural) are making sense of theirs. Thus, the study has an orientation that allows for in-depth analysis of narratives, in order to document uniqueness. The open interviewing strategy, the rationale of which is thoroughly discussed in Chapter 3, allows for rich, contradictory accounts with potential discrepancies between what, how and why things are said.

It is, as already pointed out, one of the temptations in qualitative research to be looking across cases and not sufficiently "within" each case, thus overlooking disconfirming cases (Booth, Carroll, Ilott, Low, & Cooper, 2013), or reading for similarities and disregarding differences in order to create wholes (Petrovskaya, 2014). An underlying premise of this study is that there is no one-to-one relation between the explicit and the implicit; rather, departing from an ontology of a defended or conflicted subject (Hollway & Jefferson, 2000), the present study takes it that there are no *a priori* grounds for assuming such a relation. Hence, effort has been made to ensure that the idiosyncrasy, the subjective, the tensions, and paradoxes inherent in the various ways the participants make sense of themselves are not lost in the process, but sufficiently accounted for in the write-up, and not difficult for the reader to identify. Allowing this amount of transparency takes an effort and requires ink and pages.

Limitations

What are regarded as the limitations of the present study depend to some degree on whether the question comes from a sociologist, a psychoanalyst, a theoretical purist, a qualitative methodologist, or someone with another point of view. The sociologist would probably point out that death trumps all other distinctions in the present study. What about gender, age, ethnicity, medical discipline, or profession? They were all inclusion criteria and served to safeguard diversity. What happened to the social distinctions in the process? They have not been ignored; even if attention is unequally distributed, they are part of the discussion. Still, the research question pursued in the following calls for particular attention to the reality of death. How the social distinctions inform the imprint left by the death of others upon the self-understanding of the professional needs to be explored in future studies.

The theoretical purist may voice concern regarding the eclectic application of theoretical perspectives. This is primarily an empirical study and theory is applied in order to elicit and interpret data. Hence, I am not exhaustively presenting or discussing any of the theoretical perspectives. Rather, parts of them are applied, not randomly, but eclectically, in order to elucidate the concerns in focus. The endeavor is to stay close to the data throughout, listening for whatever question, paradox, or contradiction that calls for elucidation and explanation. I concluded that the findings could not be adequately addressed from within any one theoretical perspective. I am neither a philosopher nor a psychoanalytic practitioner; thus, the theoretical perspectives were applied on the understanding that this is the terrain of other professionals, and thus may lack the competence of a more seasoned practitioner.

The psychoanalyst, perhaps, would voice concern that I am not sufficiently acknowledging my own contribution in the encounters with the interviewees, or in what gains importance in the analysis. It is true that there is no place from which I can speak about the other that is not inhabited by me. This insight tempers all my claims about others in the present study. There should be no doubt that whatever partial "truth" is illuminated, it is so by the particular "lantern" I choose to use, and the fact that it is I using it. My interests, inclinations, and values inform the choices I made along the way, from the very first drafts of the project proposal, through the interviews, to the final concluding remarks. It is equally true that there have been ongoing discussions with my supervisors, colleagues, and end-of-life care professionals from different disciplines, in order to challenge my understandings.

The narrative accounts offered by the interviewees may be regarded as a multitude of invitations, or open doors, to which the researcher is invited to return and explore further. I have responded to some of these invitations; different researchers would perhaps have responded to others. I have explicitly discussed my presence in the project where I thought it helpful to do so. I provide below a rationale for not engaging in further discussion of transference and countertransference. It rests on notions about the different character of research and analysis.

Biographical Interpretive Narrative Method sits well both with the nature of the study, and with my interest in narratives. There are strengths and limitations to any method; some of these are discussed in Chapter 3. As is evident in the present study, twelve in-depth interviews provide a richness to which it is difficult to do justice in the limited time and space provided. Still, the potential value of several shorter subsequent encounters is lost, though one benefit of such would be the chance to consider how the interviews themselves informed the interviewees. The multiple benefits of one long interview are presented in Chapter 3.

A gestalt analysis of four-star cases has been combined with an existential-psychosocial reading across twelve cases. What is implied in the latter is discussed in Chapters 9 and 10. "Star case" simply denotes a narrative case that is given specific attention through particularly in-depth analysis. There are obvious challenges and equally obvious benefits to such an endeavor. The write-ups of the star cases involve an immense amount of detail with the benefit that the voice of the interviewee comes through very strongly. The downside is that the elaborate engagement with the narrative implies taking the reader on tours and detours, with the danger that she/he gets lost or impatient and misses the voice of the narrator. However, with an exclusively thematic reading, one easily errs on the other side, by making idiosyncrasy less evident.

Finally, the most obvious objection to any study with this restricted number of participants is its limited generalizability. The reasons for the limited number of interviewees relates to the in-depth orientation of the study. Adding to the limited generalizability is a heterogeneity that comes with diversity serving as a selective principle. Diversity was the working principle when recruiting interviewees, choosing star cases and when allowing for disconfirming cases.

When building the philosophical scientific ground for the study in the next two chapters, the issue of generalizability is addressed in a discussion of what kind of truth claims one makes when engaging in hermeneutic phenomenology. The case was made that the present study should be read as part of a larger hermeneutical endeavor, an ongoing patchwork, an emerging understanding of the personal in the professional. As the findings are discussed, connections are made to other related studies. This has not eradicated the heterogeneity and non-generalizability of researching "wicked" scientific problems, but rather proved that it is possible to have a fruitful conversation between qualitative studies.

One way of moving beyond the limitation of generalizability is to generalize inductively through theory (Thagaard, 2013). This implies that what I identify as the most central findings within this limited study are assumed to be transferable to other similar situations and contexts; further research will bring this assumption to the test. Still, when discussing my findings with professionals in end-of-life care, they say that what I have identified through this study resonates with their own experience. This is true in my discussions with individuals and when presenting to nursing students or professionals from other disciplines. Thus, it is my experience that the concerns raised and identified through the present study resonate with a wider more general audience than the twelve participants who were kind enough to offer their narrative accounts for research purposes.

A Brief Outline

Chapter 1 presents the field of interest for this research and the research question, and argues the case for new knowledge. The need for new knowledge is related to the fact that end-of-life care has shifted away from the domestic sphere and has become a professional task within hospitals, nursing homes, and hospices. The study is then located within a broader field, and related strands of research are briefly outlined: 1. research that documents the impact of significant events and situations on health professionals' personal and professional change; 2. research connected to the concepts of Secondary Traumatization and Vicarious Traumatization, understood as direct and indirect traumatization upon encountering the threat of one's own or anothers' death, and 3. psychosocial studies that emphasize the mutual constituency of the subjective and the social, and how the two intrinsically interrelate. Similarities and differences are pointed out, and it is made evident that the present study can bridge gaps in the current literature.

Chapter 2 is a theoretical engagement with dimensions of subjectivity specifically represented in the research question. Drawing on relevant theories, the psychophysical and the psychosocial constitution of the research subject are discussed, laying the groundwork for an existential-psychosocial reading of the narrative accounts. Another point elaborated here is how the research subject is a narrative self with a personal "idiom", a characteristic way in which she/he is disposed to receive and organize experience. There is discussion of how there might be a discrepancy between the experiential and the narrative self, particularly in relation to narratives of emotionally charged situations.

The understanding of the research subject established in Chapter 2 serves as a rationale for the methodological choices, which will be thoroughly discussed in Chapter 3. The first part of this chapter establishes hermeneutic phenomenological grounds for the study, before undertaking a methodological operationalization of the understanding reached in Chapters 2 and 3. A rationale is outlined for why, after having considered different methods, I decided that biographical-narrative interviews were the appropriate means to achieve the aim of the project. Methodological and ethical concerns presented when researching previously untold narratives, and subjective realities not yet articulated, are explored and discussed.

An analysis of the narrative accounts lays the ground for the latter part of the book. It is undertaken in three separate, but related, steps in Chapters 4 through 9. The first step (Chapters 4–7) is an in-depth analysis of four individual star cases (Jacob, Eric, Karla, and Dina). The second part of the analysis (Chapter 8), which builds on the one before, is an existential-psychosocial reading across all cases. Finally, there is a convergence of the research question and the findings in a theoretical discussion of the dominant concerns identified (Chapter 9). Chapter 10, the last, rounds off the book by suggesting possible implications. The case is made that the knowledge gained can serve not only the professional and the patient, but also policy makers, educational institutions and employing organizations in whose interest it is to prepare, support, and contribute to the development of health professionals serving at the bedside of patients facing their own death.

Stavanger, Norway Kjetil Moen

References

Booth, A., Carroll, C., Ilott, I., Low, L. L., & Cooper, K. (2013). Desperately seeking dissonance: Identifying the disconfirming case in qualitative evidence synthesis. *Qualitative Health Research, 23*(1), 126–141. https://doi.org/10.1177/1049732312466295.

Draucker, C. B. (1999). The critique of Heideggerian hermeneutical nursing research. *Journal of Advanced Nursing, 30*(2), 360–373. https://doi.org/10.1046/j.1365-2648.1999.01091.x.

Hollway, W., & Jefferson, T. (2000). *Doing qualitative research differently: Free association, narrative and the interview method.* London: Sage.

Petrovskaya, O. (2014). Is there nursing phenomenology after Paley? Essay on rigorous reading. *Nursing Philosophy, 15*(1), 60–71. https://doi.org/10.1111/nup.12045.

Stubblefield, C., & Murray, R. L. (2002). A phenomenological framework for psychiatric nursing research. *Archives of Psychiatric Nursing, 16*, 149–155.

Thagaard, T. (2013). *Systematikk og innlevelse. En innføring i kvalitativ metode* [An introduction to qualitative method] (4th ed.). Bergen: Fagbokforlaget.

Acknowledgements

I want to thank the editorial board for Studies in the Psychosocial for their faith in the text—without which there would be no book. Thanks also to Grace Jackson and Joanna O'Neill at Palgrave Macmillan for guiding me—in a most professional manner—through the publishing process.

I am most grateful to the healthcare professionals who shared their narratives with me and thus made it possible to explore the central research questions pursued in this study. I sincerely treasure their contributions, and hope they find that I have treated their stories with the respect they deserve.

Though I am entirely responsible for this text, I am indebted to all those willing to discuss matters large and small whose generous and constructive feedback contributed to the evolving and maturing of the project and the text. In particular, I would like to express my sincere gratitude to Ellen Ramvi, advisor on the thesis upon which this book rests, for sharing so generously of her time, knowledge and enthusiasm. Lynn Froggett, my second advisor, similarly engaged with me on issues both small and large and generously offered her perceptiveness and insights. Their stimulating questions as well as their ability to see the promise in my half-baked and imperfect drafts were invaluable.

Tom Wengraf introduced me to narrative research in the most inspiring way. I very much appreciate his generous and valuable inputs early in the process, as well as his comments on the final draft. Thomas Skovholt offered input and was a most valued mentor as I turned the thesis into a book. Due to Thomas' hospitality, I enjoyed a fruitful stay at the University of Minnesota in Minneapolis, USA, as part of this adventure. Minneapolis is also where I did my chaplaincy training almost two decades ago and, I believe, where some of the first seeds of this book where sown. In particular, I treasure the contributions of Richard D. Sellers and Laura J. Kelley, my supervisors at Abbott Northwestern Hospital and Fairview-University Hospital, respectively.

I am grateful to all those who took time away from their own projects to engage in mine, not least those participating in the panels. My research group, Professional Relations in Welfare Professions, at the University of Stavanger provided me with an academic home during this journey. Thanks are due especially to two members of this group: Marta Høyland Lavik for reading through the whole text and offering valuable inputs that undoubtedly improved it, and Birgitta Haga Gripsrud for helping to discuss key aspects of its form. The research group in Psychology of Religion also provided valuable encouragement and critical readings along the way. Thanks are due in particular to Gry Stålsett for reading and commenting on the whole text.

Thanks to the University of Stavanger, and in particular to the Faculty of Health Sciences, for funding the thesis and also for contributing to it becoming a book. I am particularly grateful to Kari Vevatne, the former dean, who provided me with the best possible work conditions. I am most grateful to Lesley Marks, who language proofed the entire text and whose contribution is invaluable.

In all the above encounters, the welcoming, gracious, and constructive spirit with which I was met left me with a sense of having encountered the very best of the academic community.

I also extend my appreciation to the Stavanger University Hospital, in particular to Sverre Uhlving and Leif Lie-Bjelland, who made it possible for me to combine research with the position as Secretary of the

Clinical Ethics Committee at the hospital. I treasure the continuous feedback to my research from the many end-of-life care professionals I encounter when I am lecturing, facilitating reflection groups, or working at the bedside—health professionals who continue to educate me about how encounters with death and dying make an impact on the professional.

Thanks to family and friends for providing me with fulfilling encounters, without expectations of quotes and references. Last, but not least, my deepest appreciation goes to my wife, Hege Kristin, and to our children Daniel August, Maria Thalia, and Markus Aleksander for being my life in so many wonderful ways.

Sandnes, Norway Kjetil Moen
March 2018

Contents

1
Introduction

Live the questions now. Perhaps you will then gradually, without noticing it, live along some distant day into the answer.

Rainer Maria Rilke

One No Longer Dies at Home

Throughout the centuries, death and dying have taken place in the context of the home and community in which the dying person's life was lived—among family, friends, and neighbors. About a hundred years ago, this gradually started to change and it can be argued, at least in Western societies, that death has moved out of the home. For most of the population, the process of dying and the actual moment of death currently take place in the contexts of hospitals, nursing homes, and hospices. End-of-life care has become an acknowledged discipline within mainstream medicine and thus predominantly the art of professionals who are dealing with death at work (Ariès, 1976).

This shift, whereby the initiative for care of the dying has been passed from community, family, and friends to professionals, is accompanied by a growing expectation that end-of-life care professionals should tend

K. Moen, *Death at Work*, Studies in the Psychosocial,
https://doi.org/10.1007/978-3-319-90326-2_1

not only to the physical, but also to the psychological and spiritual needs of the patient (Kearney, 2000; WHO, 2016). Consequently, facilitating processes that used to take place in the home, initiated by the family, now engender an expectation of "use of self" (Froggett, Ramvi, & Davies, 2014) on the part of the professional. One might say this is a personal investment, required and constitutive in all relational-intense professions. Yet, there are reasons to question whether not encounters with death and dying actualize the personal in the professional in particular ways that call for further investigation.

Literature, both prose (Frankl, 1964; Kubler-Ross, 1973; Noyes, 1980; Van Laarhoven, Schilderman, Vissers, Verhagen, & Prins, 2010; Yalom, 1998, 2008) and fiction (Tolstoy, 1989; Gustafsson, 1981; Skelton, 2003), testifies to how encountering one's own imminent death, or realizing one's own mortality due to near-death experiences, can inform or alter a human being's understanding of self and life. From this, a case can be made suggesting that death informs life, sometimes in subtle and profound ways (Baumeister, 1986, 189–207; Becker, 1973; Kiser, 2015; Snyder & Forsyth, 1991). The present study explores whether daily encounters with the death of others, as part of one's professional work, may offer comparable experiences and similarly profound impacts.

Questions of Social Importance

Studies indicate that health professionals in end-of-life care are subject not only to meaningful encounters with dying patients and their relatives, but also to emotional and existential stress. There is an implicit risk of experiencing burnout (Candrian, 2014; Kalicińska, Chylińska, & Wilczek-Różyczka, 2012; Martins Pereira, Fonseca, & Sofia Carvalho, 2011; Van Mol, Kompanje, Benoit, Bakker, & Nijkamp, 2015) that might make the professionals consider leaving their jobs (Cummings, 2011), or encourage them to distance themselves emotionally (Menzies-Lyth, 1988), or leave them in emotional states that affect their ability to recognize the emotional and existential needs of the patient (Agledahl, Førde, & Wifstad, 2011). How the above reactions may relate to what is particular to end-of-life care, namely encountering death at work, is a most relevant, yet largely unaddressed, question.

An exploration of the potential impact upon the professional of encountering death is important to society. First, because the population is growing older with an accompanying rise in the prevalence of cancer (Engeland, Bjørge, & Brunborg, 2015; Kaasa, 2008). Hence, there will likely be an increasing need for health professionals willing to make their living in the "boundary" zone between life and death. Second, because understanding the impact of encountering death on the professional is crucial when considering what measures are required to prepare, sustain, and develop the end-of-life care professionals; such measures must be grounded on empirically based knowledge.

Following the above, there is one pressing question that must be subject to empirical investigation namely: How, if at all, do daily encounters with the death of patients inform the personal and professional self-understanding of the end-of-life care professional?

The aim of this study is to pursue this question and contribute to empirically based knowledge of how encounters with dying patients might inform the health professional's understanding of his/her personal self *and* professional role. Empirical investigation will examine whether and how daily encounters with the death of patients inform the personal and professional self-understanding of the end-of-life care professional and how the informant's past and present social contexts inform individual existential and emotional processes. I will use an existential-psychosocial approach, understood as simultaneous focus on the mandatory basic conditions and psychosocial constitutions of the subject, to pursue the following research question: **How do encounters with the death of others inform the health professionals' understanding of themselves as well as their professional role?**

In order to investigate the research question, two accompanying, interrelated, questions serve to frame the enquiry. The first underscores the hermeneutic phenomenological character of the endeavor and the interest for the experiencing professional. This is not limited to focusing on what is told, but also on the manner of telling: How do health professionals describe and reflect upon encounters with patients and families who are confronted with their own death? The second, like the first, is an explication of the contextualist position of the study, outlined in the next chapter, namely: How do discourses present in the social contexts in which the health professional is situated inform both the experiences at the boundary between life and death and the narration of the same?

I will elaborate and discuss these questions in the following chapters. The point made here is that the questions imply two interrelated hypotheses that can and will be subject to empirical investigation, namely that the descriptions and understandings of the health professionals implicate both subjective dispositions and contextual factors. This dual aspect and challenge—to try to grasp both the inner experience and the prevailing context—place this study within the larger emergent field of psychosocial studies (Clarke, Hahn, & Hoggett, 2008; Froggett, 2002; Hollway & Jefferson, 2000; Ramvi, 2007), which will be introduced more thoroughly below.

Professional Contexts in Focus

The study relates to the medical disciplines of palliative care and acute care. According to the WHO, "Palliative care is an approach that improves the quality of life of patients and their families facing the problem associated with life-threatening illness, through the prevention and relief of suffering by means of early identification and treatment of pain and other problems, physical, psychosocial and spiritual" (WHO, 2016). Acute care, on the other hand, is about providing emergency services and general medical and surgical treatment for acute disorders rather than long-term residential care for chronic or long-term illness. Acute care is provided as pre-hospital care, in emergency rooms and different kinds of intensive care units (general, pediatric, cardiac, etc.).

The main reason for choosing to locate my research in these particular contexts is that both have as a constitutive element, to a larger degree than other medical fields, professional encounters with patients faced with their own death. At the same time, they are quite different in character. In acute care, the focus is primarily on saving lives. When there is a shift toward end-of-life care, the health professionals will most often relate to family members, not the sedated patient. In the palliative unit, the focus is more on end-of-life care than curative care, and the health professionals relate more often directly to the patient. Each setting facilitates different kinds of professional relationships with patients in boundary situations. Even though the present work is not a comparative study, I find that including both provides an empirical breadth and descriptive "thickness" (Geertz, 1973) to the exploration of how encountering death and dying of patients might inform the self-understanding of the professional.

Empirical Setting and Criteria for Selection

I recruited interviewees that fit the following categories: four nurses, four physicians, and four chaplains, of whom six are male and six female; all participants have a minimum of one year's experience in their respective roles. The interviewees represent three professions that are all present, in different roles, by the bed of the terminally ill and dying patient. Different professions are included in order to provide a thick description of the phenomena in focus. The rationale for including three professions and both genders is that information is found in differences (Bateson, 1972).

A nurse, a physician, and a chaplain in end-of-life care will all be exposed to the death of others, but will potentially have different experiences and understandings due to their different professional disciplines. For example, it could be argued that the physicians' understandings and experiences are colored by their biomedical training, the nurses' by their focus on care for the whole patient, and the chaplains' by their primary attention to spiritual issues. What these professional roles have in common is the expectation that they relate actively to the fact that the patient is dying and to the meaning this carries for the individual. This would also be true of other professions, not least social work (Murty, Sanders, & Stensland, 2015), and to some degree also physical therapy and occupational therapy (Pizzi, 2014). Yet, the in-depth orientation of the project requires a limitation of its scope.

Methodologial Considerations

Phenomenology is an appropriate approach when the objective is exploring the self-understanding of health workers engaged in end-of-life care. It takes the subjective experience as a point of departure, has a first-person approach, seeks "the native's point of view" (Geertz, 1973), and is committed to describing reality as experienced by, and in the terms of, the interviewee (Gallagher & Zahavi, 2008; Thagaard, 2013).

However, my project is not solely aimed at description, but also understanding, which brings hermeneutics into the picture. Hermeneutics is more than a methodological approach, it is more of an attitude and has as a basic assumption that the only way to understanding is through interpretation. Understanding is created in circular movements, in a dialogue between the whole and its parts, in which understandings are challenged by new information and in which the researcher's own preconceived ideas and understandings must be taken into consideration (Gadamer, 1989; Heidegger, 2002; Thagaard, 2013).

Linked to this is another basic assumption, namely that understanding and meaning can only be reached through taking into consideration the interviewee's prevailing context(s), resting on the notion that the psychic and the social are mutually constitutive. A psychosocial approach entails both the application of psychoanalytic theory, but also any theoretical endeavor acknowledging the mutual constituency of the psychic and the social. In the case of this study, it particularly implies inclusion of the fundamental ontology of Martin Heidegger. The philosophical and theoretical basis for the hermeneutic phenomenological design will be elaborated and discussed in Chapters 2 and 3. Its application will be made evident in Chapters 4 through 10.

Locating the Study Within a Broader Field

Although the current literature is not devoid of significant individual voices addressing the concerns of the end-of-life care professional—not least related to the notion of "Whole Person Care" (Hutchinson, 2011; Kearney, 2000)—I have not identified any established line of empirical research pertaining to how the death of others informs the self-understanding of professionals. In order to place this study within a larger field of research and address questions pertaining to how it will contribute to knowledge, I have identified fields of research that are similar in scope.

There are significant strands within the field of professional development, not least those pertaining to *The Reflective Practitioner* (Schön, 1991) and *Situated Learning* (Lave & Wenger, 1991) which are relevant. In what follows though, particular attention will be given to studies within the helping professions that explore issues key to this study, namely relations between clinical experience and the evolving subjectivity of the professional. Initially, I will give attention to two such lines of research: those of Benner and of Skovholt and Rønnestad, both of which relate to concerns in my study.

In addition, by discussing the concept of trauma and its relation to death, I will explore how this endeavor both resembles and differs from research on secondary traumatization. Finally, at the core of this inquiry, there is a recognition of inter-subjectivity. Psychosocial studies (Clarke et al., 2008; Hollway & Jefferson, 2000; Walkerdine, 2008) is an emerging field of research that both theoretically and methodologically encompasses this central point. Again, I elaborate not only the points of connection, but also those serving to distinguish my study from others in this particular field.

Personal and Professional Change

The work of Patricia Benner, nursing theorist and educator, serves as a starting point for the exploration of two lines of research on professional development relevant to this study. Benner has a particular interest in the nurse (Benner, 1984), as well as in learning across the health professions (Benner & Sutphen, 2007). In addition, she has an interpretive phenomenological orientation that corresponds with this study (Benner, 1994) and, similar to this study, aims to gain insights that can provide principles for the formation of students in health care professions (Benner, 2011).

A particular point of correspondence is that, in her groundbreaking study *From Novice to Expert* (1984), Benner invites health professionals to share events and situations that have been particularly important to them. "Paradigm cases", as she calls the kind of experiences that become precedents for later practice, are foundational incidents marked by challenge, success, failure, or emotions that make the health professional reflect in a way that changes assumptions, values, and beliefs (Benner, 1984). Benner thus links meaning-making—changes in assumptions, values, and beliefs—to emotionally charged professional situations. This study has a similar interest in particular incident narratives (PIN), but provides the interviewees with an open-ended invitation. This is a distinguishing point and relates to the interest demonstrated here for considering the professional in a biographical context—a point elaborated in Chapter 3.

Another line of research on professional development, situated in another relation-intense field, namely within the professional context of psychotherapy and counseling, is for a shared interest in the life span of the professional. The research and accumulated insights of Professor Thomas Skovholt and Professor Helge Rønnestad on professional development (Rønnestad & Skovholt, 2013) are applied in various fields and professions around the world (Skovholt & Trotter-Mathison, 2011). The authors point out that, since their initial work almost 25 years ago and up until their last book, "few studies have emerged that have provided empirically based models for professional development with the focus on the entire professional life cycle of the practitioner" (Rønnestad & Skovholt, 2013, 4).

What specifically links their line of research to the present study is a shared understanding of professional development, not least in that the authors argue the importance of use of self for the quality of professional work. Their main interest is not merely on *how* the professional is functioning in executing the professional tasks, but *who* it is that inhabits the professional role. Learning to know the professional self should take priority, because the "who" informs the "how", according to the authors. In the discussion within their field on the question of "common factors versus specific factors of psychotherapy", they side with the importance of "the contribution of the therapist to the therapy/counseling outcome" (ibid.). As in this study, they place the professional self center-stage and "appreciate the deeply personal nature of being a practitioner" (ibid.).

Building on Lerner's comprehensive review of the theory of psychological development, they make the case that claims can be made about practitioners' development. Lerner states that the common features of development, "regardless of philosophical and theoretical orientation (a) development always implies change of some sort, (b) the change is organized systematically, and (c) the change involves succession over time" (Rønnestad & Skovholt, 2013, 10).

This study is also about extrapolating from narrative accounts an evolving subjectivity that is organized systematically and that involves succession over time. However, the main inclusion criterion for this study is heterogeneity: Interviewees of different gender and age, from different empirical fields, professions, and even countries, are included such that complexity and heterogeneity mark the endeavor. Kaplan states that "if the preconceptions are many and complex, and if the findings are similarly complex and diverse, then determining whether the changes can meaningfully be described as developmental becomes more difficult" (Kaplan in Lerner, 1983, 185–227).

Benner is presenting a model of developmental phases (novice—advanced beginner—competent—proficient—expert), so too Rønnestad and Skovholt ("phases of practitioner development") (Rønnestad & Skovholt, 2013, 55). They all share an interest in "skilled performance", "expertise", "the know how acquired through experience" (Benner, 1984, 3), and what may be called professional competencies and levels of functioning (Jennings & Skovholt, 1999; Rønnestad & Skovholt, 2013, 9; Skovholt, 2012).

This does not imply a lack of recognition by any of the researchers of the individual, idiosyncratic, complex, or contradictory elements (Benner, 2011; Skovholt, Hage, Kachgal, & Gama, 2007; Trotter-Mathison, Koch, Sanger, & Skovholt, 2010).

There are multiple points of connection to the above lines of research. What distinguishes this study from the above is that, more than being interested in developmental stages and levels of professional functioning, it is seeking to identify existential concerns that may, or may not, relate to the existential phenomena of death encountered in professional practice. This orientation brings us to an exploration of a second relevant line of research, namely that of secondary traumatization.

Secondary Traumatization

In the *Diagnostic and Statistical Manual of Mental Disorders*, trauma is understood as involving actual, or threat of, death. In order to earn the designation "traumatic", events must create reactions of intense fear, intense helplessness, or intense horror. Hence, when Ronnie Janoff-Bulman offers an understanding of trauma as "an event that shatters people's assumptions", she allows for one being traumatized by life as well as by death. Janoff-Bulman thus provides legitimacy to the concept of secondary traumatization (Brewin, 2003).

Mirroring this dual-dimensional thinking regarding trauma, Susanne Bang claims that traumatization of professionals can come directly following either the attack on, or threat to, the life of the professional, or indirectly by being exposed to the traumatization of others (Bang, 2003, 143ff). Secondary traumatization is a phenomenon that affects the professional helper as a result of an indirect existential shock through exposure to the client's experience or narrative (ibid., 89). It is the latter and the notion of an indirect trauma which makes secondary trauma a relevant concept for this study. Burnout, which partially overlaps with respect to symptoms (contact fatigue, compassion fatigue), is a result of the extent of contact with all sorts of people, while secondary traumatization is exclusively related to work with traumatized clients.

Vicarious trauma (VT) is often used interchangeably with secondary traumatization, compassion fatigue, burnout, and emotional contagion. What VT shares with the other phenomena is its concern with the process through which the helper's inner experience is negatively transformed through empathic engagement with the client's traumatic material. However, Pearlman and Cann suggest that VT is unique in that its focus is on the impact trauma has on the individual's psychological development, adaption, and identity rather than on symptoms, which is more applicable to other concepts encompassing secondary traumatization.

According to Pearlman and Saakvitne, people's unique individual experiences of trauma include, "changes in the individual's (1) frame of reference, or usual way of understanding self and the world, including spirituality, (2) capacity to modulate affect and maintain benevolent inner connection with self and others" (Pearlman & Saakvitne, 1995, 60–61). The first point echoes Janoff-Bulman's understanding of trauma. The second mirrors Pearlman and Saakvitne's claim that definitions of trauma often have a cognitive, behavioral, or biological orientation, and thus "often underemphasized the interaction between the traumatic event and the particular individual experiencing it" (ibid., 36).

Similarly to the present study, VT, as outlined by Pearlman and Saakvitne, includes both the affective and the cognitive effects of exposure to trauma. The authors point out how psychoanalytic theory, not least object-relational theories, has contributed to trauma therapy. They identify significant parallel lines of development central to both psychoanalysis and current trauma theory (ibid., 37). These include the relation between childhood trauma and adult symptomatology, recognition of various states of consciousness such as repression and dissociation, and finally, the concept of transference and counter-transference.

The term "vicarious traumatization" was introduced by Pearlman and Saakvitne in relation to therapists working with sexually traumatized individuals, but how does it correspond to other relation-intense fields? Does the profound impact of the other's trauma on professionals in psychotherapy correspond to what is the central interest of this study, namely the impact of encountering the other's death on professionals in end-of-life care? Sabin-Farrell and Turpin make the point that the degree of application to other occupational groups is unclear, as research on VT has primarily been carried out exclusively with professionals working with trauma victims (Sabin-Farrell & Turpin, 2003, 474).

In a more recent study, Sinclair and Hamill suggest that vicarious traumatization is a relevant concept not only for mental health, but also for understanding the experiences of oncology nurses (Sinclair & Hamill, 2007). Their argument rests on the fact that in 1994 Post Traumatic Stress Disorder (PTSD) was expanded to include reactions to diagnosis and life-threatening illness. In addition, they point to other studies showing that PTSD symptomatology is a significant concern in cancer populations (McGrath, 1999), and finally, they add what they themselves have observed of changes taking place in colleagues at their oncology ward (Sinclair & Hamill, 2007, 354).

A recent systematic review of literature (Van Mol et al., 2015), related to emotional distress among health care professionals in the ICU, included over 1600 studies reporting the prevalence of VT, alongside burnout, compassion fatigue, and secondary traumatic stress. Despite acknowledging the risk of emotional distress, the authors conclude that "the true magnitude" of the above "remains unclear". They relate this to the fact that "the reported prevalence of emotional distress differed based on the applied measurement instruments". Hence, they call for a "gold standard" to be used in future research (Van Mol et al., 2015, 14ff).

This corresponds with Sabin-Farrell and Turpin who conclude their literature review in a quite sobering way, stating, "the evidence for VT in trauma workers is inconsistent and ambiguous" (Sabin-Farrell & Turpin, 2003, 472). They too relate the inconsistency to "difficulties surrounding the research methods, instruments, and selection of participants within the studies of VT" (ibid., 467). However, they also suggest that to "label the distress as PTSD-related symptoms might also further stretch the diagnostic limits regarding PTSD and the requirement that, generally, individuals need to be exposed directly to trauma". The authors thus implicitly question the value of expanding the notion of trauma. In their discussion, they attempt to "disentangle VT and its proposed PTSD symptoms from alternative explanations involving normal distress to trauma and occupational stress arising within the workplace" (ibid., 452).

There are obvious points of connection between the present study and research on VT. An understanding of trauma that relates to both death and life, as outlined above, serves as one such possible example. The focus on in-depth research that encompasses both the cognitive and the emotional, the explicit and the implicit, is another; mutual recognition for the intersubjective and the relevance made of psychoanalytic theory add to the relatedness. The constructivist self-development theory (CSDT), on which Pearlman and Saakvitne rely, encompasses both the self-capacities of the subject and the cultural context(s) in which she/he lives. This resembles the understanding and centrality of the psychosocial that marks the present study and will be elaborated further when engaging the last line of research presented and discussed below.

Nonetheless, the differences from this endeavor are significant. Death, not trauma, is the central term in the present study which calls for a more open-ended, phenomenological exploration of experience, and subjectivity, rather than a search for stress and trauma. Finally, the empirical field does not overlap sufficiently to regard VT as anything more than a related line of research.

Psychosocial Studies

Psychosocial studies, the last strand of research discussed in this part of the chapter, shares an interest with the present study in the subjective and the social, and how they intrinsically relate, as well as in the application of psychoanalytic theory outside the clinic (Fotaki, Long, & Schwartz, 2012; Frosh, 2010). This points to the relational turn that has taken place within psychoanalysis (Clarke et al., 2008, xiii), relating to "the development of a constructivist two-person vs. one-person psychology" (ibid., 4). In a psychoanalytic context, the relational turn rests on the idea that the family is only one of the systems affecting the psyche. It is marked by a merging of perspectives of sociology and psychoanalytic theory (ibid., 113ff) and informed by important psychoanalytical forebears, systems theory, structuralism and other paradigms, as well as social movements between the 1950s and 1970s. The next chapter will elaborate on the theoretical foundations and in particular on object-relational theory.

A psychosocial approach views the subjective experience as simultaneously individual, embodied, relational, and social. Eschewing reductionism vis-à-vis both the psychic and the social, psychosocial studies are committed to finding ways to explore the mutual dependency of the two (Hollway & Froggett, 2013; Olesen, 2013), thus making the relational and the mutual constituency of the subjective and the social their distinguishing focus:

> It is a combination of this kind, between a rigorous awareness of the constructing activity of social processes and an equally potent analysis of the agentic struggles of individual subjects, that is needed in order to be able to explore how specific subject positions come to be held. (Frosh, Phoenix, & Pattman, 2003)

Thus, this approach disrupts binary thinking and focuses on exploring ways of understanding that do not reduce explanations to either the psychological or the social; nor does it locate these explanations in "the individual" or "society", or in "internal" or "external" worlds (Hollway & Froggett, 2013). It fundamentally challenges constructivist and solipsist notions of subjectivity by eliciting how fundamentally and intersubjectively constituted even the most self-proclaimed individualist is (Roseneil, 2009). This corresponds with the "contextualist" position central to this study and outlined in the next chapter. It moves beyond the impasses of either constructionism or essentialism, a conception that provides space for self-reflection in which to consider what is mine and what belongs to the other.

Psychosocial studies is a relevant line of research to the present study, not least because it entails in-depth hermeneutics that draw attention to a psychodynamic dimension of symbolic activity, meaning-making, and social agency. It is open to the notion that "even autobiographical narratives or other subjective accounts of learning and experience unintendedly involve psychodynamic aspects such as selective memory, idealizing, self-presentations and unconscious emotional engagements" (Olesen, 2013).

Finally, within the field of psychosocial studies, there is concern for the professional in relation-intense welfare professions (Clarke et al., 2008; Froggett, 2002)—a concern that corresponds with those central to the present study, namely the relations between the outer and inner, the social and the psychic. Taking postwar Britain as a point of departure, Paul Hoggett, Professor of Social Policy, problematizes the implicit understandings of the subject in the various ideological underpinnings of the social welfare system, particularly the lack of recognition for the other as an experiencing subject—either she/he is viewed as an autonomous agent or lacking agency. Hoggett also addresses the reductionism of the "professional" subject either into an "expert" or "a servant": "What is missing is a concept of a loving and hating subject with an internal world that comprises real and imagined relations" (Clarke et al., 2008, 70).

Lynn Froggett, Professor of Psychosocial Welfare, in her study "Love, Hate and Welfare: Psychosocial Approaches to Policy and Practice", also addresses the problem of who the subject becomes in past and present social welfare systems. She underscores the "thinness" and reductionism, the implicit problems of "othering" and being "done to" (Froggett, 2002, 93), that come not only with former paternalistic approaches, but also with the new more "empowering" strategies. Froggett proposes the importance of a more relational model than is presently available to underpin practice. She states: "what appears to be lacking in much current practice is an understanding of the generative intersubjective space… one that implies seeing the other as an equivalent centre of subjective experience… one that involves the ability to apprehend the separate positions of self and other, while acknowledging the interdependence between both parties" (ibid., 89ff).

An Existential-Psychosocial Approach

In significant ways, this study relates to the lines of research briefly outlined above. I find in all a shared interest for the personal in the professional and the impact of relational work. Yet, engaging them separately also elicits what distinguishes this study from these fields of research and thus also what its particular contribution may be. Specifically, I have yet to identify within any of the bodies of research referred to, the central concern of this endeavor, namely how working with the death of others in palliative care or intensive care may inform the self-understanding of end-of-life care professionals.

This study is interested in both how the trauma and terror of life itself (Hayes, Schimel, Arndt, & Faucher, 2010) and the social situatedness are incorporated in the narrative accounts of the interviewees. Thus, there is an interest in both existential and psychosocial perspectives. The phenomenological endeavor is to identify how "existential concerns" (Tillich, 1951, 2000) are informed by both. This calls for a complementary expansion of the perspectives briefly outlined above to include not only more voices within psychoanalytic theory, but existential philosophy (Heidegger, 2010), and existential psychology (Becker, 1973; Stolorow, 2011; Tillich, 1951; Yalom, 2008); traditions and voices held together in what I call an existential-psychosocial perspective, the theoretical grounds for which are elaborated in the next chapter and applied in my reading of the narrative accounts.

References

Agledahl, K. M., Førde, R., & Wifstad, Å. (2011). Courteous but not curious: How doctors' politeness masks their existential neglect. A qualitative study of video-recorded patient consultations. *Journal of Medical Ethics, 37*, 650–654.

Ariès, P. (1976). *Western attitudes toward death: From the middle ages to the present.* London: Marion Boyars.

Bang, S. (2003). *Rørt, rammet og rystet: faglig vekst gjennom veiledning* [Professional growth through supervision]. Oslo: Gyldendal akademisk.

Bateson, G. (1972). *Steps to an ecology of mind.* Chicago and London: The University of Chicago Press.

Baumeister, R. F. (1986). *Public self and private self.* New York: Springer.

Becker, E. (1973). *The denial of death.* New York: Free Press.

Benner, P. (1984). *From novice to expert: Excellence and power in clinical nursing practice.* Upper Saddle River, NJ: Prentice Hall.

Benner, P. (1994). *Interpretive phenomenology: Embodiment, caring, and ethics in health and illness.* Thousand Oaks, CA: Sage.

Benner, P. (2011). Formation in professional education: An examination of the relationship between theories of meaning and theories of the self. *Journal of Medicine and Philosophy, 36*(4), 342–353.

Benner, P., & Sutphen, M. (2007). Learning across the professions: The clergy, a case in point. *Journal of Nursing Education, 46*(3), 103–108.

Brewin, C. R. (2003). *Posttraumatic stress disorder: Malady or myth?* New Haven, CT: Yale University Press.

Candrian, C. (2014). Taming death and the consequences of discourse. *Human Relations, 67*(1), 53–69, 17p. https://doi.org/10.1177/0018726713485472.

Clarke, S., Hahn, H., & Hoggett, P. (2008). *Object relations and social relations: The implications of the relational turn in psychoanalysis.* London: Karnac.

Cummings, C. L. (2011). What factors affect nursing retention in the acute care setting. *Journal of Research in Nursing, 16*(6), 489–500.

Engeland, A., Bjørge, T., & Brunborg, G. (2015, April 9). *Kreft i Norge - Folkehelserapporten 2014* [Cancer in Norway—The public health report 2014]. Retrieved from http://www.fhi.no/eway/default.aspx?pid=239&trg=Content_7242&Main_6157=7239:0:25,8904&MainContent_7239=7242:0:25,8906&Content_7242=7244:110413::0:7243:3:::0:0#eHandbook1104133.

Fotaki, M., Long, S., & Schwartz, H. S. (2012). What can psychoanalysis offer organization studies today? Taking stock of current developments and thinking about future directions. *Organization Studies, 33*(9), 1105–1120. https://doi.org/10.1177/0170840612448152.

Frankl, V. E. (1964). *Man's search for meaning: An introduction to logotherapy.* London: Hodder & Stoughton.

Froggett, L. (2002). *Love, hate and welfare—Psycho-social approaches to policy and practice.* Great Britain: The Policy Press.

Froggett, L., Ramvi, E., & Davies, L. (2014). Thinking from experience in psycho-social practice: Reclaiming and teaching 'Use of Self'. *Journal of Social Work Practice*. https://doi.org/10.1080/02650533.2014.923389.
Frosh, S. (2010). *Psychoanalysis outside the clinic: Interventions in psycho-social studies*. Basingstoke: Palgrave Macmillan.
Frosh, S., Phoenix, A., & Pattman, R. (2003). Taking a stand: Using psychoanalysis to explore the positioning of subjects in discourse. *British Journal of Social Psychology, 42*(1), 39–53. https://doi.org/10.1348/014466603763276117.
Gadamer, H.-G. (1989). *Truth and method* (2nd, rev. ed. translation revised by J. Weinsheimer and D. G. Marshall). London: Sheed & Ward.
Gallagher, S., & Zahavi, D. (2008). *The phenomenological mind: An introduction to philosophy of mind and cognitive science*. London and New York: Routledge.
Geertz, C. (1973). *The interpretation of culture*. London: Fontana Press.
Gifford, S. (1969). Some psychoanalytic theories about death: A selective historical review. *Annals of the New York Academy of Sciences, 164*(3), 638–668.
Gustafsson, L. (1981). *The death of a beekeeper*. New York: New Directions.
Hayes, J., Schimel, J., Arndt, J., & Faucher, E. H. (2010). A theoretical and empirical review of the death-thought accessibility concept in terror management research. *Psychological Bulletin, 136*(5), 699–739. https://doi.org/10.1037/a0020524.
Heidegger, M. (2002). *On time and being*. Chicago: University of Chicago Press.
Heidegger, M. (2010). *On time and being*. Albany: State University of New York Press.
Hollway, W., & Froggett, L. (2013). Researching in-between subjective experience and reality. *Historical Social Research, 38*(2), 140–157.
Hollway, W., & Jefferson, T. (2000). *Doing qualitative research differently: Free association, narrative and the interview method*. London: Sage.
Hutchinson, T. A. (2011). *Whole person care*. New York: Springer.
Jennings, L., & Skovholt, T. M. (1999). The cognitive, emotional, and relational characteristics of master therapists. *Journal of Counseling Psychology, 46*(1), 3–11. https://doi.org/10.1037/0022-0167.46.1.3.
Kaasa, S. (2008). *Palliasjon: Nordisk lærebok* [Palliation: Nordic textbook]. Oslo: Gyldendal akademisk.
Kalicińska, M., Chylińska, J., & Wilczek-Różyczka, E. (2012). Professional burnout and social support in the workplace among hospice nurses and midwives in Poland. *International Journal of Nursing Practice, 18*(6), 595–603, 599p. https://doi.org/10.1111/ijn.12003.

Kearney, M. (2000). *A place of healing: Working with suffering in living and dying*. Oxford: Oxford University Press.

Kiser, B. (2015). The worm at the core: On the role of death in life. *Nature, 522*(7544), 33.

Kubler-Ross, E. (1973). *On death and dying*. Hoboken: Taylor & Francis.

Lave, J., & Wenger, E. (1991). *Situated learning: Legitimate peripheral participation*. Cambridge: Cambridge University Press.

Lerner, R. M. (1983). *Developmental psychology: Historical and philosophical perspectives*. Mahwah, NJ: L. Erlbaum Associates.

Martins Pereira, S., Fonseca, A. M., & Sofia Carvalho, A. (2011). Burnout in palliative care: A systematic review. *Nursing Ethics, 18*(3), 317–326. https://doi.org/10.1177/0969733011398092.

McGrath, P. (1999, July 1). Posttraumatic stress and the experience of cancer: A literature review. *Journal of Rehabilitation, 65*(3), 17.

Menzies-Lyth, I. ([1960] 1988). The function of social systems as a defence against anxiety in selected essays: *Containing anxiety in institutions* (vol. 1, pp. 43–48). London: Free Association Books. (The function of social systems as a defence against anxiety: A report on a study of the nursing service of a general hospital, first published in *Human Relations* (1960) 13: 95–121.)

Murty, S. A., Sanders, S., & Stensland, M. (2015). End-of-life care as a field of practice in the social work curriculum. *Journal of Social Work in End-of-Life and Palliative Care, 11*(1), 11–26. https://doi.org/10.1080/15524256.2015.1021071.

Noyes, R., Jr. (1980). Attitude change following near-death experiences. *Psychiatry, 43*(3), 234–242.

Olesen, H. S. (2013). The societal nature of subjectivity: An interdisciplinary methodological challenge. *Historical Social Research, 38*(2), 7–25.

Pearlman, L. A., & Saakvitne, K. W. (1995). *Trauma and the therapist: Countertransference and vicarious traumatization in psychotherapy with incest survivors*. New York: Norton.

Pizzi, M. A. (2014). Promoting health, wellness, and quality of life at the end-of-life. *Journal of Allied Health, 43*(4), 212–220, 219p.

Ramvi, E. (2007). *Læring av erfaring? et psykoanalytisk blikk på læreres læring*. Forskerskolen i livslang læring [Learning from experience? A psychoanalytic perspective on teachers' learning]. Roskilde: Roskilde universitetscenter.

Rønnestad, M. H., & Skovholt, T. M. (2013). *The developing practitioner: Growth and stagnation of therapists and counselors*. New York: Routledge.

Roseneil, S. (2009). Haunting in an age of individualization: Subjectivity, relationality and the traces of the lives of others. *European Societies, 11*(3), 411–430. https://doi.org/10.1080/14616690902764823.

Sabin-Farrell, R., & Turpin, G. (2003). Vicarious traumatization: Implications for the mental health of health workers? *Clinical Psychology Review, 23*(3), 449–480. https://doi.org/10.1016/S0272-7358(03)00030-8.

Schön, D. A. (1991). *The reflective practitioner: How professionals think in action*. Aldershot: Avebury.

Sinclair, H. A. H., & Hamill, C. (2007). Does vicarious traumatisation affect oncology nurses? A literature review. *European Journal of Oncology Nursing, 11*(4), 348–356. https://doi.org/10.1016/j.ejon.2007.02.007.

Skelton, J. (2003). Death and dying in literature. *Advances in Psychiatric Treatment, 9*(3), 211–217.

Skovholt, T. M. (2012). *Becoming a therapist: On the path to mastery*. Hoboken, NJ: Wiley.

Skovholt, T. M., & Trotter-Mathison, M. J. (2011). *The resilient practitioner: Burnout prevention and self-care strategies for counselors, therapists, teachers, and health professionals*. New York: Routledge.

Skovholt, T. S., Hage, S. M., Kachgal, M. M., & Gama, E. P. (2007). An interview with Sunny Hansen: Pioneer and innovator in counseling and career development. *Journal of Counseling & Development, 85*(2), 216–226.

Snyder, C. R., & Forsyth, D. R. (1991). *Handbook of social and clinical psychology: The health perspective* (Vol. 162). New York: Pergamon Press.

Stolorow, R. D. (2011). *World, affectivity, trauma: Heidegger and post-cartesian psychoanalysis*. New York: Routledge.

Thagaard, T. (2013). *Systematikk og innlevelse. En innføring i kvalitativ metode* (4rd ed.) [An introduction to qualitative method]. Bergen: Fagbokforlaget.

Tillich, P. (1951). *Systematic theology* (Vol. 1). Chicago: The University of Chicago Press.

Tillich, P. (2000). *The courage to be* (2nd ed.). Yale: Yale University Press.

Tolstoy, L. (1989). *The death of Ivan Ilych*. London: Penguin Books Ltd.

Trotter-Mathison, M., Koch, J. M., Sanger, S., & Skovholt, T. M. (2010). *Voices from the field: Defining moments in counselor and therapist development*. New York and London: Taylor & Francis.

Van Laarhoven, H. W. M., Schilderman, J., Vissers, K. C., Verhagen, C. A. H. H. V. M., & Prins, J. (2010). Images of god in relation to coping strategies of palliative cancer patients. *Journal of Pain and Symptom Management, 40*(4), 495–501. https://doi.org/10.1016/j.jpainsymman.2010.02.021.

Van Mol, M. M. C., Kompanje, E. J. O., Benoit, D. D., Bakker, J., & Nijkamp, M. D. (2015). The prevalence of compassion fatigue and burnout among healthcare professionals in intensive care units: A systematic review. *PLoS One, 10*(8), e0136955–e0136955. https://doi.org/10.1371/journal.pone.0136955.

Walkerdine, V. (2008). Contextualizing debates about psycho-social studies. *Psychoanalysis, Culture and Society, 13,* 341–345.

WHO. (2011, 2016). http://www.who.int/cancer/palliative/definition/en/.

Yalom, I. D. (1998). *The Yalom reader: Selections from the work of a master therapist and storyteller*. New York: Basic Books.

Yalom, I. D. (2008). *Staring at the sun: Overcoming the terror of death*. San Francisco: Jossey-Bass.

2

The Narrative Subject—A Theoretical Positioning

Leave your theory, as Joseph his coat in the hand of the harlot, and flee
Ralph Waldo Emerson (in Self-Reliance)

Merging Theoretical Perspectives

When subjecting human beings to the scrutiny of science, it is of paramount importance that whoever does so can articulate his or her understanding of the other, of subjectivity, as well as the limits and implications of one's understanding. This chapter represents such an endeavor. In any field of academic discourse within which the question emerges, subjectivity is a concept that delineates contested ground. It is a term that lies at the intersection of philosophy, theology, psychology, cultural studies, and the social sciences, and each discipline has offered its own, frequently conflicting, understandings of what it means to be a subject. At the heart of all these theoretical endeavors are vital questions regarding self-awareness, identity, agency, and the subjective construction of one's experience of the world.

In order to limit the scope of the inquiry, the focus will be on engaging dimensions of subjectivity inherent in the research question pursued

K. Moen, *Death at Work*, Studies in the Psychosocial,
https://doi.org/10.1007/978-3-319-90326-2_2

in this book: how encountering the death of others may, or may not, inform the self-understanding of health professionals in end-of-life care. The question depicts several dimensions of subjectivity between which there are no solid walls. The first is that of man's relation to death, which is called "the psycho-physical problem". This relates to the human subject being a biologically instinctive "animal" informed by its existential condition of finitude. The second dimension addressed in the following is the inherent intersubjectivity of the subject, called the "psychosocial subject" (Hollway & Jefferson, 2000). This makes for an existential-psychosocial reading of the narrative subject.

The first part of the chapter will be devoted to a philosophical discussion of what may be regarded as the most obvious dimension of the narrative subject, namely the narrative self (Ricoeur, 1988). Drawing on discussions within philosophy of science, it will focus on the relation between the narrative self and the experiential self, and in particular on the experience of "mandatory basic conditions"—a term central to existential philosophy—and the potential discrepancy between how human beings experience and narrate them.

A central question pursued in the following is: in what sense and to what degree do experiences of our own ontology become semantic objects that can be recognized and interpreted? The case is made that there can be discrepancies between life experienced and life told. It is argued that there are certain experiences, particularly those related to death, that due to their character are easily suppressed and defended against, left on the borders of language beyond immediate reach as semantic objects for the narrative self. Encounters with death, at the very center of the present study, can be catalysts for deep reflection and self-knowledge, but can also provide experiences that are suppressed and defended against, and therefore not integrated parts of the health professional's narrative self (Yalom, 1998, 2008).

One may say that what distinguishes humans from other living beings is not mortality per se, but the paradoxical situation of being both body and self, both hopelessly in nature and self-consciously out of it, determined and free, eventually becoming food for worms—and being aware of it. Existential philosophical, psychoanalytic, and cultural-anthropological thinkers (Becker, 1973; Heidegger, 2010) argue that death may be an interpretive principle when trying to understand the human subject and social phenomena.

Thus, the following is a theoretical investigation of how the psychophysical and the psychosocial dimensions of the narrative subject can be related. It is undertaken in order to provide a conceptual frame which can facilitate the thinking of the research question pursued in this study. Attention will be given in particular to object relations and how this concept offers ways to understand the thinking of the unthought, that which is not yet articulated, including experiences of basic human conditions, such as death.

It is argued that for precognitive experiences—including one's finitude—to become semantic, human beings are dependent on the containing capability of another, an intersubjectively constituted space in which the individual may relate to and "digest" (Bion, 1962). Hence, in "individuality in finitude" (Becker, 1973) there is an implied "kinship-in-finitude" (Stolorow, 2011).

Nonetheless, it is argued that an inquiry into the experience of basic existential conditions, including death, is possible, because even if expressions of the angst of non-being may not be immediately accessible to the individual narrative self, they may be recognized "at a distance" by the listener, the observer, the researcher. The above points suggest that in researching the personal in the professional in end-of-life care one needs to take into consideration elements (hints and omissions) not necessarily found in the already-structured stories of the narrative self. What follows, therefore, makes a hermeneutics of suspicion plausible. The ethical implications of such a position, and how it should be balanced by a "reparative reading", are discussed at the end of the chapter.

Self—A Theorist's Fiction?

A view of self that has become increasingly popular is that of self being constructed in and through narrative self-interpretations (Gallagher, 2008). French philosopher Paul Ricoeur, who has given substantial attention to the concept of the narrative self (Ricoeur, 1992, 1988), states that posed self-reflectively, or in regard to another, we respond to the question of self by telling stories. Ricoeur shows how a narrative identity is made up of historical components which can be verified, as well as fictional components that can change. He points out how narrative identity is not "stable and seamless", but evolves around different plots, and throughout life it "continues to make and unmake itself" (Ricoeur, 1988). Ricoeur introduces the term "hermeneutics of self", which signifies the dialectic between what he calls *idem* and *ipse*. The former is related to self as a primitive unity in time and space. It is a more constant concept than the latter, which signifies the making of personal identity as selfhood as the person relates to self and becomes a person with a narrative (Rendtorff, 2000, 133f).

Does the analogy of an evolving text imply that we are sovereign authors of the story of our own self? Gallagher and Zahavi question such a solipsistic understanding of the narrative self by pointing out that we always narrate ourselves in culturally acceptable terms (Gallagher, 2008). In that sense one is not the sole author, and the narrative is only partly his or her's. In other words, there is a social dimension to narrative selfhood, which starts from the very beginning of a human life and involves complex social interactions.

The experiences in life belong to the individual, but the meaning of the experiences is socially and discursively appropriated. The subjective and the contextual are distinct entities, yet also profoundly intertwined (Gallagher, 2008, 200), which implies that a "hermeneutics of self" needs to take more than the intrapsychic entities of the subject into consideration, suggesting not only a psycho, but a psychosocial reading when trying to come to terms with one self or another (Nicholson, 2013). Before addressing the question to what degree we actually have access to ourselves, and whether all our experiences can be regarded as semantic entities, let us further explore the constitution of the narrative self.

Narrative Self—Constructed or Embedded?

Whether we understand narrative self as subjectively or socially constructed, or both, we are still left with the question whether it is just fiction and an empty abstraction? Daniel Dennett, in his text "The Self as a Center of Narrative Gravity", claims just that: because the self in the first place is "nothing substantially real" (Dennett, 1992, 200), the coherence we experience in relation to having a self is an illusion and solely a product of language, not related to a neurological, or any other recognizable entity, in our brain or any other part of the body. Like the impossibility of locating the center of gravity in any physical object, self is also a purely abstract phenomenon, "a theorist's fiction". To believe otherwise would be equal to mistaking a fictional figure in a novel for a real person.

Dennett states that the process of the evolving story of my next-door neighbor is no different in character from that of Dostoevsky's Raskolnikov—in both cases "the selves are constantly being made more determinate as we go along in response to the way the world impinges on us" (Dennett, 1992, 4). The familiarity of the ideas of both gravity and self easily leaves us with the impression that they are real, which they are not, according to Dennett. Believing one can get to know what the self really is, is a categorical mistake. Turning to Hume, who states that "I never can catch myself at any time without a perception and never can observe anything but the perception", Dennett points to the fact that just as nobody has seen a center of gravity, neither has anyone seen a self. That is not due to an inability to grasp metaphysical reality, but rather related to the fact that "there is no conscious self that is unproblematically in command of the mind's resources" (Dennett, 1992, 7). Perhaps he would be willing to admit to what I find crucial, that the concept of self is valuable in that, like the concept of center of gravity, it serves to simplify and explain an "essential", but hard-to-grasp aspect of our "reality".

In "Contemporary Philosophy of Social Science" (Fay, 1996), Professor of Philosophy Brian Fay speaks about the legitimacy of understanding self in terms of narrative, but challenges both narrative constructionism, as illustrated above (Dennett), and "narrative realism". The latter understands narratives as true stories that are discovered, not constructed. What Fay opposes is the naturalistic idea found among narrative realists that the narrative self can be likened to "objects reflected in a mirror"; that there should be a one-to-one relation between lived life and told story. However, according to Fay, the narrative constructionist idea, reflected in Dennett's statements above, whereby historians and (self) biographers alike "impose narrative structures on a formless flow of events" is just as erroneous. The notion that the narrative self is only an afterthought, constructed rather than discovered, has some value, but it is one-sided and does not grasp the narrative self (Fay, 1996, 190).

Fay's own position, with which I agree, is to insist on the dual character (both realistic and constructionist) by acknowledging that narratives occur in life and are about life: "we tell stories in acting and we continue to tell stories afterwards about the actions we have performed". Narrators are not only authors, they also live as actors "within ongoing stories which we must constantly tell ourselves as a condition for being able to perform any intentional actions whatsoever" (ibid., 191).

Narrative Self and Experiential Self

One pressing question concerning Fay's narrativism is, where does he stand in regard to the relation between narrative and experience? Fay seems to oppose the idea that there should be any experience prior to the narration of it: "it is not as if some material exists which is not structured narratively" (ibid., 197). Gallhagher and Zahavi, taking a phenomenological stand, challenge this view. They regard the notion of "experiential self" as something other than narrative self and fundamental "in the sense that nothing that lacks this dimension deserves to be called a self" (Gallagher & Zahavi, 2008, 204).

The notion of the "experiential self" implies that the self is conceived as the invariant dimension of first-personal givenness in the multitude of changing experiences. The authors take into consideration the universal experience of "sameness" and a continuously felt subjectivity through a sense of me-ness encountering different experiences. In other words, all experiences have a common feature, namely that they are all felt as mine and in that sense carry "a subtle presence of self"—the experiential self (ibid., 204).

As Dennett points out above, even though it is difficult to conceive of this sameness as "something which can, itself, be given as an object for experience", it is a necessary condition for the possibility of (coherent) experience (ibid., 200). However, the authors do not think of the experiential self as unchangeable, as a distinct principle of identity that stands apart from and above the stream of changing experiences, as an ontological given and pure identity pole; rather, they understand it as a "pre-linguistic presupposition for any narrative practice" (ibid., 205).

This understanding of a "core", "minimal", or "experiential self" challenges the reductionist Cartesian notion of *cogito ergo sum* and suggests, as will be discussed below, that there is a quality of "mine-ness" that is pre-reflexive, which implies that there can be a discrepancy between the experience of life and its narrative. What Gallagher and Zahavi suggest—and this is central to how the research subject is understood here—is the idea that the subjective is not identical to a Cartesian notion of consciousness; that our subjectivity is not limited to our thinking capacity; that there are experiences on the boundaries of language that may not be immediately accessible to the narrative self.

Human beings are ontologically determined by forces they do not control. The individual does not only act, she/he is acted upon; the fact that one does not make a conscious and deliberate choice in all situations attests to this. That one is always tuned emotionally by inner forces that one cannot monitor, speaks to the same (Vetlesen & Stänicke, 1999, 245). There are, in other words, prelingual experiences of basic conditions beyond the immediate reach of the narrative self. This suggests that Sigmund Freud's insight that we are driven should be regarded as significant and not rejected with his more speculative non-verifiable claims that we are driven by desires. The latter understanding has been critiqued both from outside and from within the psychoanalytic community.

The relation between influences of which one is neither aware nor able to change and consciousness, self-determination, goal-setting, continuity of identity and values is not addressed exhaustively here. Yet, a key point is made in regard to the rationale of this study, namely that we are informed by something that cannot be manipulated, measured, or used; this is our nature which dwells within us and influences us by its powers (ibid.). In what follows, this will be referred to as the "mandatory basic conditions".

Mandatory Basic Conditions

The mandatory basic conditions, that each of us is subject to, are named in different ways by different philosophers: existentiales in Heidegger's fundamental ontology (Heidegger, 2010) and life utterances in Løgstrup's moral philosophy (Løgstrup, 1997). Vetlesen and Stänicke name the mandatory basic conditions more specifically as dependency, vulnerability, the fragility of relations, existential loneliness, and mortality (Vetlesen & Stänicke, 1999, 340), underlining their claim that the givens of existence are not necessarily subject to our influence.

Ivin D. Yalom, emeritus professor of psychiatry, who has given much attention to mandatory basic conditions, seems to deal with them more in line with an existentialist notion suggesting that every individual is free and therefore in a position to choose and monitor their effect (ibid., 341). His main concept, *ultimate concerns*, is specified as meaninglessness, existential isolation, freedom, and death (Yalom, 1998, 172). We will be exploring the mandatory basic condition most relevant to the present study, namely death, which is at the core of humankind's psychophysical problem.

The Psychophysical Problem

The psychophysical problem is a term encountered in Otto Rank's book *The Trauma of Birth* (Rank, 1973). Rank, an Austrian psychoanalyst, was one of Freud's closest disciples before he became a critic. In line with classic psychoanalytic thought, he made the "universally valid psycho-biological law" central to understanding not only the individual human being, but "the whole development of mankind" (ibid., xxv).

At the center of this "biologically based law of the form which determines the content" (ibid., xxv) is the finitude of man, what Martin Heidegger calls man's "own-most possibility" (Heidegger, 2002). Ernest Becker (Becker, 1973), building on Rank's authorship, undertakes a cultural analysis based on the insight pointed out above and shared by many existential philosophers and psychoanalytic theorists alike, that the inherent finitude and dependency of human beings are most crucial for understanding human behavior. Part of what distinguishes the human being is what Becker calls "the experiential burden". Like no other creature, the human being is confronted with the painful realization that she/he is not able to avoid death: "Everything that man does in his symbolic world is an attempt to deny and overcome his grotesque fate" (ibid., 27).

Becker interprets the basic human problem as an existential paradox, and he reinterprets basic Freudian psychoanalytic concepts accordingly. Instead of a sexual framework he introduces an existential one, making the point that the inherent conflict the individual is struggling to come to terms with is not related to a prehistorical event of which the impact is lingering in human nature, but rather to man's paradoxical existential condition here and now. The conflict between body and self, nature and symbol, death and life is constantly playing out.

The foundational anxieties that make their imprint on every child, man, and woman are related to the terror of life itself, its fragility, unpredictability, and death. The tragic existential situation, actualized from the very beginning of life, calls for the child to adapt, to shield itself against the full realization of its terrifying paradoxical situation, what Freud names "the great necessities of fate, against which there is no remedy" (ibid., 53), the realization of being a "god-worm" (ibid., 58).

Death as a key interpretive principle to understanding human, individual, and collective behavior aligns with the anthropology conveyed within existential psychology. This is a body with many members. Seldom speaking univocally, yet coherently enough to be regarded as a distinguishable strand within psychology, it is marked by an interest in the big questions of philosophy and what it means to be human, which often implies a phenomenological approach when investigating the human.

A shared trait among existential psychologists is engaging the inevitable non-negotiables of life, the basic human conditions. William James, Rollo May, Victor Frankl, Paul Tillich and, Irvin Yalom, all major contributors within existential psychology, have in common the application of perspectives from existential philosophy. Their writings convey the philosophical anthropologies of Kierkegaard, Nietzsche, Heidegger, and

Sartre. This rather "broad brush" introduction to a major field will be complemented by a finer touch, in the discussion in Chapter 9. In what follows, we will engage a remaining and pressing question regarding the relation between the experiential self and the narrative self, namely whether precognitive experiences can become semantic entities and thus subject to research?

A Question of Semantics

In the above, a philosophical rationale is established for any potential discrepancy between subjective experience and narrative self, particularly in regard to the experience of mandatory basic conditions. That raises the pressing epistemological question, which has hermeneutical implications, namely whether the individual's experience of mandatory basic conditions, which may evade both consciousness and language of the narrative self, is within reach of the other, the observer, the researcher?

Heidegger's phenomenological project is to detect the origin of pre-representational phenomena (Vetlesen & Stänicke, 1999, 251). He makes the case that in order to understand "being" in an ontological sense the only point of departure is what is present (ontic) to the individual human being. Through an everyday phenomenological hermeneutic of the how of "being-in-the-world", one can access the "what" of being, which is the aim of a "*Dasein* analysis". The German *Dasein* is a central Heideggarian term, which can be translated as "being-there" or "being-here".

In Heidegger's conceptual universe, it replaces terms like "subject" and "ego" and encompasses an understanding that there is no subject by itself, but only "in-the-world" (Cerbone, 2008). *Das Man*, or "the they", on the other hand, denotes the talk, the ways, and the manners of the "world" in which *Dasein* is embedded. In the Heideggarian universe, there is a tension between the two, actualized in matters pertaining to authenticity and inauthenticity.

According to Fløistad, Heidegger has no formula other than the hermeneutical circle for how to move from the concrete existential experience of the individual to the existensiales upon which it rests. To catch a glimpse of the "prism" through which meaning, death, freedom, existential loneliness, authenticity, inauthenticity, and other "givens" become visible entities for the individual, one has to engage him or her in a (deep) hermeneutical dialogue (Fløistad, 1968, 83).

According to this rationale, it takes another to identify how life experiences become parts of the narrative self. The personal "idiom" or "gestalt", the characteristic way in which an individual receives and organizes experience—why a life is told in a particular way—is better spotted at a distance. This brings us to the psychosocial, the intrinsic intersubjectivity of human life, and more specifically to the dynamics of emotional communication explicated in Wilfred R. Bion's concepts (Bion, 1962).

A Psychosocial Response

Wilfred Bion, an influential British psychoanalyst, is a central figure in the development of object relations, a theoretical framework addressing both emotions and relations. The theory is particularly relevant in that it can illuminate how the subject's environment—and particularly the relationships within it—are internalized by that subject in idiomatic ways, while also accounting for how the subject acts affectively and behaviorally within the social environment. Hence, it offers a theoretical framework possibly encompassing both dimensions of the subject, the psychophysical and the psychosocial, actualized in the research question.

A Model for Thinking the Unthought

Bion's point of departure that "an emotional experience cannot be conceived of in isolation from a relationship" (Bion, 1962, 42) places him in a broader community of thinkers emphasizing the intersubjectivity of the human subject. Many, both outside and inside the psychoanalytic tradition, have pointed out the importance of the other in order for the subject to be able to experience, feel, think, and hence make life comprehensible (Bowlby, 1997; Honneth, 1995; Rogers, 1965). Bion was particularly interested in how humans understand and relate to their life experiences. His interest in how we make sense of our experiences and make them our own was triggered in his encounters with psychotic patients in his practice. One of Bion's main contributions was to offer concepts that elicit how unthought, precognitive experiences are transformed into semantic entities.

Projective Identification, Container-Contained, Negative Capability, and Reverie

Bion uses the alimentary system as model when trying to come to terms with what takes place in mental and emotional processing of precognitive experiences. The process of "digesting" is related to the child's projections and introjections of emotional and mental material. It is initiated through "projective identification", which denotes the child identifying her/his own unbearable emotions in the mother after having projected them into her. The need to project relates and increases in proportion to, the degree of tolerance for frustration.

In short, projective identification describes how unconscious emotional material is projected from one person to another; how, for instance, emotional pain is transported between two human beings (Haugsgjerd, 1990; Holm, 2005). Projective identification was a concept introduced by Melanie Klein, Bion's mentor. She was Bion's, but primarily understood by her as a defense mechanism that occurred in the child's mind. Bion understood the phenomenon more as a form of communication, by which the mother is also moved both communicatively and emotionally (Stokkeland, 2011).

Central to Bion's theory of learning from experience is the model of "container-contained", which is related to projective identification. It denotes the foundational intersubjectivity of becoming an experiencing being. The prototype of container-contained is found in the mother–infant relationship. This "activity", in which the sense impressions of the infant are "digested" and then re-introjected by the infant, thus becomes part of the alpha-function, foundational for its learning capacity. The "activity" becomes "progressively more complex as it constantly recurs throughout mental development" (Bion, 1962, 93). Bion points out how the receptive qualities of the container, tolerance of doubt and tolerance of a sense of infinity, are preconditions for the development of the thinking found in complex scientific deductive systems (ibid., 94). "Containment" is a term relating to the capacity at the receiving end of the communication, and the question of whether the receiver is able, or willing, to contain the (unacceptable) emotions projected by the other and bear the weight of the frustrations they carry (Ramvi, 2007, 28ff). In early life, the mother is the "container"; later in life this primary process takes place in other relations, including in professional contexts.

"Negative capability", a term borrowed by Bion from Keats, is another characteristic of the container that refers to the capacity of the individual to tolerate uncertainties, chaos and not-knowing, to be patient and not act on impulse (ibid., 32).

The outcome of this relational process is linked to the ability of the receiver to tolerate rather than respond to the individual's frustrations, and to offer "reverie" and "containment" for what Bion calls "beta elements". The latter is Bion's term for the unthought, precognitive, unbearable experiences that have not yet been translated into meaning but which still have impact. In order for them to become part of the individual's experience, what Bion terms "alpha elements", they have to be "digested" by another before being returned to and internalized by the individual:

> A central part is played by the alpha-function in transforming an emotional experience into alpha-elements because a sense of reality matters to the individual in the way that food, drink, air and excretion of waste products matter. Failure to eat, drink or breathe properly has disastrous consequences for life itself. Failure to use the emotional experience produces a comparable disaster in the development of the personality; I include amongst these disasters degrees of psychotic deterioration that could be described as death of the personality. As always, the use of a model, as I am using the model of the digestive system here, is open to the dangers I discuss. (Bion, 1962, 42)

The context for Bion's writing is psychoanalysis, yet the author states explicitly: "the theory of functions and alpha-function are not a part of psychoanalytic theory. They are working tools for the practicing psychoanalyst to ease problems of thinking about something that is unknown" (ibid., 89). His empirical references when outlining his model are "a small number of… highly abnormal" phenomena, namely psychotic thinking, but, according to Bion, the "rudimentary equipment for thinking thoughts" is not limited to mental illness, but a shared inherent weakness, present with "the most advanced human beings" and in particular "when the object for investigation is the phenomenon of life itself" (ibid., 13).

Bion's interest, the "immediate concern", is thus not merely that of mental illness, but the phenomenon of comprehension, the capacity for thinking, and "the apparatus needed for thought" (ibid., 56), implied in "learning from experience". Hence, the relevance and possible application of Bion's theory go beyond a particular context. Bion provides a conceptual frame in which both the foundational intersubjectivity of the experiencing and interpreting subject is explicated, and the thinking and experiencing of the narrator can be "thought". To me, the model's validity lies in the fact that it enables one to grasp and understand what is taking place in human learning from experience, not least when transforming elements at the borders of language into semantic entities.

Having established the inherent intersubjectivity of the subject, and how it takes another to transform precognitive experience into thoughts, death, and finitude will take center-stage through an exploration of how Stolorow, a representative of the relational turn in psychoanalysis (Stolorow & Atwood, 1992; Stolorow, Atwood, & Brandchaft, 1994), comes to terms with the reality of death.

A Merging of Perspectives: Existential Kinship-in-Finitude

Stolorow's project is to explore "how Heidegger's existential philosophy enriches post-Cartesian psychoanalysis" (Stolorow, 2011, 1) and vice–versa. He identifies a profound and shared interest between the hermeneutic phenomenology of Heidegger and a psychoanalytic thinking that has moved beyond "the Cartesian myth of the isolated mind" (ibid., 24), that is "a self-enclosed wordless subject" (ibid., 20). The shared interest is a move towards what Stolorow calls "phenomenological contextualism" (ibid., 19), which denotes the inherent intersubjectivity of the subject.

Both hermeneutic phenomenology and psychoanalytic theory are interested in emotional experience, which is understood by both as always contextually informed, to a large part implicit and made apparent through hermeneutic interpretive means:

> Our dedication to illuminating personal phenomenology had led us from mind to world and thus from mental contents to relational contexts, from the intra-psychic to the inter-subjective. (ibid., 22)

The latter very much rests on the presuppositions outlined above in the discussion about the psychosocial subject. But what about mortality and finitude?

A key part of how Heidegger "enriches post-Cartesian psychoanalysis" is his descriptive phenomenology and complex ontological account of anxiety which, according to Stolorow, is "unsurpassed in the psychoanalytic literature" (ibid., 37). The absence or presence of anxiety is very much related to the inherent finitude of the subject. The psychophysical problem, "the ownmostness and non-relationality of the possibility of death" (ibid., 40), is placed at the very center of Heidegger's hermeneutic phenomenological inquiry, but interpreted existentially.

It is not primarily a matter of the future termination of physical life, but rather an ever-present "possibility of the impossibility of being", the realization of which is triggered by breakdowns in the everydayness of life "in-the-world". Stolorow argues that "emotional trauma produces an affective state whose features bear a close similarity to the central elements in Heidegger's description of anxiety, and that it accomplishes this by plunging the traumatized person into a form of authentic Being-toward-death" (ibid., 42).

Following Heidegger's existential interpretation of death and his own experience, Stolorow claims that "emotional trauma is built into the basic constitution of human existence" (ibid., 63), and that we are "deeply connected with one another by virtue of our common finitude" (ibid., 64). According to the above argument, Being-in-the-world and Being-toward-death, "the universally valid psycho-biological law" (Rank, 1973) and intersubjectivity, are thus not only foundational elements of being a human subject, but also very much interconnected.

Stolorow speaks of the importance of:

> A relational home… within which traumatized states can evolve into painful emotional experiences that can be more fully felt and articulated, better tolerated and eventually fully integrated. Authentic existing presupposes a capacity to dwell in the emotional pain (e.g. the existential anxiety) that accompanies a non-evasive recognition of finitude, and this capacity, in turn, requires that such pain find a relational context in which it can be held. (Stolorow, 2011, 51)

Thus, he emphasizes that the intersubjectivity of the subject always implies "an existential kinship in finitude". The psychophysical problem is thus placed within an intersubjective context. In different ways Bion and Stolorow are naming the importance of a holding space in which precognitive experiences can be processed. Implicit is an ethical demand, which will be elaborated below, of not making the other into an object, but allowing him or her to remain an experiencing subject (Skjervheim, 1974).

Hermeneutics of Suspicion—And a Critique

We should, according to the argument outlined above, keep in mind that we can fool ourselves with every statement we make about our being. Ricoeur, in his discussion on the narrative self, stresses the importance of not committing the mistake of mixing up what is necessarily so, *cogito ergo sum*, with a statement of adequacy, namely that I am just the way I think myself to be.

In his discussion on Freud, Ricoeur introduces the term "hermeneutics of suspicion" as opposed to "exegetical hermeneutics". The latter implies a relationship to the text marked by reverence, respect, and faith in its perfect, inner consistency and meaningfulness—qualities that are just waiting to be discovered by the interpreter. Hermeneutics of suspicion, on the other hand, are marked by a critical approach, suspecting that the text, or the narrative self, is also a layer of pretension, perhaps seemingly perfect and consistent, but in reality possibly hiding a range of inconsistencies (Vetlesen & Stänicke, 1999, 117).

Freud, together with Marx and Nietzsche, is among the first suspicious hermeneutics. He relates his suspicion of the conscious to the presence of the unconscious and to pre-linguistic, non-discursive forces, drives, and desires against which the subject defends herself. In other words, one should not take the narrative of the other at face value, but rather question the narrating consciousness, and think of it as blurring and hiding the subjectivity of the narrative self. In a hermeneutics of self, or other, attention therefore should be brought to what is not put into words, to hints and omissions.

Sedgwick argues how "hermeneutics of suspicion" has "become synonymous with criticism itself", and "the very signature of smartness", and that "to theorize out of anything but a paranoid critical stance has come to seem naive pious or complaisant" (Sedgwick & Frank, 2003). Being a feminist author, she is not seeking to totally discard suspicious readings, rather she makes the case for the importance of understanding "paranoia in such a way as to situate it as one kind of epistemological practice among other, alternative ones" (ibid., 7).

She proposes an alternative and reparative reading in which the other is not left as a static entity due to a "dogged, defensive narrative stiffness of a paranoid temporality, in which yesterday can't be allowed to have differed from today" (ibid., 23). This reading offers what Winnicott may call "transitional space" and Benjamin "thirdness" (Benjamin, 2004). This space is in contrast to the paranoia often inherent in the hermeneutics of suspicion, which is reductionist because it seeks to eliminate surprise and "is closely tied to a notion of the inevitable" (Sedgwick & Frank, 2003), "orders more and more remote phenomena to a single formulation" and thus risks being "strongly tautological" (ibid., 12).

The latter are characteristics of strong theories. The case can be made that psychoanalytic theory and existential philosophy can, and even should, be understood as strong theories, followed by a normative reading. Becker, making fear of death the sole interpretive principle for his cultural analysis, may be an example of just that.

The aim is not necessarily ridding oneself of the concepts offered by these strong theoretical positions, but rather to be conscientious about how they sensitize the reading of the narratives, and in particular ensuring that they do not do so in a tautological manner. The latter would imply as much of an error as reading the interviewees' self-reports exegetically. A first step against slipping into the temptation of explaining the other, the patient, the interviewee, or the student in a reductionist way is to embrace the other as a unique center of experience and practice—a not-knowing position in contrast to that of being the exponent of a normative expert system of knowledge (Skjervheim, 1974). The latter has been the critique of traditional psychoanalysis (Frosh, 2010, 216); the former a mark of the relational turn in the same tradition, and hopefully also of the present study.

References

Becker, E. (1973). *The denial of death.* New York: Free Press.

Benjamin, J. (2004, January). Beyond doer and done to: An intersubjective view of thirdness. *The Psychoanalytic Quarterly, LXXIII*(1), 5–46.

Bion, W. R. (1962). *Learning from experience* (3rd ed.). Oxford: Rowman & Littlefield.

Bowlby, J. (1997). *Attachment and loss.* London: Pimlico.

Cerbone, D. R. (2008). Heidegger: A guide for the perplexed. *Guides for the perplexed.* London: Continuum International Publishing Group.

Dennett, D. (1992). The self as a center of narrative gravity. In F. Kessel, P. Cole, & D. Johnson (Eds.), *Self and consciousness: Multiple perspectives.* Hillsdale, NJ: Erlbaum.

Fay, B. (1996). *Contemporary philosophy of social science: A multicultural approach.* Oxford: Blackwell.

Fløistad, G. (1968). *Heidegger: En innføring i hans filosofi ved Guttorm Fløistad* (2nd ed.) [Heidegger: An introduction to his philosophy by Guttorm Fløistad]. Oslo: Pax forlag AS.

Frosh, S. (2010). *Psychoanalysis outside the clinic: Interventions in psycho-social studies*. Basingstoke: Palgrave Macmillan.
Gallagher, S., & Zahavi, D. (2008). *The phenomenological mind: An introduction to philosophy of mind and cognitive science*. London and New York: Routledge.
Haugsgjerd, S. (1990). *Lidelsens karakter i ny psykiatri* [The character of suffering in psychiatry]. Oslo: Pax forlag.
Heidegger, M. (2002). *On time and being*. Chicago: University of Chicago Press.
Heidegger, M. (2010). *On time and being*. Albany: State University of New York Press.
Hollway, W., & Jefferson, T. (2000). *Doing qualitative research differently: Free association, narrative and the interview method*. London: Sage.
Holm, U. (2005). *Empati* [Empathy]. Oslo: Gyldendal Norsk Forlag AS.
Honneth, A. (1995). *The struggle for recognition: The moral grammar of social conflicts*. Cambridge: Polity Press.
Løgstrup, K. E. (1997). *The ethical demand*. Notre Dame, IL: University of Notre Dame Press.
Nicholson, C. (2013, September). Holding it together: A psycho-social exploration of living with frailty in old age. *International Journal of Nursing Studies, 50*(9), 1172–1179. https://doi.org/10.1016/j.ijnurstu.2012.01.006. Epub 2012 February 4.
Ramvi, E. (2007). *Læring av erfaring? et psykoanalytisk blikk på læreres læring*. Forskerskolen i livslang læring [Learning from experience? A psychoanalytic perspective on teachers' learning]. Roskilde: Roskilde universitetscenter.
Rank, O. (1973). *The trauma of birth*. New York: Harper Torchbooks.
Rendtorff, J. D. (2000). *Paul Ricoeurs filosofi* [The philosophy of Paul Ricoeur]. København: Hans Reitzels Forlag.
Ricoeur, P. (1988). *Time and narrative* (Vol. 3). Chicago: University of Chicago Press.
Ricoeur, P. (1992). *Oneself as another*. Chicago: University of Chicago Press.
Rogers, C. R. (1965). *Client-centered therapy*. Boston, MA: Houghton Mifflin Company.
Sedgwick, E. K., & Frank, A. (2003). *Touching feeling: Affect, pedagogy, performativity*. Durham, NC: Duke University Press.
Skjervheim, H. (1974). Objectivism and the study of man. *Inquiry: An Interdisciplinary Journal of Philosophy, 17*, 1974.
Stokkeland, J. M. (2011). *Å gi og å ta imot: Donald Meltzers psykoanalytiske tenkning i tradisjonen fra Melanie Klein og Wilfred Bion* [To give and

to receive: Donald Meltzer's psychoanalytic thinking in the tradition of Melanie Klein and Wilfred Bion]. Tromsø: Universitetet i Tromsø, Fakultet for humaniora, samfunnsvitenskap og lærerutdanning, Institutt for lærerutdanning og pedagogikk.

Stolorow, R. D. (2011). *World, affectivity, trauma: Heidegger and post-Cartesian psychoanalysis*. New York: Routledge.

Stolorow, R. D., & Atwood, G. E. (1992). *Contexts of being: The intersubjective foundations of psychological life*. Hillsdale, NJ: Analytic Press.

Stolorow, R. D., Atwood, G. E., & Brandchaft, B. (1994). *The intersubjective perspective*. Northvale, NJ: J. Aronson.

Vetlesen, A. J., & Stänicke, E. (1999). *Fra hermeneutikk til psykoanalyse: muligheter og grenser i filosofiens møte med psykoanalysen* [From hermeneutics to psychoanalysis: Possibilities and limitations in the encounter between philosophy and psychoanalysis]. Oslo: Ad notam Gyldendal.

Yalom, I. D. (1998). *The Yalom reader: Selections from the work of a master therapist and storyteller*. New York: Basic Books.

Yalom, I. D. (2008). *Staring at the sun: Overcoming the terror of death*. San Francisco: Jossey-Bass.

3
Research Beneath the Surface—A Methodological Positioning

"Below the surface-stream, shallow and light,
Of what we say we feel – below the stream
As light, of what we think we feel, there flows
With noiseless current strong, obscure and deep,
The central stream of what we feel indeed"
(Mathew Arnold, *Saint Paul and Protestantism*)

The Art of Living with "Wicked Questions"

Scientific questions and problems may be categorized as "tame" or "wicked" (Rittel & Webber, 1973). Social science is home to many wicked questions and what changes occur in self-understanding due to encounters with terminally ill and dying patients is definitely among them. Tame problems share the fact that they can be solved; wicked scientific problems, on the other hand, are not evil, but unsolvable. They are slippery in that they can be explained in indefinite ways and are designated differently by different times, places, and people. These are the kind of questions that call for laborious, in-depth, scientific work without the promise of clear unequivocal answers. Engaging wicked

K. Moen, *Death at Work*, Studies in the Psychosocial,
https://doi.org/10.1007/978-3-319-90326-2_3

questions is all about shedding light on complex parts of our existence, which often lie at the borders of language.

The wickedness of the research questions in this study was introduced in the previous chapter. Any associations between the present study and things that can be counted and measured should by now have been countered. When claiming to undertake an empirical study, it is particularly important to make clear what kind of truth claims one is making regarding the object of study, how understanding is reached, and what is understood. Hence, in the following paragraphs, the study will be located within a hermeneutic phenomenological frame. The study is phenomenological as the objective is to explore the experience of health professionals engaged in boundary situations. It thus takes the subjective experience as its point of departure, has a first-person approach, seeks "the native's point of view" (Geertz, 1973), and is committed to describing reality as experienced by the narrator (Gallagher & Zahavi, 2008; Thagaard, 2013). However, the project is not aiming solely at description but also understanding, which brings hermeneutics into the picture. The relation between the two will be outlined in the following.

This chapter is thus not only a presentation of the Biographical Narrative Interpretive Method (BNIM) (Wengraf, 2011), but also a discussion of the rationale, the *logos*, behind the particular methodological choices. It serves as a response to the critique voiced in the Preface—that "a problem with many qualitative studies is the absence of linkage between the method used and a clear statement of the philosophical underpinnings that should guide the method" (Stubblefield & Murray, 2002).

After a presentation of the particularities of BNIM, and before presenting the process of constructing data, space is made for a critical appraisal of the *sine qua non* of BNIM, namely the uninterrupted telling of narratives. In particular, the following looks at how the method is potentially challenged by social constructionist positions, such as those voiced by Kathy Charmaz, professor of sociology and a significant contributor to Grounded Theory (Charmaz, 2006), and psychologist and therapist Harlene Anderson (Anderson, 1997). I pursue questions relating to how the fundamental social constructionist insight that "meanings are not automatically shared" works with the "minimalist" approach of BNIM. The case is made that an uninterrupted telling of life stories helps to elicit what appears to be omitted in constructionist narrativism, namely that the narrative self is both "in life" and "about life". I claim that it is within reach to identify not only the latter, but also the embedded narrative; thereafter, I show how BNIM, through its analytical protocols, facilitates such an extrapolation.

A Matter of Hermeneutics

Not many have engaged the wicked problem of understanding as thoroughly as the German philosopher Hans-Georg Gadamer. Hence, in the following paragraphs, I will engage him in my discussion of issues central to this project. Gadamer traces not only the history and the characteristics of *Geisteswissenschaft*, but also the various principles of interpretation and scientific pretensions that have accompanied it. He makes the point that when applying "method" to *Geisteswissenschaft*, it is easily subjected to the foreign measuring sticks of natural sciences (Gadamer, 1989, 24), as if it were resting on a positivist paradigm seeking univocal explanations and Truths about the other, rather than what is closer to truth, namely that it is a study in which truth(s) is individual (Gadamer & Holm-Hansen, 2010, 23). This does not refer to Truth grasped at a distance, from the detached position of a "neutral" scientist, but rather truth which is grasped through participation. Understanding narratives is like playing a game—or speaking a new language. You must enter the world of the game and go where it takes you, which may be far from where you started or intended to go (ibid., 19). Whatever one is trying to understand determines the method, not the other way around.

This is an understanding of truth that doesn't imply pretensions of generalizability or predictability, but rather what Gadamer calls "truth-events", an "uncovering" (*aletheia*) of why something appears to be true (ibid., 12). The truth thus understood resembles what happens when encountering art and great classical texts. It is not about confirming or expanding common experience to attain knowledge of "a law" about "how men, peoples and states evolve – but rather to understand how this man, this people, or this state has become what it is, or, more generally, how it happened that it is so" (Gadamer, 1989, 5).

The ideal is to understand the subject itself in its unique and concrete historical appearance. Acknowledging the indefinite "qualitativeness" of any biographical narrative is never about evaluating the truth in what is being stated, but rather searching for an explanation for why something is stated. This way of understanding research experience corresponds very well with the intentions of the BNIM, which informs the methodological approach of this study and is introduced below.

Hermeneutics is thus more an attitude than a methodological approach; one of its basic assumptions is that the only way to understanding is through interpretation. Understanding is created in circular movements, in a dialogue between the whole and its parts, a process Heidegger called "the hermeneutical circle", in which understandings are challenged by new information and the researcher's own preconceived ideas and understandings must be taken into consideration (Thagaard, 2013). Another related basic assumption, discussed below, is that understanding and meaning can only be reached through taking into consideration the context of which the object of study is a part.

According to Gadamer, researching history, unlike the natural sciences, is not about revealing the laws behind it; experiments cannot be undertaken. Nonetheless, understanding is reached, not so much by observing events at a distance as by engaging questions related to the narratives of individuals. When there is no universal scheme by which to understand world history or biographical narratives, there is still a historical dynamic that can be identified (Gadamer, 1989, 203). Implied in this understanding, and very much informed by Hegel's dialectic philosophy, are the notions of "power" and "necessity": "Beside freedom stands necessity. It consists in what has already been formed and cannot be destroyed, which is the basis of all new activity" (ibid., 204).

What is thus acknowledged in the new science of history, a lingering truth informing my engagement with biographical narratives, is that "the power that makes history is not mechanical power", because "any acting individual could have acted differently" (ibid., 206). Hence, there is a power (*dynamis*) that "possesses potentiality… [as it]… is not only the cause of a particular effect but the capacity, wherever it is used, to have that effect" (ibid., 205). Freedom thus coexists dynamically with necessity. It is the dynamic between the two that drives history, according to Hegel, and this is a premise for the approach taken here to biographical narratives.

Being as Understanding

The position of the present study is that hermeneutics are not something we apply to being. It is rather part of being itself. The German philosopher Wilhelm Dilthey's main contribution to hermeneutics was his identification of it as life's central trait. "Life interprets itself. Life itself has a hermeneutical structure. Thus life constitutes the real ground of the human sciences" (ibid., 226). According to Dilthey, this explains "intention" and "significance", which to him were dynamic phenomena through which individuality—which he didn't regard as a power in itself—makes itself manifest.

Both Dilthey and Edmund Husserl, regarded as the founder of phenomenology, see *life*—understood as something more than particular experience—as what constitutes the phenomenological "object". *Life*, *horizon*, *Lebenswelt* have thus become terms that in particular signify what the subject is relating to, and which are always situated in a *world*. The latter is understood more as a continuous changing stream than a static entity, relative yet shared, but which can never really become an object for the individual.

Martin Heidegger, whose fundamental ontology was in part introduced in the previous chapter and will be explored further in Chapter 9, claims that the "facticity of hermeneutics" is neither related to the subject's reflexivity, nor its consciousness, in contrast to the naiveté of unreflecting life. It is rather that understanding is "the original form of the realization of Dasein"; hence, it makes up Dasein's mode of being "before any differentiation of understanding into the various directions of pragmatic or theoretical interest" (ibid., 259).

Heidegger stresses that one cannot investigate the way of being of Dasein merely by ontical description, a narration of objects or activities; rather, it must be through delineating the ontological dimension of the latter (activities), that is, "making explicit the understanding of being at work in Dasein's activity". In Heidegger's terms:

> For us phenomenological reduction means leading phenomeno-logical vision back from the apprehension of a being, whatever may be the character of that apprehension, to the understanding of the being of this being. (Heidegger, 2010, 21)

"The understanding of the being of this being", the individual's self-understanding, requires a hermeneutic phenomenological endeavor, according to Heidegger. This is due to Dasein's understanding of her own being; it is not something she "has in mind"; rather, it is about how she acts in her "world", her "referential totality" (Cerbone, 2008, 41). Hence, understanding Dasein and the world (the referential totality) as two independently intelligible notions is a fallacy. "Being-in-the-world" is rather a "unitary phenomenon".

The latter can be stated in terms of philosopher Charles Taylor's communitarian anthropology. "Strong evaluations" (Taylor, 1989) is Taylor's way of naming what takes place in meaning making (and identity development), i.e., how we make qualitative, moral distinctions and choose our fundamental, categorical values—categories through which we negotiate the meaningless from the meaningful, the admirable from the contemptible (Taylor, 1989, 21).

Taylor states that, "it is impossible to learn strong evaluations without learning a language and it is impossible to learn a language outside a collective. It is therefore unthinkable to develop an identity independent of a community" (Nyeng & Taylor, 2000, 30–31). He also says that "the subject does not permit language which escapes personal resonance" (Taylor, 1989, 511). Meaning making then, according to Taylor, is both personal and contextual. This resembles the psychosocial position established in the previous chapter.

Addressing the contextual in terms of discourse, Pierre Bourdieu uses phrases like "the universe of the undisputed", "that which goes without saying", "learned ignorance", "the taken for granted". Thus, he communicates how the subjectivity of the interviewee is always embedded in socially constructed language (Bourdieu, 1977, 18ff). He recognizes the influence of the cultural and linguistic rules (ibid., 24), but he refuses to give into an objectivist determinism.

Bourdieu is not willing to understand practice simply as the "product of obedience to rules", and he challenges an understanding of cultural structures as "capable of acting as agents responsible for historical actions or as a power capable of constraining practices" (Bourdieu, 1977, 171). Bourdieu, as Taylor, leads us to understand that there is a social dimension to narrative selfhood, which starts from the very beginning of a human life and involves complex social interactions. I am not the sole author and the narrative is only partly mine. The experiences in life are mine, but the meaning of the experiences is socially and discursively appropriated. To have an eye for only one dimension is to be one-eyed, according to Bourdieu.

Taylor points out that neither moral frame nor autobiographical elements may be consciously present to the individual:

> ...their lives may be entirely structured by supremely important qualitative distinctions, in relation to which they literally live and die... But it may be left entirely to us, observers... to try to formulate explicitly what goods, qualities or ends are here discriminated. (Taylor, 1989)

The existential-psychosocial understanding of self-understanding outlined above calls for a methodological approach that offers interpretive means to explore how being in idiosyncratic ways is an issue for Dasein through her engagement with her "world". BNIM, with its strong link to phenomenological research traditions (Wengraf, 2001), is one such methodological pathway. It has been used in several studies in recent years (Casey, Proudfoot, & Corbally, 2016; Chamberlayne, Bornat & Wengraf, 2002; Wengraf, 2011, 892ff).

Inclusion of the rather detailed discussion of the method below first and foremost ensures the level of transparency promised, but also acknowledges that this part of the book may be for those readers most interested in the methodology.

A Biographical Narrative Approach

Implicit in BNIM is a notion of "being-in-the-world" similar to the one we find in *Being and Time* (Heidegger, 2010). There is a recognition of the mutual constituency of the individual being and its world, and BNIM aims at grasping the "situated subjectivity" by "thinking in a more than usually focused way about the socio-historical context, situatedness in time and social space… and then thinking in a more than usually focused way about subjective experiencing" (Wengraf, 2011, 136). This dual aspect resembles and encompasses also what is at the heart of the object-relations theoretical perspective outlined in the previous chapter.

According to Tom Wengraf, one of the main exponents of the method, the interviewee is a narrative self with a personal "idiom" or "gestalt", which inhabits a "selective principle", the characteristic way in which he/she is disposed to receive and organize experience (Wengraf, 2001, 69). These anthropological notions resemble those of Heidegger stated above: "a being whose being is an issue for it" and for whom "things show up" and "matter" to it (Cerbone, 2008, 31). To extrapolate such a self-understanding calls for a non-interruptive, minimalist-passive approach to interviewing. According to Wengraf, "the gestalt principle… requires the spontaneous pattern of the speaker to complete itself fully and so be fully exposed for analysis" (ibid., 113).

Three Sub-Sessions

The BNIM interview is made up of three sub-sessions, of which the first two are covered in one interview. The first starts with an open question framed by the research question, a single question inducing narrative (SQUIN). In the second sub-session, the interviewer takes the long narration from the first session as a point of departure and pushes for particular incident narratives (PINs). Instead of being satisfied with a thematically whole narrative, BNIM continuously takes steps to get as close as possible to the situated subjectivity, the experiences of the interviewee in particular situations, by focusing on the PINs. The rationale for this is further explained below.

When searching for PINs, the interviewer asks deepening questions, respecting the order and language of the narratives told, without introducing themes or terms that were not raised by the interviewee. The third stage (sub-session three), which can be a separate semi-structured interview, is optional. It can be based on the need for further clarification, or as an opportunity to introduce themes key to the project that were omitted or not covered sufficiently in the first two sub-sessions. The focus in the following will be on the first two sub-sessions, as there was no need for a third.

What to Ask: Forming a SQUIN

Fundamental to forming the SQUIN was of course the research question, which was directed toward the professional but voiced with the realization that there is no strict boundary between the personal and the professional in relation-intense professions (Skovholt & Trotter-Mathison, 2011). The SQUINs needed to reflect this and be framed in such a way so as not to trigger too much sorting out of the professional from the personal by the interviewee. Hence, there were good reasons not to frame the SQUIN too much in terms of "Tell me the story of your life as an X", because a rehearsed response is easily evoked (Wengraf, 2011, 654). In such cases, the interviewee is asked to filter out events and experiences not relevant to being an "X", and to search for those which are. This requires a theorizing and filtering that may result in "thinner" descriptions.

Hence, I decided to refrain from any reference to "x-ness" and leave the SQUIN open-ended. To make sure that the professional context for the study was conveyed, I included a reference to it in the introduction. The single question inducing narrative, read twice to the interviewees, was thus as follows:

> As you know, I am interested in how physicians/nurses/chaplains as persons have changed, or not changed, due to working with terminally ill and dying patients.
>
> Therefore, can you please tell me your life story: all those events and experiences, which were important for you personally?

> Please take the time you need! I will just listen and won't interrupt you with questions. I will just take notes so that I can remember what I want to ask you about when you have finished telling me about it all. Take the time you need. Start wherever you like.

A Position of Not-Knowing

Harlene Anderson makes a claim in regard to the client in therapy with which I identify as a researcher, namely that:

> I have access to limited information, never can fully understand another human being, continuously am in the process of being informed and always need to learn more about what is being said or that which may not have been said. (Anderson, 1997)

Anderson names this the "not-knowing" position of the professional (Anderson, 1997, 175), which rests on the assumption that "meanings are not automatically shared" (Charmaz, 2006), but must be explored and negotiated.

An attitude of not-knowing fosters curiosity and dialogue, according to Anderson. The obvious main methodological implication of a not-knowing position is that the interviewer has to ask! One may claim that engagement through questions is the *sine qua non* of interviewing. This also seems to be the strategy of Kathy Charmaz in what she calls "intensive interviewing", which is her approach to deep exploration. Charmaz stresses how the interviewer's role consists in listening, observing with sensitivity, but also encouraging responses from the interviewee. According to Charmaz, "intensive interviewing" ensures "in-depth" exploration as "the in-depth nature of an intensive interview fosters eliciting each participant's interpretation of his or her experience" (Charmaz, 2006, 25). The eliciting, as understood by Charmaz, follows a different etiquette than conventional conversation as:

> conversational rules may dictate that you listen, not ask for clarification, agree with the speaker – at least tacitly – but not question, let the speaker

direct conversational flow, rather stop it to explore an earlier point, and hear a story, but not repeat it in your words to recapture the other person's. (ibid., 26)

An intensive interview to the contrary stops and explores, whereas conventional interviewing might include "uh-huh's" or nodding as if meanings are shared, and in this case, an interviewer might say, "that is interesting, tell me more about it" (Charmaz, 2006, 26).

At the same time, Charmaz voices the importance of limiting the number of questions, encouraging the interviewer to "choose questions carefully and ask them slowly to foster the participant's reflections", as well as acknowledging that "a few broad, open-ended, non-judgmental questions… encourages unanticipated statements and stories to emerge". Finally, she points out that "your first question may suffice for the whole interview if stories tumble out" (ibid., 29).

Responding to a Social Constructionist Perspective

BNIM rests on "an extreme end of the research interview intervention spectrum" (Wengraf, 2001, 13) and responds to the not-knowing position slightly differently. This particular trait may be regarded as the *sine qua non* of the SQUIN-BNIM approach, namely its insistence on the uninterrupted telling of stories, allowing for silences in order for the unsaid to surface, for the sake of "a full gestalt to emerge". This will be further discussed in what follows. However, by giving voice to social constructionist perspectives, I will also explore whether a SQUIN-BNIM approach goes with an understanding of qualitative knowledge as co-created.

To explain a social constructionist position, and particularly its implications in relation to conversations and research interviews, I lend an ear to Kathy Charmaz (Charmaz, 2006) and her thoughts on "intensive interviewing", as compared to the "intensive listening" (Wengraf) approach of BNIM. In addition, I refer to professor of social psychology Elliot Mishler's critique of traditional interview methods (Mishler, 1986) and Harlene Anderson's discussion of a social constructionist position in regard to her collaborative therapy approach (Anderson, 1997). Since it is beyond the scope of this study to give a full presentation of each of these theoretical standpoints, discussion will be limited to those parts that elaborate a social constructionist critique of BNIM. I will then show how BNIM both incorporates fundamental social constructionist insights and challenges a too narrow constructionist reading of biographical narratives.

BNIM takes what Charmaz calls "a careful approach" a step further. Whereas she speaks of the importance of the list of questions being as short as possible, BNIM emphasizes the importance of posing only one question, namely the SQUIN. This is in order to attain the same goal as Charmaz, namely to ensure one of the main "conversational prerogatives" of the interviewee—to "choose what to tell and how to tell it" (Charmaz, 2006, 27). This prerogative is echoed by Anderson, who also has in-depth ambitions when she states the importance of "risking letting the client be at the center, let them author their stories the way they want to without being supported by what the therapist finds important" (Anderson, 1997, 177).

According to BNIM, confirming "uh-huh's" and nods—careful gestures of positive regard (Rogers, 1965)—suffices in the initial phase of the interview (sub-session one). Thereafter, having listened, it is time to take seriously what is agreed upon and stated above, namely that meanings are not automatically shared, and elicit each participant's interpretation of his or her experience. The very legitimate response "that's interesting, tell me more about it" is communicated in good time and in a way that does not break the telling of a story, but rather deepens it in the order, and on the terms, offered by the interviewee. This ensures that a legitimate question is not asked prematurely, which would risk the interviewee not being allowed to decide what to tell and how to tell it. Sub-session two is when the "dominant story" is complemented and "thickened" by experience-near stories, PINs, thus allowing space for the complex experience and contradictory narrative accounts.

One obvious reason for letting the interviewee talk uninterruptedly at length during sub-session one of a BNIM interview—"to hold the floor beyond the limits of a usual turn" (Mishler, 1986, 74)—is in order to allow the narrative, whether a life story or critical incident, to flow.

We make sense of ourselves and the other through narratives (Ricoeur, 1988). Still, the narratives are often suppressed by the standard survey interview (Mishler, 1986, 69) and also potentially by semi-structured interviews. In order to understand how individuals perceive, organize, give meaning to, and express their understandings and their world, we, as researchers, must allow stories to be told without interruption. BNIM facilitates for this through its insistence on uninterrupted telling.

The constructionist notion of plural meanings is taken seriously, not primarily by inviting intellectual reflections about the experience, phenomenon, or terms, but rather eliciting them by listening for the other's experience and actual use of the terms. Using the BNIM protocol for pushing PINs: "you said they became furious… do you remember anything more from that incident?", the interviewer takes seriously that meanings (furious) are not automatically shared, and undertakes an in-depth exploration about the meaning of a particular term, situation, or phenomenon by exploring how the interviewee applies it to a concrete situation.

The emphasis on withholding one's own inclinations and probing questions, and instead staying with the flow of speech and use of the other's language, resonates to a large degree with what Anderson regards as the implications of a not-knowing position. Her emphasis on "staying with" the other's narrative and facilitating a conversation which is led as little as possible by the prejudices and "knowledge" of the therapist (Anderson, 1997) resembles Mishler's claims about the narrative-inducing research interview:

> We are more likely to find stories reported in studies using relatively unstructured interviews where respondents are invited to speak in their own voices, allowed to control the introduction and flow of topics, and encouraged to extend their responses. (Mishler, 1986, 69)

Still, the question remains whether the uninterrupted telling of narratives does not challenge the more particular social constructionist notion of the interview as "a joint production of what interviewer and interviewee talk about together and how they talk to each other" (Mishler, 1986, 1). Is sub-session one a stimulus-response situation in which the questions evoke a predetermined and shared meaning, a narrative that mirrors "reality", rather than a speech event in which shared meaning must be negotiated and not be taken for granted? Before elaborating further on a BNIM rationale for the uninterrupted telling of the story, we will elicit the understanding of reality, truth, and knowledge as a social construction, as invented rather than discovered.

The Social Construction of Data and BNIM

Distancing herself from the original, more positivist, and objectivist foundations of Grounded Theory and laying stronger emphasis on constructivism, (Charmaz, 2006, 180) states that "whether participants recount their concerns without interruption or researchers request specific information, the result is a construction – or reconstruction of a reality" (ibid., 27).

Harlene Anderson, claiming a postmodern position in therapy, argues along the same lines as Charmaz regarding what can be counted as "real" and the limited potential for getting beyond the narrative construction of the other to a "real" event. Hence, the therapeutic process is not about discovering, revealing, or detecting a hidden reality about which the expert has privileged knowledge, but rather it fosters a conversation in which new narratives emerge.

Therapy becomes a lingual event in which people engage in a cooperating relation and conversation—a common struggle toward possibility, not the tracing back to an original point of departure (Anderson, 1997, 160; 2003, 160), but a generative event through which new meaning and new possibilities occur. In a similar fashion, the research interview has an element of cooperation and negotiation of meanings. Mishler elaborates on this in his book on research interviewing, in which the main point is that "interviews are speech events" and that "the discourse of interviews is constructed jointly by interviewers and respondents" (Mishler, 1986, ix).

The question lingers whether the "minimalist passive reception of interview narrative" (Wengraf, 2001, 113) as we find it in BNIM rests on assumptions other than those elaborated on above?

What I hear Wengraf claim is that through the research interview one can get knowledge about "discourse, objective referents and subjectivity" (Wengraf, 2001, 7), not *ding an sich*. BNIM claims that providing space for an uninterrupted telling of the individual's narratives is a means of grasping the evolving subjectivity of the interviewee *and* the discursive context in which it is embedded, the mutual constituency of the psycho and the social. The in-depth exploration of both rests with the space and suggestion for telling of the narratives, as it gives space for the interviewee's discourse to surface in a more intuitive way than in an interview marked by the interviewer's probing questions.

I have made the case that BNIM's insistence on the uninterrupted telling of narratives does not preclude a social constructionist insistence on understanding the subjective in its discursive context. What follows is an examination of situated subjectivity and the way it may be elicited by the uninterrupted telling of narratives.

Embedded Narratives

According to Wengraf, "one way of understanding the philosophy behind a minimalist-passive reception of interview narrative is that of "the Gestalt principle… which requires the spontaneous pattern of the speaker to complete itself fully and so be fully exposed for analysis" (Wengraf, 2001, 113). The interviewee is a narrative self with a personal "idiom" or "gestalt"— a characteristic way in which she/he is disposed to receive and organize experience. The argument is made that "the more free behavior was from external constraint, the more completely the internal dynamic could be expressed, and the more intelligible to the researcher that internal dynamic would then become" (Wengraf, 2001, 69).

Sub-session one, with its emphasis on the free-associative telling of narratives, rests in part on the arguments above and on the understanding that the observation of "free behavior would reveal to the researcher the current 'structuring principle' (gestalt) of all the particular behaviors being expressed" (ibid., 69). Hence, the more basic rationale for the uninterrupted telling of the stories is that premature questions exploring meaning can potentially produce an emerging image of the "situated subjectivity" of the interviewee. This is what Wengraf refers to as the "gestalt" (ibid., 113, 125, 137), and Christopher Bollas, professor of English, psychoanalyst, and author of *Being a Character*, calls "idiom" (Bollas, 1989, 9, 10, 212) and I would call the "embedded narrative" (cf. discussion above).

Bollas uses psychoanalytical theory, and in particular object relations, to relate "idiom" to "true self". According to the author, the true self "cannot be fully described", as "it is less like the articulation of meaning through words which allow one to isolate a unit of meaning as in the location of a signifier, and more akin to the movement of symphonic music" (ibid., 109f). Even though I am a researcher and not a psychoanalyst, I believe it is within my reach to identify through interpretation.

> 'The unique presence of being' (idiom) as opposed to other unique presences of being as we are singular complexities of human being – as different in makeup of our characters as in our physiognomies; our person design finds its expression in the discrete living villages (composed of all those objects we select to cultivate our needs, wishes and interests) that we create during our lifetime. (ibid., 9)

To me the notions of "idiom", "gestalt", and "embedded narrative" are not essentialist claims; rather, they imply that the self is conceived as the invariant dimension of first-personal givenness in the multitude of changing experiences, a continuous felt subjectivity through a sense of me-ness encountering different experiences. In other words, all experiences have one common feature, namely that they are all felt as mine and in that sense carry "a subtle presence of self"—the experiential self (Gallagher & Zahavi, 2008).

Thus, BNIM does not have to be understood as opposing the idea of narrations being constructed. Rather, it could be understood as a proper way of taking the social constructionist notion of narratives seriously as it provides a space in which the researcher can recognize the particular ways the interviewee is constructing his/her narratives and narrating his/her experiences subjectively. BNIM provides a methodological approach that elicits the research subject's acquired gestalt, her habitual projective and receptive dispositions, which interpose themselves between primary experience and meaning making. The "gestalt", "idiom", and "embedded narratives"—the changing individual structuring principle of experience elaborated above—can best be identified through the non-directed, free-associative telling of stories.

An uninterrupted telling facilitates the emergence of what might be omitted from constructionist narrativism, namely that the narrative self is both "in life" and "about life", and that it is possible to identify not only the latter, but also the embedded narrative. The fundamental social constructionist insight that "meanings are not automatically shared" calls for positive curiosity and questions on the part of the researcher, which a BNIM interview also encompasses and gives space to, but in due course during sub-session two.

Analysis: From Data to a Thin Sense of Subjectivity

Analytical Aim and Process

The aim of the analysis is to come to terms with the research question, and in order to do so, I engaged the data in a fourfold analytic process. Thus, the analysis chapter is divided into four parts, with an introduction to each:

1. A biographical narrative analysis of four individual "star" cases—Jacob, Dina, Eric, and Karla.
2. A write-up of themes across the star cases.
3. A reading across non-star cases based on identified themes in star cases.
4. Discussion of findings in relation to the central research question and relevant theory.

Each part is related, yet distinct, from one another. Rather than using the initial research questions as bait to fish randomly among the various transcribed interviews, seeking "proof" for one hypothesis or another, the SQUIN-BNIM analysis embodied a process that eventually led to an understanding of the four individual star cases. The reading across non-star cases resembles that of the star cases. Finally, in the last part of the analysis, I relate the findings across all cases to the research question and to theoretical perspectives that may shed light on it all. I will explain the different steps in the model more fully in the respective introductions to the four sub-chapters.

Interrelational Dynamics

Narrative accounts must be read with an eye on the context in which they are delivered:

> *If it is the case that psychological knowledge is constructed in the context of an interchange between 'researcher' and 'researched', then understanding the determining characteristics of that interaction – including what the researcher brings to it – is crucial for evaluating the significance of any research 'findings'.* (Frosh, 2010)

The first step in a SQUIN-BNIM analysis is thus analyzing the communicative interaction with the interviewee. In order to understand how my presence may have informed the account, it was important "to objectify the act of objectification". I have done so realizing that the way the interviewee objectifies me informs the telling of the story.

Psychoanalytic theory provides the conceptual means to grasp intersubjective dynamics. Addressing transference and countertransference in the therapy room and speaking about analysts, Bollas claims that "our presence is an action and the patient responds" (Bollas, 1992, 242), and "it is the analyst that becomes the patient's object not the other way around" (ibid., 196). The analyst becomes an object for the transference of undesirable or challenging parts of the client, or her history. The therapist's reaction to this is called countertransference. In general, a main feature of clinical work and relation-intense professions (Skovholt & Trotter-Mathison, 2011) is for the professional to reflect on who he is becoming for the patient or the client; Bollas argues that this "unthought known" may be sensed during the encounter, but can only be articulated in hindsight.

The debriefing notes made immediately after the interview are important in this regard. In these, I tried to grasp my sense of the interrelational dynamics, what the other provoked in me, and my experience of the encounter. I made use of this, as well as a transcription of my verbal and nonverbal contributions to the interview and reflective journaling during the process, to interpret how the interviewees may have been informed by my presence.

Prior to undertaking the interviews, I talked to my supervisors about whether I should disclose my professional background as a chaplain, or not. We agreed that I should primarily present myself as a researcher, which I did in the invitation letter. However, when asked what my professional background was while face-to-face with the interviewees, this proved difficult to sustain; hence, when asked I chose to be open about it.

The data suggest, to varying degrees, how my presence informed the interviewee's account. In Dina's case, the data revealed the relevance of my background and position, which suggests that this may have been a factor in the other accounts, though possibly to a lesser degree. In several passages, Dina relates my profession to her narrative and the telling of her story. Talking with a man affiliated to the church would have been much more difficult, if not impossible, for Dina, in a not too distant past:

> *(.) the worst for me was (.) hehe ((laughs!)) (.) you have to know (.) you can be glad that you are here now (.) a male pastor in the Norwegian church (.) that was the enemy - - (.) do you understand - -*

The fact that Dina sought out male pastors to process her own experiences of oppressive religiosity suggested that encountering a man who was also a chaplain could take precedence over other roles a man might have, such as being a researcher. Dina showing particular interest in my professional background, and explicitly probing whether or not I was ordained or not, could have suggested prior to the interview that she was about to be "coerced into some interpersonal environment" (Bollas, 1992, 200) of her past and that "*what first came to mind*", and arose subsequently, might have been a response to my presence. This is not to say that Dina's narrative account was not embedded, or that the selective principle of the telling was not of her own choosing, but rather that my presence, as compared to that of another researcher, informed the telling to some degree.

Being a sociologist of self is not an easy task, particularly when delineating the unconscious dynamics playing out between the researcher and the researched. The therapy room has its own traditions and practices to regulate the clinical encounters in which the language of transference and countertransference is established; in research encounters, these are different. This implies that one should be cautious of bringing the vocabulary (read transference and countertransference) of the former into the latter (Frosh, 2010, 215).

The Use of Panels

The use of panels is a key, but not unique, aspect of BNIM. I had full day panels for each of the star cases. The panel is supposed to comprise a heterogeneous group of people and provide a space for the individual researcher and group members to develop hypotheses dialogically. The intention of the panel is:

> *...to ensure the surfacing of sleeping assumptions, blind spots and misrecognition on the part of the researcher as an interpretive group is likely to be less defended and more insightful than any one of its members.* (Wengraf, 2001, 231)

The rationale for a panel accords with the realization that "the researchers are part of what they study, not separate from it" (Charmaz, 2006, 178) and provides a space in which the dynamics between interviewer and interviewee can be explored. The use of interpretive panels in the analysis phase of BNIM takes two elements seriously: that experiences in life are mine (cf. discussion above), and that the meaning of the experiences is socially and discursively appropriated, informed by cultural discourses and relative to the situation.

What is particular with BNIM's use of panels is the developing of future-blind hypotheses, counterhypotheses, and tangible hypotheses;

the latter implying a third option, in order to prevent dualistic thinking. Panels then contribute to making the research process into a simulation of the subject's own future-blind experiencing and future-forming decisions and selections. The emphasis on hypothesizing rests on certain anthropological premises. One is that life is lived future-blind: we can guess what will happen, but none of us know for certain. The panel discussion thus challenges the idea that what became the dominant storyline was the only possible storyline, and embraces the idea that the meaning of any action lies in the foregone alternatives.

The job of the panel is not to provide better lines of action, but actual lines of actions. Not "wild hypothesizing", but rather safeguarding against just that. What becomes apparent through a panel discussion is a multitude of possible subjective responses to the same situation, thus ensuring that my initial hypotheses are challenged (or confirmed), and my own subjectivity (and that of the panel members) elicited.

Researching Under the Surface

Self-understanding, as outlined in the previous chapter, the way a human being understands his or her own being, is implicit, which implies that one has to move beyond discursive means to make it explicit. This calls for a minute and systematic attention to not only *what* is said, but also *how* it is said.

BNIM offers protocols that extrapolate the implicit emotionality of the biographical account by considering the sequence, length, and manner in which the different topics are treated by the narrator. Subjectivity, understood as "the way the events and actions were experienced as well as are presently being understood, at the point of the interview, by the interviewee" (Wengraf, 2001, 239), on the other hand, implies more creative work by the researcher. It requires engaging the verbatim transcript in a way that extracts meaning and makes visible elements that highlight the particular subjectivity suggested in a told story. Wengraf argues that the starting point for this exploration should be a description of the textual structure: "a full description – full, that is, from the point of view of the instrumentation theory – of the textual structure created freely by the interviewee is a precondition of interpreting its significance" (ibid).

Embedded in the interview text are the patterns of speech, the perspectives on factual biographical elements, and hence the gestalt particular to the narrator at the point of the interview. However, the pressing question remains, namely what structural elements in a story can, by identification, represent a first step toward moving the researcher closer to understanding the subjectivity of the interviewee? Speaker, topic, and text type are all fundamental structural elements in an interview text, and change in any of them should be systematically noted and identified: "*a change in the way that somebody talks about an old or new topic is held to be significant*" (Wengraf, 2001, 243). Changes in regard to the following text types in the narrative accounts are identified and analyzed: descriptions, reports, argumentation, PINs, and evaluations. The text types often appear in the accounts as mixed categories (Wengraf, 2011, 888).

The changes are systematized in what is called a text structure sequentialization (TSS) and inform the chunking of the data for the panel. The TSS is a process that not only serves to make the transcripts more comprehensible, but more importantly progresses the researcher's analysis of them. This is because they shed light on how the interviewee spontaneously creates a coherent life story. The interpretation of the following lines, in which Dina is speaking about how she relates to death, serves as an illustration of how attention to text types can elicit the emotionality, and thus the subjectivity, of the text:

> *I am looking at everything in my life (.) turn every stone in a way to find out of things (.) then death was the next question (.) look at this thing about death (.) and this I also think is very important as a doctor (.) that you are capable of talking with people (.) that you have a natural relation to death and illness and all this right (.) and not be afraid of it yourself.*

There is a significant change in Dina's telling when she engages the topic of death. She goes from speaking in first person throughout her account to speaking in general, from "I" to "you", from Dasein to das Man. Considering the whole account thus facilitates an extrapolation of the "evolving subjectivity", the possible altered ways of perceiving and acting in the world, and hence the changed ways of making one's own being an issue.

In other words, BNIM offers methodological interpretive means to undertake an extrapolation of what lies beneath the surface. By holding together the "biographical data analysis" and the "teller flow analysis", the interpretive method facilitates a construction of the "phases of mutating subjectivity" and hence extrapolates from the biographical narrative "how the informant has changed perspectives and priorities about self, her life, her world and how best to understand and act in it" (Wengraf, 2011, 558).

The Particular and the General

A "Good Enough" Number of Cases?

Analysis is a responsive process that may go on as long as there are perspectives not yet applied to the material. In other words, it can go on forever. So how do I know when enough is enough? As a qualitative researcher, I am not looking for the point at which I feel confident enough to make a generalizable truth regarding physicians in palliative care, or nurses in intensive care. On the contrary, my initial focus is very much on the particular, not on universal laws, but on individual patterns. Hence, in the SQUIN-BNIM analysis, the first of the four analytic parts, "enough" is when, having interpreted the whole interview, I get a clear emergent gestalt, an image of the interviewees' situated subjectivity, and of their respective ways of perceiving and acting.

Although committed to exploring the particular, the study has a broader aim than eliciting the accounts of the individual subjects. Hence, having worked on identifying an emerging gestalt, I read across the four star cases to identify common themes, and then, I consider the remaining accounts for the same purpose. After using a creative written process to identify themes that seem to be common across the material, I generalize further using substantial theories.

Choosing Four Star Cases

First Case

The process is not concerned with undertaking an in-depth exploration of a representative case, as there is no such thing. In order not to be tempted into any unconscious positivism, I decided that my first star case should be the interview that stood out as the most surprising, the one that most challenged my prejudices and made me most curious. It had to be Dina. Her "unexpected" account challenged my preconceived ideas the most, and there was an audible call to explore theoretical and methodological issues fundamental to my project from the inherent "problems" in this case.

Second Case

To identify the second case I used "difference" as a selective principle, choosing the one that stood in starkest contrast to Dina. I chose Jacob (55), a physician who heads an ICU unit, for several reasons. He was the same age as Dina, had a similar amount of experience and the same education, but yet he delivered a very different account; this called for an exploration.

Maybe the most important point distinguishing the two accounts was that Dina situated her narrative primarily outside the clinic, whereas Jacob stayed almost exclusively within it. When talking about his son's illness and his mother's declining health, he apologized for bringing in "my own world". Although there were other personal references, his references to his son, mother, and father-in-law were all told in relation to, and to describe, clinical issues. This is both similar to and very different from Dina, who told clinical stories to illuminate her own personal issues.

Dina almost exclusively spoke in first person, while Jacob used very few "I" statements. Thematically, in various ways, Jacob mentioned guilt—not in relation to a higher being or significant others, as in Dina's case, but rather to being in a position to make life and death decisions (and the possibility of being accused of misconduct by "the system").

Another reason for making Jacob the second case was that his account was not as structured as that of his female colleague. In Dina's case, there was a stronger sense of rehearsed story. Jacob's sharing, on the other hand, of close to 30 mainly clinical incidents, is almost impossible to rehearse. He also voiced the concern at the end that he had not been coherent enough. In other words, it was my impression that he had no clear idea of where he was going with his account.

In a sense, by focusing his account on the clinical, Jacob was the more conventional of the two. He responded to the SQUIN as one might expect from a physician. Still, his personal engagement was very much felt throughout. What made this personal tone and emotional engagement different from Dina's? I had the impression that as she recounted her narrative during the interview, Dina's focus was more on care for self and her own personal development, whereas in various ways Jacob was telling stories about patients and families and hence—seemingly—displayed more care for others. This was challenged through my interpretive work, but was definitely a point that made me want to explore his narrative account in more depth.

Finally, my experience of speaking with them was very different. In Dina's case, I was on the edge of my chair throughout. In contrast, during my own debrief after the interview with Jacob, I noted that I had never felt as tired during any other interview. In addition, I noted that I didn't feel there was much to say after the interview, or much material for the debriefing. Listening to the recorded interview some months later, my experience of listening to him was quite different—which makes me wonder what was happening at the time.

Karla (33), an intensive care nurse, was another strong second candidate. I chose Jacob because Karla, like Dina, had a structured, more linear, and "rehearsed" account. Jacob, on the other hand, was not as linear in his narrative construction. Jacob's account was as void of personal references as Dina's account was full of them. In Dina's case, the pressing issue was to demonstrate how encounters with other people's death may have informed her self-understanding when there were so few references to such encounters. In Jacob's case, there was no lack of references to encounters with the deaths of others. The pressing methodological question was how to extrapolate self-understanding at all when the account so lacked first-person statements and biographical elements (a question also raised by Karla's account).

Third Case

In the name of diversity, what should then be my third case? Which of the remaining ten seemed to be only marginally related thematically, but could still potentially enrich the study? Karla could for reasons elaborated above. Gail, a chaplain from a university hospital in the USA, was also a viable candidate. She was different from the first two in that she was situated in another cultural context, held a different professional role, and was about to retire from her position. Exploring what leaving professional life implied for her narrative was a very interesting question. It seemed to incentivize her more than Dina or Jacob to tell a total story (as compared to one which is more focused), in which she reflected upon how her personal life and professional life were intertwined. She even made a comment about the interview providing her with the opportunity to do so.

The telling mirrored this as it took her back and forth between her childhood years at the farm to working at the boundary between life and death for 30 years, and now as she looks ahead to the "promised land" (she retired a few months after the interview to go home to take over the farm). More than Dina and Jacob, Gail explicitly reflected upon how her personal life and professional life were intertwined. As in Dina's and Jacob's accounts, there was strong ambivalence toward both the role and the health service in general. The toll the work had taken on her was even more explicitly addressed, and in more detail than the previous two interviewees. There was significantly more overt anger and strong negative statements regarding her own profession. She voiced a strong sense that the job and particularly the neoliberal turn within health care were a threat to her life.

Eric, another chaplain (Norwegian) and also a candidate for third interviewee, voiced a much more positive attitude to his current professional role and context. Like Karla, this may have been related to him having had only limited experience in the hospital context. Maybe he was a candidate because more than any of the others (with the possible exception of Fiona), he talked extensively about his own relation to death and how it had changed over the years. Eric was placed between Dina and Jacob in terms of including PINs from both his professional and his personal life. Eric's account represented continuity in regard to themes already raised in the other two accounts. Hence, to some extent, Eric's biography and account both related to, and contradicted, those of Dina and Jacob.

Carl, the third chaplain, provided a less spontaneous account than Eric. It appeared more as a theological testament/rationale. Like Gail, it was as if he used the opportunity of the interview to author "a testament". Eric, on the other hand, came across as more spontaneous. After the interview, he voiced surprise that he had talked so much about his father, and recognized that the interview had triggered new interest in how this relationship had influenced him. There was both a width and a thickness to Eric's account. He spanned the clinical and the personal, and he lingered over particularly important incidents. Death was very much the red thread that ran throughout it all.

Hence, more than Dina and Jacob, Eric's account seemed to relate in a slightly different way to my central research question, as death and the fear of it was much more explicitly addressed; it not just mentioned at the borders of the narrative, as was the case with Dina, Gail, and Jacob. Fiona, another anesthesiologist, also spent the first part of her account talking about the presence of death in her upbringing (somebody commented: "Gee, you are really growing up in a hospice"). Fiona talked about death in a more distant manner, while Eric shared more intimately his exposure to his father's fear of death, his own fear of death, him being sick of hospitals and of caring for his mother, as well as how he experienced death and dying in the hospital. I decided that Eric would be my third case, not least because it was hard to overlook the centrality of death in his account.

Fourth Case

The first three cases were selected according to the differences identified in the narrative accounts. The side effect of this was that all three narrators shared one important biographical trait, namely age. They had all turned 50 by the time of the interview. Another equally important point was that so far none of the nurses' accounts had been analyzed. Karla, the young female intensive care nurse, was thus a strong candidate to go fourth; so was Leah, a female nurse in her late twenties working at a palliative unit.

Like Jacob, Karla's first narrative was situated solely in the clinic. Unlike Jacob, however, Karla focused on five PINs; most of the time was spent exploring two of these (one took ten minutes, the other forty!). The PINs seemed to have been chosen as a result of their particular and profound impact on her. Karla, more than any of the other interviewees, was very detailed in her telling of the clinical incidents. At the same time, her manner of speech differed significantly from the first-person style adopted by Dina and Eric. Karla seemed to be reporting diligently and thoroughly. She also made use of more technical language, more so than Jacob, seemingly letting her talk be informed by the professional context she inhabited, but which she had not yet made her own. This was different to Dina whose account was more informed by the therapeutic process she had recently undergone. Again, as in Jacob's account, the themes Karla raised seemed to both overlap and supplement those of the previous three.

Ethics and Validity

I don't know you (.4) ehm (.2) so some of it just makes me feel very vulnerable (.) a little exposed (.) so I am putting my heart in your hands (.1) so I am thinking () here and there I thought 'who is going to be able to listen this'.

(Iris, one of the interviewees responding to my question about how it was for her to do the interview.)

A primary concern in a qualitative study is to safeguard the integrity of the interviewees. Another is to safeguard the integrity of the text. The two are closely related and at times seemingly at odds with one another, as when trying to maximize participant anonymity, "managing identifying details" (Saunders, Kitzinger, & Kitzinger, 2015, 617), and at the same time maintaining the integrity of the data. The following shows how the choices of method gave rise to ethical issues, and elaborates the particular criteria applied to safeguard the integrity of both the interviewees and the text.

Felt Dilemmas

The open invitation articulated in a single question does not force the interviewee to share any sensitive material, but at the same time it may bring forgotten—and potentially challenging—material to the surface. Having trained and worked as a chaplain, supervisor, and family therapist, I have experience in being sensitive to the vulnerability of the other, to power issues, taking responsibility for the relational process, and supporting the autonomy of the client and his or her right to say, "No, I don't want to do this".

It is my experience that the non-interruptive interview approach both facilitated and challenged the above. It supported the interviewee's autonomy in that the researcher didn't guide the narrative. Yet, we are always caught in feedback loops that emerge from the explicit or implicit messages from our surroundings. Wengraf makes the point that interviewees shouldn't know the details of the SQUIN, the precise invitation, prior to the interview. The rationale for this is that a prepared, rehearsed, story doesn't provide the full gestalt to the same degree as a spontaneous telling.

It is my understanding that knowing only part of what is expected can breed a strong sense of insecurity and powerlessness. Hence, it was of paramount importance for me to provide the interviewees with an information letter in good time prior to the actual interview. In every case, I also offered time for questions before starting the tape recorder. In some instances, for unknown reasons, the interviewees had not read the letter. In these cases, I talked about the project and introduced the interview process before we started the actual interview. None of the participants raised concerns regarding the lack of guidance, either immediately after the interview or in the follow-up call a week later.

There were certain points though at which I felt an uneasiness in not being "allowed" to respond to an interviewee's request for instruction. Typically, when I had the sense that the interviewee was coming toward the end of the initial account, after a long pause, to ensure they felt free to add more, I repeated at least part of the SQUIN. Like the kind of clarification, or not, that took place about half an hour into my interview with Eric:

Eric yes (.) I do not know if I have that much more to say (.7)
Interviewer Other events or experiences… (.)
E **((interrupts me))** Personal experiences (.)
I …which are important to you personally (.)
E related to death then (.1) and those things knotted to death (.) **((is probing, possible to trace an insecurity in his voice?))**
I Ehh (.) other events (.) experiences that are important to you personally in the the story of your life (.5)
E which are not necessarily related to what has to do with death (.) or which have a consequence in regard to it or influencing it or are relevant in relation to it (.6)
I I think it is how you hear it. (.) actually really an open (.) an open question…. ((Eric is expressing that he understands)) (.7)
E but with relevance in regard to what has to do with chaplaincy (.) or did you think it totally open (.)
I So can you tell me the story of your life - - (.) tell me about all those events and experiences that are important to you - - (.) personally (.) - - then I don't help you more than that

Listening to this part of the interview, while transcribing, made me sweat. It was uncomfortable witnessing the way I was refusing to lead, not providing help, leaving the floor open. Neither my own discomfort, nor Eric's, however, necessarily implied that what was taking place was ethically questionable. It can be argued that I was just fulfilling our "contract" by not interrupting his telling, and not, at this point, providing guiding questions.

Before giving attention to the particular issue of anonymity, and the ethical obligations toward the individual, let us move toward an outline of criteria supporting the validity of the project, and thus also its ethical soundness.

Validity

Validity is a debated and controversial concept within qualitative research. The term may be broadly defined as "*the state or quality of being sound, just and well-founded*" (Webster, 1989), which I would assume is the aim of most research, quantitative and qualitative. Still, the process of "assuring validity" (Whittemore, Chase, & Mandle, 2001, 527) looks quite different within these two different research orientations. This rests in part on the different ontological and epistemological assumptions underpinning them and how one relates to what Hacking terms "elevator words"—truth, reality, knowledge—and I would add quality (Braun & Clarke, 2013, 278).

It has been difficult to establish a set of generally accepted criteria for qualitative research. This is partly related to both the heterogeneity in regard to the objects of study and the variety of philosophical grounds on which researchers stand. Qualitative knowledge is temporally and interpersonally situated, and thus "contingent, strategic and provisional", co-constructed by researcher and researched. When acknowledging language as performative, it doesn't make sense to speak of "having knowledge about a subject" (Frosh, 2010, 210).

Whittemore et al., following Maxwell, suggest an understanding of validity both as a regulative *and* as a relative ideal (Whittemore et al., 2001, 528). Opting for only one of these measures on the basis that validity is comprised of only one set of legitimate and normative criteria would not take sufficient account of the wickedness of qualitative research, or the fact that it is defined by heterogeneity, uncertainty, fluidity, and emergent ideas. This realization invites a flexible and relativist position rather than one which is rigid. Still, few would support purging any criteria or leaving the individual researcher to define them. This speaks to the importance of understanding validity both as a regulative *and* a relative ideal.

Primary Criteria of Validity

Whittemore et al. (2001) explore the main issues in the debate about validity in qualitative research during the last decades and propose a synthesis in which they distinguish between primary and secondary criteria. According to the authors, primary criteria are credibility, authenticity, criticality, and integrity. Secondary criteria are explicitness, vividness, creativity, thoroughness, congruence, and sensitivity. They caution against blind faith and suggest that both the criteria and how they are prioritized must be informed by the research question, study design, and the philosophical position of the investigator. The following paragraphs are an attempt to come to terms with such an endeavor vis-à-vis my own project.

Credibility	Do the results of the research reflect the experience of participants or the context in a believable way?
Authenticity	Does a representation of the emic perspective exhibit awareness of the subtle differences in the voices of all participants?
Criticality	Does the research process demonstrate evidence of critical appraisal?
Integrity	Does the research reflect recursive and repetitive checks of validity as well as a humble presentation of findings?

The above-listed criteria served as guidelines for my project. Credibility—the trustworthiness of the research—cannot be claimed, it must be earned, and it is up to the reader and those from the clinical communities in which I have been interviewing to decide whether they view my findings as credible. That does not necessarily imply agreement. I have worked to show explicitly how I relate my interpretations to the data. In addition, not least in this chapter, I have been transparent about how the transcribed texts were worked with, transformed and synthesized. I have made the methodological choices explicit. Hopefully, this was done in vivid and creative ways so the reader is able to deem the process trustworthy or not.

BNIM works to elicit the subjective by paying minute attention to what is particular in each case, working toward, and continuously testing, structural hypotheses. This is to ensure authenticity and an extrapolation of the sometimes subtle differences between individual voices. Doing an interpretive study implies that there might be a discrepancy between the etic and the emic—the researcher's interpreted understanding and the self-reported understanding of the interviewee. What must be present, in order for the reader to assess the degree of authenticity, is an explication of where one ends and the other begins, as well as of the underpinnings that guide the interpretation. This has been my purpose throughout and is pursued in the write-up of the individual star cases as well as in the more thematic engagement with the non-star cases.

Criticality indicates a self-reflective and critical appraisal of my own process. I have pursued this through ongoing discussions about choices and findings with my supervisors, as well as with colleagues at home and abroad. The panels, whose contribution I outlined above, also served this purpose, challenging my preconceived ideas about the accounts and the "enchantment" of the first listening. I hope a self-critical attitude will be apparent to the reader throughout the text.

The final primary criterion on which the validity of my project rests is integrity. The degree to which this has been met is informed by the presence, or absence, of the first three criteria. It rests on the willingness to be self-critical as well as transparent, allowing others to question the process as it moves forward. I have pursued self-critical transparency by participating in conferences and seminars, and subjecting unfinished thoughts and texts to other scholars for assessment.

Secondary Criteria of Validity

The secondary criteria relate to one another: the degree of "thoroughness" and "sensitivity" relates to "explicitness" and "vividness". Whether the latter two are met relates to the degree that "creativity" and "congruence" are present in the study. These secondary criteria are as stringent as the primary. Again, the reader will be the final judge.

Explicitness	Have methodological decisions, interpretations, and investigator biases been addressed?
Vividness	Have thick and faithful descriptions been portrayed with vibrancy and clarity?
Creativity	Have imaginative ways of organizing, presenting, and analyzing data been incorporated?
Thoroughness	Do the findings convincingly address the questions posed through completeness and saturation?
Congruence	Are the process and the findings congruent? Do all the themes fit together? Do findings fit into a context outside the study situation?
Sensitivity	Sensitivity to context of existing research, of participant's perspectives, of ethical issues, of owning my own perspective.

Anonymity

> As a general principle, those who are made the subjects of research are entitled to have their personal information treated confidentially. The researcher must prevent any use and communication of information that might inflict damage on individuals who are the subjects of research. Irrespective of the duty of confidentiality, researchers have a legal obligation to avoid punishable offences. The researcher must decide when and in what way the participant should be informed about limitations of the duty of confidentiality.
>
> (The Norwegian National Committees for Research Ethics)

In the letter of consent to the participants of the present study, I made the claim that I "will do what I can to ensure anonymity". How does one simultaneously safeguard the anonymity of participants without compromising the integrity and authenticity of their narratives? Replacing key features of the interviewees' biographical and narrative constitution to protect them against identification may in fact undermine their descriptions and transform them in ways they would not want. This is a central problem to the issue of anonymizing qualitative data. The key point made is that "anonymizing is not, in practice, something that can be done on automatic pilot with a 'one size fits all' or 'find and replace' approach" (Saunders et al., 2015, 627). It is a continuum with no sure indicator of which direction to take.

Many will argue for the importance of anonymity, while at the same time acknowledging that complete anonymity is beyond reach in most qualitative studies (Clark, 2006). Some will question the "culturally embedded assumption that anonymity is an ethical prerequisite". They will bring attention to the "underestimated likelihood of research participants wishing to be acknowledged in published research thus enabling them to retain ownership of their stories" (Grinyer, 2002) and offer the participant non-confidentiality in the name of autonomy (Giordano, O'Reilly, Taylor, & Dogra, 2007). My primary argument for anonymity is to prevent harm to the participants. Nonetheless, ethics preclude undertaking protective means in a paternalistic manner (Moore, 2012).

All interviewees' names—and the names of those they include in their narratives—have been changed at the point of transcription. However, other opportunities for identification remain. Changing religion, gender, cultural, and ethnic affiliation is not unproblematic, because in many instances these are not simply background information, but rather integral and integrative parts of the interviewees' lives and narratives. "Such data… provides context for deeper, and fuller, understanding of the empirical data" (Clark, 2006, 6). Change may result in decontextualizing the accounts, depriving the narrators of their idiosyncratic voices and thus threatening integrity and limiting the analyses.

Hence, I have tried to balance concern for the vulnerability that comes with naming with that which comes with losing one's name. Identifiers have only been removed when no serious harm is done as a result either to the integrity of the narrative account or to the communication of the narrator's subjectivity. At the same time, what the individual interviewee experiences as vulnerability is not solely for me to judge, and this poses the question whether to negotiate anonymity issues directly with the interviewees (Saunders et al., 2015), a question that relates to the issue of "member checking".

Member checking usually implies presenting the research, or parts of it, in written or oral form, to some or all of the participants at various times for their validation (Braun & Clarke, 2013, 282). I contacted all the interviewees within the first week of the interview (except for Jacob and Karla, whom I contacted at a later date), to make sure they were comfortable with the outcome of the interviews. A dialogue with the participants concerning the validity of my interpretations and analysis was not part of our contract.

The choice not to include such a process relates in part to the understanding of both the research subject and research process outlined in this and the previous chapter. The study is primarily about interpreting rather than representing the experiences of others. It does not rest on the assumption that the participants always have full insight; therefore, I avoided any dialogue that might suggest the opposite or leave the impression that together we could reach some kind of objective truth. This was not built into the design of the study, and thus, interviewees were never invited to such a discussion.

Still, this argument does not settle the question of anonymity, and whether the steps I took to protect interviewees were sufficient. For a while I deliberated whether to invite the four star case participants to read the section which dealt with their respective narrative accounts. There were substantial arguments for and against; I discussed the matter with several experienced, qualitative researchers, including narrative researchers.

One reason for this step would be to enable them to detect information that might reveal their identity to people who knew them. It would also be an opportunity for them to comment on changed information they would rather keep authentic. An important reason against including this step was that it was not part of our initial contract; none of them had expressed a desire to read the analysis. One did ask for a copy when the project was finished, but that did not imply a desire to undertake quality assurance along the way.

Thus, the expectation was that it was my responsibility to handle their narratives and the matter of anonymity in a respectful and professional fashion. Asking them to decide whether to read or not could easily foster insecurity. This was also the key argument used by the researchers I consulted. Not finding sufficiently compelling reasons to change the contract, I left things as they were. However, I did take further steps to anonymize the text.

A Reader's Map for the Star Cases

The following is a map of the SQUIN-BNIM analysis of the four star cases which appear in the next four chapters. It is an in-depth analysis in order to elicit the implicit thin lines of evolving subjectivity identified in the narrative accounts, what is referred to as "the first narrative"—the free-associative, uninterrupted telling in sub-session one. It is aiming at getting an understanding of the structure of the cases, giving voice to the idiosyncratic, before considering, in Chapter 8, what these four and eventually all the cases share thematically. The endeavor follows the protocols introduced in the previous chapter, considering both what is told and the manner of telling it.

The write-up of the star cases is the last reading in a process that includes several analytic steps. The methodological steps and their rationale are outlined above; nonetheless, it is worth describing the layers of analysis upon which the last reading rests.

The SQUIN-BNIM analysis is framed by a two-track model guided by two theoretical questions: (1) What is the structure/pattern of the lived life? and (2) What is the structure/pattern of the told story/the self-presentation? These lead to a third question: (3) What is the relationship between the structure of the lived life and the told story? The elaboration of what is conveyed here briefly is presented under the heading "The telling of the story in detail", an analysis of the relation between parts and whole leading toward the researcher's understanding of the situated subjectivity.

After having constructed a transcribed text, the first analytic step was to present the data in chunks to a panel of four to six members. There were four different panels each spent a full workday (seven to eight hours) discussing the lived life and then the told story of each individual star case. Their insights and comments, which challenged my own reading of the data, will be included in the write-up of each case.

In order to respond to the first question above regarding the structure of the lived life, I have undertaken an enriched biographical data analysis. This elicits the lived life, considering the sociohistoric context and speculating on different possible ways of experiencing and acting, and arriving at a hypothesis. Similarly, regarding the told story, I was informed by the notion that meaning lies in the forgone alternatives and thus undertook a teller flow analysis, which identifies and interprets changes in topic, manner, and speaker. I asked why the narrative account is developing this way, trying to sense an emotional shape and assuming the flow primarily to be created by the interviewee.

In the history of the case's evolution, which is the researcher's account, the reader is presented with the merger of the two perspectives and inputs from the different panels. The teller flow analysis is at the core of the final write-up, but cultural–historical factors discussed in the enriched biographical data analysis are included only to the degree required by the telling. Hence, the reader will recognize that the number of cultural–historical references differs in the four write-ups.

Based on the flow analysis, I undertook a thematic field analysis. The thematic fields are a way of naming what appear to be the "undercurrents" that inform what emerges in the telling, what structures the flow, the "subtle choreography between subject and object" (Wengraf, 2011, 520). It can be singular or plural, often contradictory. This is done to identify the pattern/patchwork of the told story and thus render intelligible those parts identified in the flow; it also moves the analysis toward a sense of the subjectivity, the gestalt emerging through my reading of the narrative account. This is captured in the last sub-chapter of each star case analysis, under the heading "A thin sense of the situated subjectivity" (at the point of the interview) .

Part of the rationale for the lengthy and detailed individual case write-ups in the following is to honor the sequence and manner of the narrator's telling, and to demonstrate the richness and complexity in a single professional's narrative account. It ensures both transparency and idiosyncrasy. Hence, there are a number of quotes included, written in italics to enhance their visibility in the text. To give the reader a feel of the narrator's speech, I have included pauses, e.g., "(.5)", which indicates a five-second pause in the telling, and "- - ", which indicates my nonverbal responses like "mhm-mhm", and **bold type** denoting a raising or intensifying of the narrator's voice.

The interpretation of the narrative accounts, which the reader may sometimes find confusing, is outlined thus so the individual gestalt can emerge in thin dotted lines. Still, both a shared and recognizable structure, the eliciting of dominant themes, and a summary of each case all help facilitate a synoptic reading and thus pave the way for a thematic reading across all cases in the next chapter.

References

Anderson, H. (1997). *Conversation, language, and possibilities: A postmodern approach to therapy*. New York: Basic Books.

Anderson, H. (2003). *Samtale, sprog og terapi: Et postmoderne perspektiv* [Conversation, language, and possibilities: A postmodern approach to therapy]. København: Hans Reitzels Forlag.

Bollas, C. (1989). *Forces of destiny: Psychoanalysis and human idiom*. London: Free Association Books.

Bollas, C. (1992). *Being a character: Psychoanalysis and self experience*. New York: Hill and Wang.

Bourdieu, P. (1977). *Outline of a theory of practice*. Cambridge: Cambridge University Press.

Braun, V., & Clarke, V. (2013). *Successful qualitative research: A practical guide for beginners*. Los Angeles, CA: Sage.

Casey, B., Proudfoot, D., & Corbally, M. (2016). Narrative in nursing research: An overview of three approaches. *Journal of Advanced Nursing*. https://doi.org/10.1111/jan.12887.

Cerbone, D. R. (2008). *Heidegger: A guide for the perplexed*. Guides for the perplexed. London: Continuum International Publishing Group.

Chamberlayne, P., Bornat, J., & Wengraf, T. (2002). *The turn to biographical methods in social science: Comparative issues and examples*. London and New York: Taylor and Francis.

Charmaz, K. (2006). *Constructing grounded theory: A practical guide through qualitative analysis*. London: Sage.

Clark, A. (2006). *Anonymising research data* (ESRC National Centre for Research Methods, Real Life Methods Working Paper Series). Retrieved from http://eprints.ncrm.ac.uk/480/1/0706_anonymising_research_data.pdf.

Frosh, S. (2010). *Psychoanalysis outside the clinic: Interventions in psycho-social studies*. Basingstoke: Palgrave Macmillan.

Gadamer, H.-G. (1989). *Truth and method* (2nd rev. ed., translation revised by Joel Weinsheimer and Donald G. Marshall). London: Sheed & Ward.

Gadamer, H.-G., & Holm-Hansen, L. (2010). *Sannhet og metode: grunntrekk i en filosofisk hermeneutikk* [Truth and method; the fundamentals of a philosophical hermeneutic]. Oslo: Pax Forlag AS.

Gallagher, S., & Zahavi, D. (2008). *The phenomenological mind: An introduction to philosophy of mind and cognitive science*. London and New York: Routledge.

Geertz, C. (1973). *The interpretation of culture*. London: Fontana Press.

Giordano, J., O'Reilly, M., Taylor, H., & Dogra, N. (2007). Confidentiality and autonomy: The challenge(s) of offering research participants a choice of disclosing their identity. *Qualitative Health Research, 17*(2), 264–275.

Grinyer, A. (2002). The anonymity of research participants: Assumptions, ethics and practicalities. *Social Research Update*. Retrieved from http://sru.soc.surrey.ac.uk/SRU36.html.

Heidegger, M. (2010). *On time and being*. Albany: State University of New York Press.

Mishler, E. G. (1986). *Research interviewing: Context and narrative*. Cambridge: Harvard University Press.

Moore, N. (2012). The politics & ethics of naming: Questioning anonymisation in (archival) research. *International Journal of Social Research Methodology, 15*(4), 331–340. https://doi.org/10.1080/13645579.2012.688330.

Nyeng, F., & Taylor, C. (2000). *Det autentiske menneske: med Charles Taylors blikk på menneskevitenskap og moral* [The authentic human being: With Charles Taylor's perspective on human sciences and morality]. Bergen: Fagbokforl.

Ricoeur, P. (1988). *Time and narrative* (Vol. 3). Chicago: University of Chicago Press.

Rittel, H., & Webber, M. (1973). Dilemmas in a general theory of planning. *Integrating Knowledge and Practice to Advance Human Dignity, 4*(2), 155–169. https://doi.org/10.1007/BF01405730.

Rogers, C. R. (1965). *Client-centered therapy*. Boston, USA: Houghton Mifflin Company.

Saunders, B., Kitzinger, J., & Kitzinger, C. (2015). Anonymising interview data: Challenges and compromise in practice. *Qualitative Research, 15*(5), 616–632. https://doi.org/10.1177/1468794114550439.
Skovholt, T. M., & Trotter-Mathison, M. J. (2011). *The resilient practitioner: Burnout prevention and self-care strategies for counselors, therapists, teachers, and health professionals*. New York: Routledge.
Stubblefield, C., & Murray, R. L. (2002). A phenomenological framework for psychiatric nursing research. *Archives of Psychiatric Nursing, 16*, 149–155.
Taylor, C. (1989). *Sources of the self: The making of the modern identity*. Cambridge: Cambridge University Press.
Webster (1989). *Webster's encyclopedic unabridged dictionary of the English language*. New York: Gramercy Books.
Thagaard, T. (2013). *Systematikk og innlevelse. En innføring i kvalitativ metode* (4rd ed.) [An introduction to qualitative method]. Bergen: Fagbokforlaget.
Wengraf, T. (2001). *Qualititative research interviewing: Biographic narrative and semi structured methods*. London: Sage.
Wengraf, T. (2011). *BNIM short guide bound with the BNIM detailed manual*. Interviewing for life-histories, lived periods and situations, and ongoing personal experiencing using the Biographic-Narrative Interpretive Method (BNIM).
Whittemore, R., Chase, S. K., & Mandle, C. L. (2001). Validity in qualitative research. *Qualitative Health Research, 11*(4), 522.

4
Jacob

Lived Life and Told Story

Setting the Scene

I called Jacob from the information desk, as we had agreed. Within a few minutes, a tall anesthesiologist in his fifties welcomed me with a warm smile and a firm handshake. He guided me to an office-door with a yellow post-it note stuck to it: "Jacob Olsen, 11–14". Jacob, having thus planned my visit, made me feel expected and welcomed. I soon learned that this level of order contrasted somewhat with his narrative account of "loose ends".

Jacob used the first couple of minutes to probe me about my professional background. Through positive comments about his son's recent confirmation, the presence of a chaplain at the hospital, and his father-in-law's religious epiphany at his deathbed, he expressed no hostility toward the fact that I am also a chaplain. On the contrary, during the interview, I had the sense that he was relating to me primarily as a researcher. He spoke as if assuming I knew nothing about his professional context. I take it that if responding to me primarily as a chaplain,

K. Moen, *Death at Work*, Studies in the Psychosocial,
https://doi.org/10.1007/978-3-319-90326-2_4

Jacob wouldn't feel any obligation to introduce me to his context, but assumed that I would know.

Jacob had already told me that his shift started at 3.00 p.m.; we broke off at around 2.55 p.m., though doubtless we could have gone for longer. There were no signs of Jacob wanting to leave. From the outset, he engaged himself in the narrative task, making no effort to hold back, but sharing generously from his 30-year career. At no point did he seem to notice the tiredness that almost overtook me at times. He engaged himself in the telling, even though he was "*not used to this*".

Lived Life—In Brief

Jacob was born in the late 1950s in a midsize city in Norway. He started his studies in medicine at around age twenty. This meant moving from his hometown to a bigger city. He married at age twenty-six, the same year he graduated. Immediately following graduation, Jacob started a year-long mandatory internship, followed by military service. At twenty-eight, in an order not determined by his account, he fathered a son, moved with his family to another city, and worked for several months as physician in one of its district offices. Soon he got a temporary position at a local hospital and started to specialize in surgery. He changed direction to pursue training as an anesthesiologist instead. Twelve years after graduating, he got a permanent position. During his early forties, Jacob married for the second time and moved to several different places before eventually returning to the same city, and the post of head physician at an intensive care unit, where he was working at the time of the interview.

Told Story—An Overview

At my invitation to "tell the story of your life", Jacob paused for six seconds then spoke uninterruptedly for about two hours. Twice toward the end of our three-hour interview, he expressed concern at having offered me an account of "loose ends". When later engaged in the analysis of the transcribed text, I tended to agree. It is hard to identify a pattern in Jacob's narrative upon first hearing it, and this may leave the impression of a lack of structure. It took time, and multiple readings and interpretations to identify potential thematic fields underlying the twists and turns of the narrative account.

Jacob's account consisted of around thirty particular incident narratives (PINs) from his career as a physician. Most were only briefly introduced before he made them into typical situations described in general, technical, or procedural terms as "*how things usually are*". I categorized "*the loose ends*" under the following thematic headings: (1) the many faces of death; (2) communicating with patients and relatives about imminent death; (3) the importance and limit of procedures; (4) guilt—that of others and Jacob's own; (5) the question of dignity—and who determines its prospect; and (6) the complexity and ambiguity of change.

Jacob's account was densely populated. There was a collage of faces, but all presented as quite distant portraits. He referred to several different people, but gave them no names, rather addressed them by means of impersonal pronouns, at times with a diagnostic label attached. This resulted in thin descriptions of those inhabiting Jacob's universe, his mother being one possible exception. An important aspect of his reflection on encounters with patients and relatives was his "reading" of the other's gaze, facial expressions, body language, and interactions. Although he did not give them faces, Jacob provided glimpses of their facial expressions and voices through quotes and dialogical enactments. Repeatedly, during his telling, he had an eye on what was at stake for the other.

A few months prior to the interview, Jacob was in a cardiac unit with stress-related chest pain. He related this to something that was barely mentioned, left on the borders of the narrative, present yet absent, and raised both before and at the very end of the interview: the "*violent organizational change*" that was taking place at the hospital. This included changes in the physician's professional role and something that might threaten, and actualize, Jacob's line of defense (professionalism): "*you are sucked in (.) whirls around with it (.) it never stops … feels life threatening*".

Detailed Reading of the Narrative

A Professional's Trajectory

> *Then I can start with my background.*

Jacob's first response to the SQUIN, "*Then I can maybe start a little bit with my background*", suggested that he was going to adhere to a typical trajectory of storytelling, starting with the past to provide a background for the present. "Background" could have implied starting at the very beginning and providing the interviewer with a glimpse of childhood, upbringing, and relationships with significant others. In evaluative terms, he could have talked about a good childhood or a challenging one. He could have recounted events or situations, even traumatic ones, that had informed his choice to become a physician, or he could have elaborated on the reasons and events that initially made him pursue medical school.

"*Background*" for Jacob implied something else. To fill it with meaning, he provided a brief report, a summarizing, of his professional trajectory. The first few minutes of the account included the frequent use of professional terms which for many signal status: *"hospital doctor", "anesthesia", "head doctor", "intensive care", "surgery", "heart thorax surgery", "highly specialized unit"*. To the panel, the brief initial report consisted of personal and professional moves in accordance with a stereotypical professional doctor's trajectory. The timing of the next steps in Jacob's life, as summarized in the brief account, left no room to see him as a man hesitating: no pauses, no breaks, no lingering, no detours. To the panel, this suggested "*ambition*", "*independence*", and "*conventionalism*". In such a case, "*natural*" next steps and moves in the same "*conventional direction*" that provide a sense of "*achievement*" could be "*house, kids, station wagon and dog*", according to the panel.

In the year Jacob changed from surgery to anesthesia, specialization was a prerequisite for getting a permanent physician's post, as it is today. Hence, pursuing specialization as early as possible in one's medical career is an expectation in line with a "normal" career path in Norway. Toward the end of the 1980s, there were thirty-eight specialization options. From one perspective, medical specializations are viewed on a hierarchy of medical conditions in which the most prestigious are those at the "spectacular" end, where treatment deploys sophisticated technology in specialized hospitals. Heart disease, cancer, thorax surgery, and anesthesiology are all toward the top of this hierarchy, whereas illness that may be related to lifestyle, old age, or mental health is at the lower end (Album & Westin, 2008).

Apparently unwavering in sticking to a professional trajectory, Jacob may thus be understood as a responsible father pursuing a permanent position in order to become a reliable breadwinner for his family. Another interpretation is that he is an ambitious professional working toward the top of the hierarchy by pursuing one of the most prestigious disciplines in the field. Was he unaware of the route demarcated for physicians, selecting his specialism according to interest and competence rather than the pursuit of status? Jacob left us in the dark concerning what moved him in this professional direction, but what followed the report may indicate other concerns more important.

Compartmentalizing Emotions

> *You don't know what to say… words became poor… you cannot ((laughs)) it becomes unnatural to kind of put your arm around them in a way… people you have never met before.*

Jacob's self-presentation soon moved beyond titles and allowed for the emergence of an experiencing, relational, emotional, and empathic person, one able to see the pain of others; this image was recognized by the panel and very likely too by patients and families in the clinic. There is a shift in the text as the report is followed by a brief description about what it meant to embody the role he had just presented: "*We see a lot of ill patients and there are very many who die at our units*". *This was* followed by an evaluative statement about how facing this reality "*is not always easy*", and how it stood in contrast to what was at the core of "*being a doctor*", namely the desire to "*help and save lives*". Jacob could have pursued and elaborated on career and positions, but he chose not to. Rather, over several hundred lines of transcribed text that comprised a large chunk of the interview, he presented various categories of the many deaths: unexpected deaths, expected deaths, expensive deaths—"*hopeless situations in which chance for survival is minimal, but cost of resources colossal*"—and the most difficult deaths—"*patients who are awake*".

In recounting these very emotionally charged situations, the engaged physician repeatedly inserted descriptions about how things usually were. Jacob thus opened a window onto his experience, but only at a distance and only in glimpses. He switched from particular incident narratives (PINs) to general incident narratives (GINs); from experience-near to experience-distant.

He could have remained with one narrative, turning over every stone of it, exploring an emotion in depth. He did not do so, and the effect was a compartmentalizing not only of the personal and the professional, but also of the emotional and the rational. In one instance, he talked about the "*brutality*" in meeting relatives after an unexpected death and the fact that he had to convey the message that "*a complication occurred and the patient died*". Instead of staying with the experience, elaborating on how the situation was experienced emotionally, he moved on to discuss the juridical aspects of it and then moved on again to tell yet another story.

Perhaps Jacob avoided engaging with the emotional experiences due to a sense of having limited time and wanting to cover a lot of ground. What seemed to counter this interpretation was the calmness he maintained throughout, allowing himself pauses of two to three seconds, eight seconds, as much as eleven seconds, as he spoke. This suggested that he had entered a reflective space. The ninth PIN recounted about forty minutes into the narrative, a recent "*dramatic ending*": "*He looked totally well… he was a healthy man (.) very young (.) and then terminally ill within two three days… strange thing*", illustrating both Jacob's willingness to be with grief-struck relatives and revisit awkward situations, yet also the difficulty he had articulating the emotional impact of the experience:

> *I sat there in the middle of the night with his father who was totally devastated... ehm... you don't know what to say... words became poor ... you cannot ((laughs)) it becomes unnatural to kind of put your arm around them in a way... people you have never met before... all of a sudden you meet them in such a stress and... situation... but did it anyway (.).*

Through sharing an awkward moment, Jacob allowed me a glimpse into the ambivalence he felt of being personally engaged in the professional role. Again it was just a peek, not an in-depth exploration, before "*the window*" closed. In sub-session two, as a result of my pushing for more experience-near telling, Jacob filled in details, and eventually also elaborated on his experience:

> *I didn't know what to do in order to comfort him... don't think he even had any questions... that I laid my arm around him was in a way a relief for me ((laughs))... not certain that physical contact was what he needed (.2).*

In both sessions, Jacob recounted his experiences in a similar manner: not very experience-near, rarely any first-person statements, mostly GINs and descriptions. In one instance, again in sub-session two, talking about a death that was particularly important to him, a six year old who had stayed at the unit for a year, he repeated four times how "*sad*" it was, but did so without explicitly stating that it was Jacob who felt sad. Similarly, when elaborating on the encounter in which he held the patient's hand and looked him in the eyes, telling the patient that "*this will work out just fine*" despite "*knowing that this won't probably work out*"—a tremendously intimate, emotionally charged moment, one would imagine—there was no display of, or elaboration on, the emotions experienced.

Is this experience-distant manner of telling an indication that bringing in his own emotions is not legitimate? A comment made further into the account may suggest just that: "we *do what we have to do without mixing in too much emotions and feelings*"; this will be revisited below. Immediately afterward Jacob spoke of how "*we physicians are not very good at debriefing... the nurses are better at it*". Thus, in both instances, Jacob was possibly making explicit the demarcation line, suggested above, between the emotional and the rational, and between the personal and professional—a demarcation which informed the telling of his account. Thus, in both instances, possibly making explicit the demarcation line suggested above between the emotional and the rational, and between the personal and professional, both informing the telling of his account.

Conveying Messages of Death—A Fate Worse Than Death Itself

> *Deep inside I knew already at that point that he was not going to make it.*

The above does not imply that these deaths did not have a profound impact on Jacob. His account suggested the contrary by voicing several dilemmas inherent in the role, actualized in encounters with dying patients and their families. He explained the dilemmas both through the PINs and in pregnant evaluative statements. A core dilemma, in which others are rooted, subtly placed in the middle of a PIN, relates to Jacob the physician knowing more about the imminence of death than the dying patients:

> *Remember one of the days before he died he took me by the hand and kind of… felt that 'we are going to overcome this'… and… deep inside I knew already at that point that he was not going to make it.*

The pressing issue *was* "*to find a frame around this then (.) how you should end*", finding a way in which the message "*this life will not be a dignified life*" could be conveyed to relatives "*clinging to every possible straw of hope*". Yet pretending, delivering a message of "*hope*" by pointing to a blood test and saying "*look here, now we know that it is that type of bacteria we have to deal with hence we can give this kind of antibiotics…*" was rather what, at times, he felt was "*expected*" of him.

He understood the relatives' hunger for good news in light of the "*incredible suffering of patients and relatives*". However, he considered that giving into a quest for hopeful news was:

> *...kind of a prolonging of (.2)* ***you prolong that death process in a way ... that is an enormous strain*** *(.) that I find to be a difficult decision at times (.) you (.) then you have to meet the relatives on their own premises (.) eh (.) they are very different (.) to try to meet them on the wavelength they are at (.) it is* ***not always easy.***

The latter evaluative statement sums up the dominant theme in this part of the interview: the narrator wants to persuade me as listener that being Jacob the anesthesiologist, encountering dying patients and their relatives is not only "*challenging*", but also "*difficult*" and "*strenuous*". What was most stressful is not death per se, but communicating with patients and relatives about death as it approaches: the "*biggest challenge as I see it is meeting them in different ways*", meeting them on "*their own terms*".

Jacob provided a global evaluation, an "I" statement, about "*the better way*" of communicating with relatives: "*I believe one profits by being honest with the relatives and telling the facts*". However, it soon became evident that his relation to truth-telling was more ambiguous. The encounter mentioned above in which he held a patient's hand, looked him in the eyes, and told him that "*this will work out just fine*" despite "*knowing that this won't probably work out*" illustrates the point. The conflict playing out within Jacob, and in encounters with relatives, seems to be between the conviction that they have the right to know and the idea that "*one is not supposed to take from them the hope*".

In sub-session two, when elaborating on this, and in particular relating it to dying patients that are "*awake*", Jacob did not side with truth:

> *Personally I don't think that it is right that one should inform a terminally ill patient that 'now you are going to die' (.) I think that is totally wrong (.) in my view.*

When asked, he could not recall one instance in which he informed a patient about imminent death, but he provided several examples of having done the opposite, namely saying that all would be fine while knowing differently. Jacob described how the BMT (bone marrow transplant) patients are met with very "*tough information*", so that "*fear is glowing in their eyes*". He questioned whether this information-giving should be mandatory, because even though "*you have a right for information... and even if the prognosis is bad (.) some (of the patients) are making it...*".

Jacob referred to a mistake made 25 years ago, which involved performing surgery on the wrong hip of an older patient: "*Nobody wrote anything or, yes I don't even think we notified the patient*". This may suggest that the sense of responsibility has grown in him. This impression was somewhat tempered in sub-session two, when I asked him to explain his claim that he was "*hardened*" through the year, and that what used to be a catastrophe no longer is. Jacob recounted early experiences of informing patients before surgery that they would wake up afterward, but then "*they die between your hands*". During the interview, he seemed to come to terms with similar situations, less burdened by a sense of responsibility, with the help of the following rationale:

> *When you move around on the outskirts of what is medically possible then you will (.2) have a greater risk of making mistakes (.) it is like a high jump right (.) when you place the bar high up then you will fail - - (.) sometimes.*

Jacob's manner of addressing the task of conveying difficult messages to dying patients and grieving relatives suggested that this was still a conflicted issue for him, which was perhaps why he did not leave the subject, but moved on to discuss different aspects.

End-of-Life Decisions—A Conflicted Responsibility

After his comment about how physicians disregard debriefings, Jacob moved on to talk about the positive and negative elements of debriefing conversations with relatives. He made the point that these sessions may arouse self-blame and feelings of guilt in the relatives, which is why he finds such conversations "*not always good*". He then shared a PIN, a story about blame directed toward him as the physician: "*'But you turned off the respirator'(.) she said to me (.)'if you had not done that he may have survived' (.6)*". Jacob interrupted himself by laughing. He took a deep audible breath, before continuing, "*yes, one becomes guilty of an answer* - -(.7)".

He then repeated the accusation again and explained how the lady offering it "*had the impression that it was similar to when one terminates animals (.3) and she couldn't forget it....*". Her claim was that he should not have turned off the machine "*even if the chances were slim*". Jacob, thoughtful, acknowledged "*that little uncertainty one can never totally get rid of (.) Nothing is 100% certain in the world in which we operate*", before again appealing to common sense. As "*the heat*" was turned up, and one might have expected an elaboration of how this challenging encounter was for Jacob, the focus shifted again, from PINs to GINs, from experience-near to experience-distant, to patients in general and a more academic discussion:

> *If you are ill enough (.) and come to an ICU and you know that five so called vital organs are failing at the same time then you know that chances of making it are minimal (.) and that people without a health professional background understand too... they are not that stupid.*

This was a move from the affective to the rational, from personal to professional, and from experience-near to a more distant telling. Yet, it became clearer that what came across as an insistence on staying within the professional realm was related to Jacob's deep personal engagement in a continuous actualization of responsibility and guilt.

As the narration proceeded, Jacob focused on concerns pertaining to care and responsibility, examining them from different angles, voicing the relatives' accusations, the health system (which asks the impossible of its employees), and himself. Jacob thus described how he was "*pressured*" from different angles. It felt like having "*one's back against the wall*", not least when having to exercise the responsibility of prioritizing:

> *This thing about use of resources (.) it it (.) very difficult... we have an ICU that is always too small (.1) it is almost like playing 'musical chairs'... and then you are asked to prioritize who is most sick.*

In a subsequent reflective passage, marked by pauses, he recounted how he felt pressured and "*pushed to make decisions you rather would have avoided (.3) because the resource situation is so limited (.3)* ***that*** I ***think is***

almost even more troubling *(.2)*". Four times he repeated how "*difficult*" it was. "*What do you do?*"

Several times Jacob expressed a strong sense of responsibility and spoke of how the patient could die due to "*you moving him out*"; how "*you may have contributed to the patient dying*", and that this may be regarded as "*blameworthy*". He became more specific in questioning himself in the PIN that followed. Several years ago, a male patient was waiting for planned heart surgery. The night before an ulcer was located and surgery was rescheduled immediately, but the man died as "*we were about to put him in narcosis*". Jacob questioned himself over this:

> *…or you could have postponed the whole surgery* ***(.2)*** *maybe until the next day* ***(.2)*** *eh* ***(.2)*** *yes (.)* ***maybe he would have survived*** *without a surgery even… you will never know (.) but think afterwards still* ***(.4)*** *did one make a mistake (.) could one have done something different… would he have died anyway (.)* ***((sighs))*** *never get an answer.*

Jacob admitted that mistakes of life and death may have been made. It was like an echo of the accusations made by the above-mentioned relative; only this time Jacob was questioning himself. Reflective pauses suggested that at this point in his telling he had moved beyond any rehearsed narrative, entering more disorganized and confusing areas on the border between life and death; this territory was out of control, but still his to patrol. There was a lot at stake, but still no display of emotions. However, he had opened the door a little more, to a pressured and vulnerable self perhaps, to someone living the question "*who is to decide what is a life of dignity (.3)*".

Jacob posed the question first in relation to witnessing his own mother's declining health, and how bringing her home after surgery made him wonder "*to what life?*" There was a lowering of his voice when the physician talked about her declining health, the surgery, how he took care of her, her fear of death, his expectation that she might die, and finally her loneliness due to having lost all her friends and the fact that her children lived in other parts of the country. The latter was expressed by Jacob quoting her in sub-session two saying: "*I don't have anyone anymore (.3) there is nobody visiting me - -* (.5)". Twice Jacob suggested that sharing about his mother was "*a little detour*". Why did he allow himself to get off track? Was it the fine red thread running through his account that took him there, the sense of feeling responsible?

As the telling proceeded, he argued for and against whether one person (the physician) can "*judge*" the degree of dignity—or its potential—in someone else's life. In between PINs related to his mother and then to his father-in-law, Jacob presented two different acute scenarios (cerebral hemorrhage and heart attack), in which both suggested considerable brain damage; then, he posed the question: "*Where do you draw the line?*" He made the last scenario personal: "*Say it was you or me who fell over with a heart attack*", thus shifting the perspective, putting himself in the patient's place and speaking of his own mortality for the first time: "*Can you and I who sit here decide that this life is undignified (.12)?*"

Jacob recounted two PINs to underscore his point that at a certain moment one must allow someone to die—in the name of dignity. The first was about his father-in-law who was "*allowed to die*"; the second was a story from when he was a young doctor and he and a colleague decided to stop resuscitation. The patient's son "*got furious because we had given up on his father and he jumped onto the bed and continued resuscitation*". Jacob appreciated the despair expressed but explained it as "*denial (.) one denies it (.) it is one kind of denial (.2) one wants life to continue (.2) one realizes not that it is (.) death comes one day (.) however we turn and twist it*".

In a multitude of ways, Jacob gave voice to the challenge, difficulty, and impossibility of his professional position. The reality of the patient's death, communicating to patients and relatives about imminent death, as well as judging which lives to save and which not, all leave a strong sense of the responsibility and potential guilt with the physician. It was as if Jacob, through persistently staying with his conflicted sense of responsibility, allowed me a glimpse into an internalized "courtroom". The accusations are outlined above, but what was his defense?

Professionalism as Defense

But anyway on (.) our unit is very professional I think (.) regarding this (.) and it is important to behave in an orderly manner (.) be professional - - (.1) that is what I think (.) ***that*** *I think is a very important message (.) that one* *has (.) one does a (.2) one does a (.) a job (.) or one does (.) one does something which one is capable of and has the education for (.4) … we have to act professionally (.2)… do what we are supposed to without mixing in too many emotions and feelings.*

According to Jacob himself, the quote was a message he made efforts to "*convey to other colleagues*". Hence, it made sense that he took time in the telling to elaborate on it extensively. What immediately caught my attention was the extraordinarily repetitive use of "*one does*". It was a manner of speaking in which the individual potentially got lost in an impersonal "one". One might ask whether it related to the above-identified demarcation line between the personal and the professional?

The intensive care physician continued, under various headings, to elaborate on what he understood "*professional*" to imply in different clinical situations: when communicating a request for autopsy, handling conflict between relatives, giving out information, responding to request for documents from relatives, responding to the same requests from authorities. What is common to these situations is the fact that they are regulated by law. The importance of staying on the right side of the divide between professional conduct and misconduct ran like a red thread throughout these passages. The degree of regulation, and thus the risk present for the professional, increased with each new typical situation outlined and eventually took Jacob to an unpleasant memory, which perhaps explained his focus on professionalism in the first place:

… () have had unnatural deaths that (.) that have been reported to the police (.2) and reported to the health authorities (.) and then a file is opened and then it becomes (.) one has to give out all the documents of course.

Even after repeated listening, I am unable to detect whether Jacob actually uttered an "*I*" in the first sentence above. In the subsequent sentences, the first-person pronoun is dropped altogether as the particular is replaced by general talk about how such cases were typically handled and how:

…one possibly gets a feedback that something is done (.1) blameworthy (.) one can get a warning (.) that sort of thing one must be prepared for (.8) … It rarely happens, but it occurs… *particularly if there are consequences (.)*

> *that the patient dies (.4) even if you can say that the prognosis for the patient was bad... one gets hung up on details... so it is very important to be orderly when it comes to such journal notes (.17).*

Claiming that he had acted according to a professional code, according to how "*one*" does it, was Jacob's best defense against accusations of misconduct. He did not say whether that was what had saved him when he was investigated by the health authorities. The quest for order offered a contrast to Jacob's account of "*loose ends*". When asked at the very end of the interview how it was for him being interviewed, it was as if he was acknowledging this paradox:

> *No I think it was okay (.2) it came out a little incoherent perhaps (.) there was not a red thread in it or any chronological sequence in a way (.6) we physicians (.) like to have a degree of overview ((both chuckle)) (.) order in our things (.13).*

In my debrief note immediately afterward, I reported feeling tired during the interview. All the descriptions of routine and procedures, general narratives, void as they were of real human beings, the speaking in general, the use of impersonal pronouns, all took its toll on me. Jacob, on the other hand, did not at any point seem to consider ending it. When interpreting it all as an important part of his defense, a pleading of his case as a professional made it easier to acknowledge and appreciate what was at stake.

Burdened by Being a Demi-God

The relation between care, responsibility, and guilt was pursued, but reframed by the narrator in the second part of the interview. At first, it was as if he was articulating a lessening of the sense of responsibility and guilt:

> *One hardens a bit through the years in a way (.) one gets experience (.) in a way wisdom of life that makes one handle situations (.2) maybe (.) what was a catastrophe or gruesome some years back is kind of (.) one now thinks is a (.2) yes (.) one takes it in another way (.)... perceives the situation differently (.6).*

One may have expected examples to illustrate Jacob's claims of change. Instead, his focus was on how the professional context had changed and how that in turn changed who he is. At first, the medical technological development that "*a medical truth doesn't last longer than ten years*" got his positive regard; then, when addressing the effect it had on him in his role, he spoke of it in much more ambiguous terms.

Jacob then revisited the issue which seemed to underpin the whole account, and again actualized the "*impossible*" of being in the physician's position, namely the conflicted sense of responsibility for making decisions at the boundary between life and death. Despite claims of change, this still seems to be experienced as a profoundly ambiguous and paradoxical part of his professional situation, described in a brief narrative about a multiply handicapped girl who was on his unit:

> *What is a life of dignity for that child… depended upon nursing and supervision twenty four seven (.2) how much resource shall we put in (.) how far are we supposed to let this go… nobody can (.) it is a totally impossible task (.).*

The girl "*miraculously made it*". Life and death are both in his hands—and yet out of them. It is not so much how Jacob as a person has changed, but rather how the context has changed by projecting expectations such as those expected of a demi-god, deified by technological "*unimagined possibilities*". Jacob, like other "gods" before him, has to stand trial when he cannot deliver what is expected of his almighty "*unimagined*" powers. People don't take no for an answer to their prayers anymore:

> *It was probably easier to be a physician before… because then one could say that 'this patient is so sick that cannot do anything more' (.11) and it was accepted.*

Revisiting Dominant Themes

"*Cooperation with other units*" was touched upon before Jacob once again turned his attention to the dominant themes, the red threads, running throughout the account, namely how to communicate with patients and relatives regarding imminent death, as well as what it meant to have a life of dignity.

In regard to the former, Jacob presented the formulas used when delivering the message to patients and relatives that there is no more curative treatment. One approach is to state that "*if there are more complications we won't step up treatment*"; another is "*treatment is at maximum*". According to Jacob, playing these cards is justified when "*chances for survival are minimal (.)*". It is one way to advance a process that is at a standstill. The effect of "*putting a roof on treatment*" as the "*relatives get the impression that treatment is now at its maximum… you have played out the last card*".

Before leaving the topic of "*cooperation with other units*", Jacob argued how the surgeons "*often have an unrealistic relation to certain things… when we have done that and that surgery the problem is solved (.) it is not*". Implied is an element of critique of a merely biomedical understanding of encounters with patients and relatives, a recognition of the relational, the existential, and ethical dimensions of end-of-life care.

Listening to Jacob, there was a sense of thoroughness, of him minutely filling in the blanks, making sure that every inch of the topic was covered. This impression did not seem to resemble Jacob's own experience, when he came to the end of yet another round of mostly posing questions about necessary, unnecessary, and legally required information, and thus also to the end of his first narrative: "*yes it may be a little incoherent this but (.) I don't know (.) it became loose threads (.) which it is going to be your task to knit together*".

The Personal in the Professional—Crossing the Demarcation Line

After about two hours of uninterrupted speech flow, Jacob paused. He was then invited once more, again in the wording of the SQUIN, to tell about events and experiences that have been important to him personally. After first double checking whether it meant "*outside my job situation or in total*", and having got no help deciding from me, Jacob provided a global evaluation. Three times he repeated how "*difficult*" those things were that: "*relate to the closest (.)* ***that which all experience*** *(.) own family (.1) children (.2) wife (.4) (.) that is always difficult*".

Despite the difficulty, Jacob proceeded to tell the story about when he had to resuscitate his own daughter—how "*he turned totally blue (.)*" and "*I thought he was going to die*"; what an incredibly "*long time*" it took before the ambulance came; how Jacob "*panicked*", was in "*despair*" and "*didn't get a word of what they [the health professionals] said*". According to Jacob, this "*worst experience*" has helped him "*understand when relatives panic and despair*". Hence, this personal narrative which was late in coming echoed the dominant themes in his account. Jacob did not dissolve the demarcation line between the personal and the professional, but he did leave substantial cracks in it.

He then recounted yet another story in which death had been personal. Years back, a colleague had died in a helicopter accident: "*I was at his funeral, there was a little boy that walked up front and put one of those roses on his father's coffin… it was terrible (.16)*". Then, another narrative about a colleague who had killed herself: "*could one have done anything to prevent it (.) comes also that self-blame - - thought in (.3) could* ***I*** *have visited the person (.8)*".

Why did Jacob recount this at this point in the interview? It was as if he was saying, in the first person, implicitly and explicitly, that there was something harder than the difficulties related to his work, namely "*that which all experience*", losing someone dear in death. He explicitly linked the panic and despair he himself felt when almost losing his daughter to that which he encountered in grieving relatives.

He soon brought his narrative back to the professional context, with the recurring, very personal, self-scrutinizing question "*could I have done more*". If language is the house of being, through this narrative account Jacob seemed to be making a courthouse for himself. The effect of this may be what was brought forth in his last global evaluation, pertaining to his professional role:

> *One says that part of the charm with being anesthesiologist is that one can be exposed to such unforeseen things (.) continuously (.) can take its toll though ((resigned laugh)) (.21) it varies how much stress one can handle too (.12) different personalities (.22).*

When asked, at the very end of sub-session two, whether he could recall a situation in which the question of how much stress one can handle was actualized for him personally, Jacob responded by telling how just a few months back he had been hospitalized due to "*pain in the chest*":

> *…remember I came into the car and was about to drive to work and then (.1) I felt kind of 'oh it is so hard to breath' () then I got flashback to my father who had angina (.) chest pain.*

Then again Jacob spoke of how his years of experience made it easier for him to handle "*these things purely professionally*", even though the recent hospitalization and the pressing themes of his account suggested otherwise. Jacob seemed torn about relating the very audible physical reaction to work-related stress: "*…cannot blame it on work either but it has a lot (.) it was a lot of work related stress during that time*", alluding to the "*violent organizational change*" in which "*you are sucked in (.) whirls around with it (.) it never stops (…) feels life threatening*". What Jacob returned to at the very end though, unprovoked by the interviewer, was the same dominant theme that had lingered throughout, "*the most difficult*":

> *It is much easier to say yes than no (.) to stop a treatment - - (.) that is to say yes and start a treatment - - (.) to get a patient into the ICU (.) that is much easier than saying no - - and stop and bring to an end and (.) reduce active treatment as we call it then (.). that is extremely difficult (.) when you have (.1) the opportunity to keep it going. (.) and that we have almost always - - () and who is to decide - - (.) is it the patient or the relative or health professionals or the physician - - (.) is it the chaplain – is it (.)or somebody outside us again - - (.5).*

Questions unresolved, court proceedings to be continued.

A Thin Sense of the Situated Subjectivity

Jacob apologized twice for bringing in "*his world*". Hence, both implicitly and explicitly he seemed to be operating with a demarcation line between the personal and the professional. There were certainly cracks in the wall Jacob had erected around personal issues, but even talking about his mother, his father-in-law, and his daughter were given legitimacy by being placed within a professional frame, informed by professional concerns (old patients, palliative care, stroke). It was as if he needed an excuse to introduce life from outside the unit into the narrative.

Despite the open invitation to tell the story of his life, in his account Jacob hardly reflected upon possible life-changing events and experiences outside the clinic. During the interview, in the free-associative non-interrupted account, there were other, more pressing issues that took precedence, informing his telling and leaving the impression of a subject very much informed by his professional context. His background was primarily outlined as a professional trajectory. When the people populating the account were introduced in Jacob's first narrative, in the first sub-session, it was exclusively in relation to his professional role or professional concerns.

As his telling progressed, Jacob moved from denoting his professional situation as "*challenging*" to "*difficult*" to "*impossible*". The selective principle of his telling thus seemed related to the challenge, difficulty, and impossibility of his professional position, the conflicting character of being part of life, and death situations. On the one hand, Jacob is a demi-god who "*can do unimaginable things*". On the other hand, he is up against "*the impossible*"—making life and death situations vis-a-vis fellow human beings, "*prolonging*" death processes or "*allowing*" someone to die.

The thin sense of subjectivity that emerged in an interpretation of the account, shared during the interview, was that of the defense of an intensive care physician "on trial". A "courtroom" surfaced through the telling. Though faceless and nameless, those summoned by the "prosecutor" and the "defense" were not without a voice. Jacob's main defense strategy against the multitude of scrutinizing eyes was a claim to professionalism.

In Jacob's understanding of professionalism, there was limited place for emotions. Yet, paradoxically enough, the time spent and the diligence used to provide a review of professional situations and dilemmas inherent in his professional role suggested that there was something at stake both personally and emotionally. Jacob's explicitly stated sense of chaos both at the unit and in regard to his own account, the laughs following the telling of difficult situations, as well as the depersonalized language used throughout the account all seemed to point in the same direction.

The lack of structure in the account, which was more like a stream of consciousness, suggested a processing, rather than the presentation of something processed. When asked, "How this was", Jacob said that he had expected more guidance and added, apologetically, that he had come unprepared. Still, he did not leave me with a sense of having wanted to hold back or having had a need to hide whatever was uncomfortable, on the contrary.

Nonetheless, underscoring how debriefing was not his cup of tea, he expressed some hesitation toward systematic reflection upon clinical experience. At no point in his telling did he refer to opportunities during his education or career for systematic consideration of life inside the clinic, life outside it, or possible connections between the two. His fragmented manner of telling seemed to reflect a lack of reflexive space and systematic considerations of emotionally charged experiences.

Reference

Album, D., & Westin, S. (2008). Do diseases have a prestige hierarchy? A survey among physicians and medical students. *Social Science and Medicine, 66*(1), 182–188. https://doi.org/10.1016/j.socscimed.2007.07.003.

5
Eric

Lived Life and Told Story

Setting the Scene

Eric and I met in the hallway just outside the chapel, close to "home" for Eric, chaplain of the hospital. As I was about to find my way to him, he turned a corner and headed straight toward me. Even though the recognizable collar gave him away, I uttered his name with a question mark. We shook hands. He had a soft, mild appearance. Still, had I only seen his hands, I would have said that he was not a man afraid of physical work. As we sat down in his office, he lit a candle at the table and offered me a glass of water. I assumed these gestures were typical of the way he hosted conversations with patients and their relatives about what was most important in their lives. This morning Eric's own narrative was the subject.

After a few minutes of small talk and introductory remarks, Eric was ready for the Single Question Inducing Narrative (SQUIN). For the next couple of hours, he shared events and experiences that were important but not necessarily favorable to him, which suggested trust,

K. Moen, *Death at Work*, Studies in the Psychosocial,
https://doi.org/10.1007/978-3-319-90326-2_5

but also a narrator used to considering the personal in the professional, and thus moving in familiar terrain. Nonetheless, in my debrief note after the interview, I noted a shift in how I perceived his experience of the interview, from being at ease at the beginning and throughout sub-session one, to becoming increasingly tense during sub-session two. I interpreted this as tiredness, but his probing after the interview about how I planned to use the data, suggested his growing insecurity about what I wanted from him.

Lived Life—In Brief

Eric grew up in an industrial city in the Eastern part of Norway during the 1960s. The first major change in his life came in his preteens, when the family moved to a smaller community. The next self-reported main event took place during confirmation class, when he had a conversion experience in the local church. He has two siblings, living in different parts of the country. His parents were both born in the early 1930s and had died by the time of the interview. Eric's father was ill during most of Eric's upbringing and died many years back. His mother, on the other hand, died not long before the interview.

Eric began theological studies in his early twenties. Some time into his studies he changed educational institution as he moved closer to where his fiancé lived. They got married and had children. Eric has worked most of the time outside the clinic. Over the course of his work life, he pursued further training to enhance relational skills.

Told Story—An Overview

Even though Eric's telling started out in a linear manner, and thus complied with what seemed like a "natural" inclination for storytelling, it soon became evident that there was a particular thematic focus driving the telling. He didn't feel obliged to tell his whole life, but provided a thematic focus from the start. Although Eric left childhood stories behind early in his telling, his early experiences remained a fundamental part of his account.

Eric provided an experience-near telling, evident in how he used emotional language, and how a range of sentiments were described in the first person. The emotionality that marked his narrative was less apparent in his narrating voice, however, which had a mellow quality to it. The evaluative language was significant in that it provided the account with a strong sense of the narrating subject. This particular subjective flavor he brought to the telling was evident not least in the consistent use of "I", but also in the fact that he did not omit paradoxical or contradictory statements. The lack of critical questioning of self during and after the interview—he did not censor himself when speaking—may suggest that he was comfortable with the situation and with sharing even emotionally charged events and experiences.

Although Eric's narration was very much experientially driven, it was not void of topical focus. There were primarily four main topics of focus in the account. The first two had subsidiary-related topics: (1) *Death*, and how experiences in both personal and professional contexts informed his understanding of it, was the first topic, which took up about half of the first session. After an interim passage in which Eric negotiated what to talk about further, he shared (2) *formative experiences in youth and adulthood*: "*having kids*", "*getting married*", "*education*", and "*friendships*". The third more briefly addressed topic was (3) "*settling down*". The last, given the least amount of time, but no less regarded by Eric as the most important, was (4) "*experiences of the transcendent*". He offered three particular incident narratives to describe the latter.

Detailed Reading of the Narrative

Death—From Paralyzing Fear to Natural Relation

> *I had such death anxiety, (afraid) the heart was going to stop during the night*

Eric gave himself twelve seconds, before providing an initial response to hearing the SQUIN twice. This was the first of multiple pauses, most of them no longer than ten seconds, integrated into the narrative that

I was about to hear. This first pause may have been, as suggested by the panel, him clearing his head after a busy morning, or buying time in order to figure out a correct response to a colleague. Eventually, the pause ended, and Eric spoke:

> *"Then I would like to start with (.9) I think I am going to say something about (.3)… this thing about death"*

Provided only with this sentence, and acknowledging that Eric could choose various routes from here, the panel pointed out that he immediately seemed to be taking on a difficult issue, which again could trigger a spectrum of different emotions in him; emotions related both to the "then" and to the "here and now". It may have been uncomfortable for different reasons, according to the panel. He may have been confronted with a sense of survival guilt, or the fact that he really wanted his father dead earlier; he may have been carrying a long-felt wish for another dad, or shame due to the death recalling his boyhood even though he was now a grown man. Or perhaps the level of discomfort would make him want to be done with the whole issue sooner rather than later. Or, it was a slip of the tongue and not the direction he intended his narrative to take. All these were speculations, not wild but related to how others—the panel members—would have responded to the surfacing of death as a first topic.

Eric continued, seemingly with confidence, along the same track, insisting on making death a dominant theme:

> *"…and the experience of death (.) and the presence of death was something that was quite (.1) challenging for me growing up and during youth (.) was very (.2) could sometimes wake up during the night out of anxiety that I could die tomorrow (.1) and that was due to my father being sick (.) he died when he was () (.) and was at the hospital several times and often there was talk that he could die (.)I (.) sometimes I had such death anxiety that the heart was going to stop during the night (.) and that is something I have been feeling for a long time ((slows down)) (.) particularly after I had children (.) had a family life of my own (.) then (.1) then (.) particularly when the kids were little I could sometimes wake up and think that "now it is over" or "now I can die" (.1) so it (.) so I have had that kind of anxiety (.) or consciousness*

that I am going to die (.) young (.) as my father died young that it is not a matter of course that I was to live particularly long (.2) so that is part of what I have been carrying with me ((voice fades)) (.5)"

Eric waived away any hesitation and stepped deliberately into the personal, when he could have taken the safer professional route. Within the first minute and a half of the interview, he introduced topics and concerns that some people do not get in a lifetime. He spoke as if he were navigating very familiar terrain. For many, even the dying, it may take time to get to life and death issues in a conversation, particularly when conversing with a stranger. Eric was right there right away. He started out in the style of a reporter, covering many years in a couple of sentences. His own narrative, and in particular the topic of death, which remains inaccessible throughout life for many, thus seemed to be very much at hand for Eric. He appeared so at ease with how the narrative went, that it triggered the panel to ask whether he was possibly not really emotionally engaged.

Regardless of what emotional state the telling evoked in him, already at this point, the panel suggested a structural hypotheses, a dot in the thin line of the situated subjectivity, namely that Eric had the ability and courage to relate life experiences in ways that created meaning and understanding. He made links between the illness and death of his father and significant emotional states of his own in childhood and adulthood. In addition, he was able to identify phases in which these experiences had been particularly pressing, thus expressing a familiarity with his own narrative.

The very first part of the account thus indicated a self-reflective capacity on the part of the narrator. Eric himself countered any notion that he was providing a rehearsed story though, which might have been suggested by the flow of the telling and the outline of processed, digested experiences. In sub-session one, in regard to addressing the topic of death in general, he stated: "*I haven't talked so much about death ever*", and in sub-session two, in regard to the imprint of his father's death on him: "*have thought some about it but not so concretely as I am doing right now*". Commenting upon the interview experience in hindsight, Eric claimed that he was particularly surprised regarding his own reflections about his relationship with his father. A comment that underscored the self-reflectiveness that was his way of inhabiting his life.

When asked whether he remembered one particular night when his fear of death was present, Eric responded that:

> *… it was so often that that I cannot remember one particular day or time (.2) it has been there throughout (.)I can still feel it (.) but I am not as preoccupied with it as I have been before.*

It made itself evident from early teenage years, but Eric could not recall a first time. One aspect of the deep impressions left from witnessing his father's heart disease was, according to Eric, a sensitized ear to his own heartbeat. To desensitize himself to the rhythm, "*a way to not hear*", Eric had a technique that consisted in moving around in bed "*until I fell asleep*". When describing in more general terms how he developed a strong sensitivity to irregularities in his own heart rhythm, he switched between past and present tense:

> *… but then I often wake up (.) very awake at once and then I stand up and then I walk around some (.2) … because it is a little upsetting - - (.8) …it was quite uncomfortable.*

The alternating between past and present tense in the telling at this point may suggest that the anxiety was still present, even as he spoke, even though Eric claimed that it had subsided about ten years ago. This change of attitude toward death led to a physical examination that ruled out any heart disease, but mostly that:

> *… this whole process (.) all these hospitals (.) all these deaths and (.) all (.) actually the job (.) made death less prominent (.) or it became so usual - - (.) so that I was not as focused on heart and heart rhythm (.).*

Eric thus completed a very pregnant introduction of what was going to be the dominant theme for the next twenty minutes of the interview, namely his relation to death and what has informed it. He did so by a paradoxical claim that exposure to numerous deaths in the professional context made the fear of it subside.

Death at Work—Living in an Absurd Situation

> *My reality and what I daily face is (.) it is a reality and a dimension that they don't know or yes or that they don't relate to.*

After a five-second pause, Eric continued to explore the impact of death in his life, in relation to various professional contexts—a turn in the telling foreseen by the panel. First, he made the point that dealing with death was very much also a dimension of his parish ministry. The presence of death that comes with his professional role was at the same time "*natural*" and "*absurd*", according to the chaplain. The absurdity was that death, which for most people would be anything but natural, had become just that for him, "natural". "*I have given this some thought*" and:

> *... I think that other people may think that this is a little strange that it can (.) or (.4) that it is maybe strange that I have it this way... that this is my reality ... (.) and that (I) may have a measuring stick on death that is not totally congruent with what most people (have).*

It was as if Eric was providing a glimpse into an ongoing inner dialogue, a conversation with himself about what exposure to the death of others was doing to him in the eyes of others, a self-critical inner talk that led him to pose the question whether he may:

> *... have lost some of the grip to understand (.) how others may have it (.) think about it (.2) that has struck me lately (.) to such a degree part of everyday though (.5) yet I know that it is emotionally difficult and sensitive.*

We are left to speculate who the "*others*" may be: patients, relatives, friends, and family? Had anyone pointed out to him that he had "*lost some of the grip*"? When asked in sub-session two whether he remembered when "*having lost some of the grip*" first struck him, Eric literally took a minute to identify the possible situation that initiated the thought. He eventually shared a story about how he had had a key role when one of his friends was dying of cancer. The feedback he got during and after was similar to what he received later as a chaplain, leaving a sense in him that:

> *... my reality and what I face daily is (.) it is a reality and a dimension that they don't know or yes or that they don't relate to.*

In the sub-session two, though, he pointed out how his frightening experiences with his father at the hospital may "*remind myself of how others can experience death*", and thus that he may not have lost his grip after all.

Eric described the social implications of having gained a natural relation to death: recognition, on the one hand, and a sense of a stigma, on the other. Again, he showed the ability to connect different parts of his life, matching experiences inside the clinic with those outside, which may indicate that he was processing as he was narrating. His sensitivity to having "lost the grip" may suggest just the opposite—a sensitivity to what was taking place between him and the other.

The Impact of Encountering the Death of Others

Eric moved on in his telling, and related the profound change in regard to death, the subsiding of fear, not merely to witnessing the death of others, but:

> *... taking part in the processes until they die (.2) and then (.2) eh (.3) and then witness what is taking place within the patients (.) it has moved me strongly (.) that I have to say (.1) moved me really strongly (.5) mhm* (.17).

When asked in the second part of the interview whether there were one or more patients that came to mind when talking about "*witnessing what happens within the patient*", Eric responded by talking about a patient he got to know about three months prior to the interview. The patient:

> *... was very articulate healthy and up and going (.) yes yes (.) healthy relative to the situation then - - (.) and talked very much and had a warm and good language and it was easy to communicate with him and then you witness the change from day to day (.) how the talk silenced (.) eh (.) how you witness in a way that the body is changing. (.3) the cheeks become more distinct (.) the cheeks are much are pressed in and the nose becomes eventually (.) more distinct*

> *features of it (.) the eyes sink in and the conversation fades and at the end it is all about holding the patient's hand (.) and just be there in relation to that - - (.) and then cannot do much more than that - - (.) and then finally you notice that he is gone (.) has entered coma and then (.) then there is no more contact anymore (.) then it is only the breath (.2) it is powerful to experience (.).*
>
> *Researcher: "What touched you in particular in this situation?"*
>
> *Eric: "The loss of no longer being allowed to be in it (.) that conversation (.) or that process then- - (.) - - to it in a way becomes silent".*

What left as strong an impression as what was going on inside the other was what was occurring between the two of them, Eric and the patient, namely the gradual fading of a relationship.

Eric then provided more PINs illustrative of the various "*inner processes*" that can take place in patients. All of which were also, at the same time, descriptive of different kinds of relationships between chaplain and patient. It may be a "*peaceful*" death or "*chaotic death*", but for the most part "good deaths".

The good death was witnessed in "*the calmness of dying patients about what comes after*", the "*beauty of palliative care*", in how "*fantastic that medicine has come this far*" and how "*fun*" it was to be part of deaths that take place at home. Considering Eric's use of adjectives, there was almost a rosy hue to the way he spoke about death. In stark contrast to the fear of death that had been so prevalent in his life, but in line with his own claim that encountering the death of others has eased his own fear of dying.

The darker side of death, to Eric, is not so much leaving life, but thinking about those being left behind:

> *That would be a tough situation to be in (.4) their grief can be very painful to bear (.) when I am gone (.2) that it will be difficult for them (.3) and that I therefore maybe also will stretch far to keep life as long as possible (.12).*

Clinging to life as long as possible in order to protect his own family members from grief is an argument Eric shared with patients and relatives he encountered. What surprised him in these encounters though was their ability to also find something in life to hold onto for themselves, a hope of another birthday, another spring, "*something small*". "*I am very surprised… maybe it will kick in for me as well*".

The lack of resentment expressed toward death, his rather rosy manner of talking about it, and his surprise at how patients cling to life at all costs, gave the impression of a more complex relation to death than what had earlier been described as "*natural*". When Eric summed up his main point, he claimed that "*death is something I will receive when it comes (.) but maybe I will fight more than I have thought before that I would*".

The use of "*receive*" may bring associations to "gift" or "guest", positive connotations that may not be far-fetched interpretations of Eric's understanding of death at the time of the interview. This perspective was perhaps informed by what immediately followed in the narrative, namely the circumstances around Eric's own mother's death. "*It was demanding*" and when she eventually died it was "*an enormous relief (.2) it was a (.) liberation*". Eric stressed how "*exhausted*" relatives can become by tending to family members who have an illness that spans years: "*that I can recognize*".

The "Beauty" of Palliative Work

After having shared a personal PIN about his mother's death, Eric took a step back, as if feeling the need for space. His telling moved from experience-near to experience-distant. He was not leaving death, but rather looking at it from further afar. He talked about how some patients were "*believers*", and could have thoughts and feelings about the hereafter and the possibility of "*two outcomes*". Eric distanced himself from such theological positions, as he considered them "*foreign*". He himself found "*an anchoring*" for exercising his role in "*thinking that none of this exists*". Even when taking a step back, engaging theological topics, Eric placed himself in the equation by evaluative "I" statements, underscoring his self-reflective inclination identified above.

Eric placed the topic about the "*two possible outcomes of life*" at the margins, but traditionally—and up until quite recently, and still for quite a few—the subject of what happens after death has been a contentious issue in the church to which Eric belongs. It divides congregations, not least in those parts of the country where Eric served as pastor. It seemed important for him to convey in the interview an understanding of "religious language" as "visible words" of religious symbols, rather than the articulation of particular beliefs.

An opposition toward particular theological and religious language made itself evident and connected with earlier parts of his biography, life outside the clinic:

> *I had such (.5) discussion with myself regarding where to take the theological education… such a big and important… and a scary decision… at the time.*

In a couple of sentences, we were made aware that there were very different, and partly opposing, voices in Eric's life at the time; that he was pulled between the "left" and "right" of his church. There seemed to have been a quite substantial move theologically and ecclesiastically: from his conversion experience in a very pietistic context at age 15 to an academic context not very much in favor of pietism.

Despite a strong sense of the potential risk concerning future jobs, he chose the *narrower path*. Eric underscored the importance of this choice even up to the present time, and explained that what is particularly important to him, and what impelled his choice, was what he calls "*folk-church theology*", implying an understanding of church as defined from below, from the people. Eric reflected on why this was, and still is, so important to him: "*I believe that it is anchored to my parents who were folk-church but not actively religious*".

The above biographical and theological threads may explain why Eric used "*beautiful*" when describing palliation. In what follows, he repeated the adjective three times. What he found beautiful was the use of "*health language*" when encountering end-of-life. He equated "*health language*", which for most would imply connotations of medical terminology, with "*an ordinary, secular, interpersonal language*", different from "*religious language*". Eric held the former in high regard and found it both "*awesome and good for the patients*". Hence, the beauty of palliative care, for the chaplain, was related to how it allows for the experiential and the relational, perhaps not that far from the unarticulated folk-church theology of his parents.

After praising the other members of the palliative team, Eric stated that he had said what he wanted to say. I invited him, as I did with all the interviewees, to consider once more whether there were "other events or experiences that have been important to him personally"?

The invitation seemed to startle him and he asked for guidance:

> *… related to death then (.) and those things related to death… which are not necessarily related to what has to do with death (.) or which have a consequence in regard to it or influencing it or are relevant in relation to it* (.6) … or did you think totally open.

It was as if he had heard the first invitation as a call to talk about death, but the second as more open.

Formative Experiences of "The Transcendent"

Eric responded to the lack of guidance by turning his focus once again to the early part of his life and to experiences of the "*transcendent*", which he regards as fundamental both for his personal and professional life. He recounted three PINs that all relate to "*transcendent experiences*"—all glimpses of light against rather dark and shadowy personal backdrops. In the last story, a young suicidal patient was the main character. In the former two, Eric was the one at center-stage. The very first experience took place when he was about fifteen and in confirmation class:

> *During confirmation age I had one such strong experience - a conversion (.) that became significant for (.) was very significant for me (.) I want to say a kind of vocational experience of me being the important (.) that I was important (.2) because I was one of the smallest in class and I was not really (.) I was small (.) I was (.) yes as said one of the smallest in class (.) and I had a very low self-image.*

The elderly female verger approached him after the service, gave him a hug and said, "*welcome home*". Both of us chuckled at this expression, as if having a shared understanding of what this implied, namely that a community of faith, for some, carries connotations of family and home. What Eric heard was a call to regard himself as valuable, a profound experience of being welcomed, and a countering of his "*low self-esteem*" at the time. Thus, for Eric, a psychological interpretation of the experience coincided with one which was more theological.

The next major experience of the transcendent took place during his adult years and was named by Eric "*the descent and ascent*":

> *We had an exercise… (.) it was pretty much a failure (.) or I felt it was a failure… in that situation I connected with a crying that just came (.) within me… and I connected with my failure then (.) the crying became so strong that I couldn't control it… overwhelming… and then nobody in a way turned away or felt it difficult but they accepted it and let (.) I was allowed to be in that experience then - - (.) long enough till it quietened down (.) and then afterwards (.) a few hours later (.) it was this ascent (.) in which I feel in a way (.) something (.) a new power (.) or something like that come to me (.) which was very powerful - -(.) I am sure I could have moved mountains (.) it lasted for a long time (.) a month afterwards really (.) it was like being on Horeb (.) or something - - (.) and after that many inner images surfaced (.) an inner life (.) visual inner life (.14) which also was very (.4) great then - - (.7).*

In sub-session two, he painted a rather dark backdrop for the "*descent and ascent*". It took place at a point when:

> *…that enormous emptiness and slowness that dragged itself over me (.) I felt like one of those trucks (.) a truck that was going uphill and faith and everything was totally dead and (.) I felt very exhausted and was really (.3) I guess I was (.2) it was such a heavy time in my life (.) but it was then that I had that experience.*

The final story about experiences of the transcendent was a "*very beautiful*" experience from the clinic. According to Eric, it is a PIN about a young patient who was hospitalized due to her second attempted suicide, and according to him, it served as an illustration of how he worked with the transcendent more professionally. When Eric entered her room, she was in a state of disappointment due to having survived.

The conversation eventually moved in a direction where Eric found it appropriate to ask whether she had had any religious experiences. She then recounted two significant such incidents. After having recounted them:

> *She totally changed character… from being down and sorry and insisting on life being meaningless… to choosing to enter therapy… looking at the possibilities in life….*

This was not very different from his own "*decent and ascent*" and resembled his own life:

> *I can see myself in the same (.) when I got in touch with those great experiences in life (.) it gives energy in a way (.) and power to remind oneself about being (.) to retrieve it (.) that you are part of something very big (.) can give hope when it is dark (.) I see it is an experience that many patients can make use of (.) so I am very concerned about that dimension then.*

The panel remarked at this point that what seemed to be going on in the telling was "*a floating in and out of the personal and the professional*", a seeming lack of clear boundaries separating the two.

All the "vertical" experiences of the transcendent were very much facilitated by "horizontal" relations involving the (acceptance of the) preacher, the verger, the chaplain (in relation to the patient), and the (accepting) group in which he had exposed his feelings. In all the stories about the transcendent, there was something relational at stake for Eric. Neither he nor the patient he talked about were at "*the mountain of Horeb*" alone. This was evident to the listener, but perhaps not to the narrator?

Home—Already and not yet

Eric shifted focus to "*the enormous expanding grand experience*" of becoming a parent, but didn't stay there long, and when invited to tell more in sub-session two, he provided only fifteen more lines. The brief reference to getting married which followed, added to this picture. The discrepancy between the claim of importance and the time spent telling may relate to various things, but it was as if in Eric's mind he was relating to events and situations on the boundary of what was required. This was a more open space than in the initial part of the interview, in which he seemed informed by the notion that his telling should relate to death in one way or another.

After the longest reflective pause this far in the interview, and having stated that:

> *(.37) Important things in my life - - (.6) I have said very much of what is important to me - - (.) experiences (.15)*

Eric remained in the open space and continued to address relational issues close to "*home*".

He seemingly ended, or attempted to end, a rather sober last part of the account on a happy note by pointing out that *"now we live in our own house in the middle of the city (.) and then we have the vacation home (.) hence I feel that I have (.) right now I am very okay". Being "very okay" seemed to be inconsistent; as if, despite the beauty of palliative care, issues remained unsettled.*

As if reading my mind, Eric again brought up the dark period in his life, ten years back, the backdrop to the "*ascent and descent*":

> *That vast emptiness and slowness that crept over me… it was such a heavy time in my life.*

In sub-session two, he elaborated:

> *I had such a fierce longing to experience God… was very absent (.) gone (.) hence it felt meaningless (.) … felt powerless.*

It was in the midst of this time that he had the energizing experience of the transcendent already addressed above:

> *Hence these transcendent experiences I must say have been important to me in my (.) in my life (.) and my way of relating to life.*

With these exact words, Eric ended his first narrative.

A Thin Sense of the Situated Subjectivity

Throughout the account, Eric displayed an ability to relate to the parts and the whole of his life. He thus came across as one pursuing understanding and coherence. His choice of further education and the vocational turns suggested an interest in the internal and the relational more than the societal and the political. It was a self-reflective account leaning toward the melancholic. Childhood experiences related to the illness of a significant other triggered fear of death and a life-long sensitivity to his own vulnerability.

What the panel pointed to as "*a floating in and out of the personal and the professional*" in life and in the telling may be related to a strong identification with patients and relatives, but also that his own issues (self-esteem, fear of death) were "resolved" through vocational interdisciplinary work. A longing for "*home*" lingered, but was partly resolved by the most recent geographical and professional move.

The strong sense of me-ness did not preclude explicit and implicit references to dialogues and interactions, both related to personal and professional contexts. His own family, friends, colleagues, patients, relatives, and other members of the interdisciplinary team thus inhabited his narrative account. This brought a certain dynamic to the narration, one that seemed to mirror one aspect of Eric's way of being in the world, namely that he was sensitive to feedback from his surroundings, that words uttered in relation to him stayed with him. There was a red thread through most of the dialogical quotes that were evaluative of Eric in one way or another. This may reflect sensitivity, but also the multiple examples of Eric being able to create a space in which he could reflect upon encounters with the other (his father at hospital, the "*fading*" patient he encountered as a professional).

Death ran through the account and informed the choice of clinical and personal incidents. This seemed very much in line with Eric's own understanding of what should drive the narrative. It was as if he needed to defend himself when he went off this track. It was the very first topic introduced, and he related it to the here and now, as well as to the there and then. It moved around in the telling like a very strong current, surfacing in various ways, but also making itself evident implicitly in parts where the link to death was not as obvious and intentional. This was so not least in the very symbolically charged "*homecoming*"—the conversion experience at age 15, and in the "*descent and ascent*" experience as an adult. Death and dying were thus not only about being alive or dead for Eric, but about being a part and/or apart. His ease with death and dying was of particular concern to him: How it may be viewed as an absurdity and separate him from others.

At several points in his life, Eric recounted incidents when he "*stayed even when it was difficult*". This was stated in relation to the very uncomfortable experience, when his father was terminally ill at the hospital. It was also appropriate in other stories in which others may have left the scene: When he supported the family after his friend died, when he stayed in the parish despite feeling like a truck going uphill, caring for his mother during her decade-long illness despite getting very exhausted, staying with a family in despair for hours after the medical equipment had been turned off as they waited for their daughter to pass.

6
Karla

Lived Life and Told Story

Setting the Scene

Karla and I made an 8.00 a.m. appointment for our interview. I met her after a good night's sleep; Karla met me after a night shift at the intensive care unit. I looked for signs that this was not a good time to embark on a three-hour interview, but I found none. She appeared awake and alert. As if silently agreeing that we should get down to business, and not wanting to postpone what would be her well-earned sleep unnecessarily, the initiating small talk was limited to about four minutes.

Almost instantly, Karla blended into my image of an intensive care nurse. The efficiency, the clear articulation of her words, and the lack of hesitation served to put me at ease, as if giving me a sense that she was in control. When I later analyzed the interview, I found that this control served to camouflage some of her issues. I marked in my debrief note after the interview that I found myself more relaxed, more spontaneous, and deliberate in my follow-up questioning with Karla—a

K. Moen, *Death at Work*, Studies in the Psychosocial,
https://doi.org/10.1007/978-3-319-90326-2_6

possible effect of having already undertaken several interviewsby this point.

When looking over the transcribed interview, I found that I had reacted in an almost patterned way, responding in a non-verbal, yet affirmative manner. This may have suggested agreement, encouraging the narrator to continue in the same vein. In hindsight, I saw that I could have been an active listener in a more subtle manner. Still, at only one point during sub-session one did I respond verbally and thus break my stance as a non-interruptive listener. When listening again to this particular part of the interview, it was as if Karla was about to express more of her own emotions. Did I stop her? Was I intervening and thus perhaps contributing to what I identified as one of the dominant themes in her telling?

Lived Life—In Brief

Karla was born in the early 1980s and is thus significantly younger than the other star cases. She grew up with older siblings in the northern part of Norway, in "*a small community in which everybody knows everybody*". Both her parents worked. When Karla was still an infant, her mother had a serious medical condition. She survived, but needed long-term rehabilitation. Karla was an active handball player from the time she started school and into her twenties. Throughout high school, she had a summer job at the local nursing home.

At high school, she took business economics, which she followed up with an education in economic and administrative sciences at a university college. In her early twenties, Karla was accepted to a prestigious school of economics, but opted for a nursing school closer to home. The very same year, she started cohabiting with her boyfriend and together they built a house for themselves. Karla's first job as a nurse was at a small local hospital. After having undertaken additional education in intensive care nursing, she made a geographical and professional move. At the time of the interview, she was almost three years into her new position, while at the same time pursuing additional education within her field.

Told Story—An Overview

Karla's first narrative was almost exclusively limited to professional contexts. She dwelt upon situations that "*stick*" and which have given her occasion for reflection and learning. Her telling of the last two clinical incidents, which were closest together in time, was particularly elaborate and detailed. The first three incidents were all more univocally negative and told in brief; they occurred at least ten years before and were her first experiences as a nursing assistant and nurse, respectively. The categorization between "*first three*" and "*last two*" may have served an unconscious purpose for the narrator, namely to describe the change that took place in her way of dealing with challenging critical situations.

A particularity of Karla's telling was her use of dialogical enactments. She conveyed the essence of what was communicated in any particular situation by including dialogue and exchange of sentences verbatim. This was a very effective move used by the narrator, intentionally or not, to convey the change that occurred in how she dealt with her main concerns regarding end-of-life care. Karla thus allowed the reader to see the changes that had taken place since she first started to relate to patients, relatives, and colleagues: She had gained a voice, and she was using it.

Gaining and giving voice, the importance of mastering her job, the sense of guilt, and the conflicted relation to truth-telling were all dominant concerns that ran through the telling, and grew in significance as Karla's account unfolded. Death, however, was the absent presence. It was implied in everything that was recounted, but it barely qualified as a principal topic. Death was implicitly present in the fact that the patients died, but as a phenomenon having an existential and/or psychological impact it was left out of Karla's explicit self-reflections. Karla described how death was usually dealt with practically at the unit, but she addressed to a lesser degree how it impacted her personally and emotionally. As a concern, it was thus placed at the margins.

Detailed Reading of the Narrative

A Surprising Professional Turn

After a five-second pause, during which she took an audible breath, Karla began her narrative by taking a leap into the past:

> *Yes mhm (.) ((takes a deep breath)) (.3) then I think that I maybe begin from when I (.) started as nursing assistant (.) ehm (.1) I had just turned 18… a nursing home that actually is at the same place as I am coming from (.) a rather small local community (.) ehm (.) had (.) and knew many of the staff who were there from other contexts.*

In sub-session two, Karla added details about her lifelong relation to the nursing home, how it was located only 300 meters from her house and how the janitor was an acquaintance of the family and became her first point of contact to what later became her workplace.

Starting her narrative at 18 meant leaving out a large chunk of lived life. To the panel, the omission that felt most pressing, and surprising, was that of Karla's mother suffering a serious medical situation a few years into Karla's life. It was an "earthquake" that one would assume had had a profound impact on a young life—emotionally, economically, and socially. Yet it was left out of her narrative account altogether. Considering the potentially devastating impact on a family of such a traumatic event, and the long rehabilitation phase following it, the panel pointed out that there was support available from public health services at that time which may have helped to relieve the challenging situation.

Karla pursued the summer job, because she "*thought it would be a good opportunity to…*". The panel, hypothesizing what the last part of this sentence would be, suggested that the summer job was a good opportunity to "*…reflect upon encounters with dying*", "*…get work experience*", "*…find out what education to pursue*", and less piously "*…make money*". Their last suggestion pinpointed the issue. Karla reported that she continued as a nursing assistant during the summers and weekends for several years and also worked with cancer patients who were living at home.

During this time, there was a change, if not a turning point, in which the reason for pursuing relation-intense work changed from the pragmatic (economic), with the attitude that she was "*not going into health care at all*", to "*this is something I could actually want to work with*". She attributed the change of attitude to an increased sense of "*mastering the game*" and a growing sense of feeling a legitimate part of the team: "*feeling that one was contributing something to those patients and (.) not least the relatives... got a good response (.) good chemistry with many" which left a sense that (quoting self) 'this is actually quite rewarding*'".

In passing, Karla mentioned that she was actually heading in a quite different professional direction and that this change of attitude toward health care took place as she was studying economics. Finishing high school marks the end of compulsory education, and for many of her fellow students, that was a time for exploring the world. Karla, however, remained within the world that she knew, deciding to make a minor, and what may be regarded as a safe, move in life.

The fact that Karla went straight from high school to pursue an education in economic and administrative sciences at a university college may indicate a strong determination that she was quite goal-oriented from early on and, having identified her goals, found no reason to postpone pursuing them. As in the interview situation, even after a night shift, she appeared to have not been easily distracted, even back then. Positioning herself for a safe job in public management may also speak of a person seeking security. According to the Bureau of Statistics in Norway, close to 40% of Norwegian women went straight from high school to higher education during 2001. In that sense, one may say that Karla placed herself in the mainstream.

This glimpse into the choice between very different professional trajectories was by-passed almost without mention. In sub-session two, in contrast, Karla used more time and made evaluative statements concerning the "*very difficult choice*" of not pursuing an education in business, but becoming a nurse instead. Having been accepted at a prestigious school of economics, several factors redirected her into health care, not least that "*I enjoy talking with people*". The fact that her boyfriend, now co-habitant, was studying in close proximity to the nursing school "*may also have been a significant factor*". Karla also mentioned "*the incredibly good atmosphere*" at the nursing home as significant to her choice:

> *...experienced that one was recognized for the questions one asked and the discussion one took – (.) they took you seriously (.) ... they gave very positive feedback... general feedback that one had (.) yes that I had good (.) had communicated well with patients - - and that I (.) that I was thorough in what I did... that I enjoyed having things to do in fact... I like that things happen - - (.1) feel useless to be at work without doing something - - (.) that being 'in action' in way (.) that I got feedback on (.) and that I enjoy.*

Pursuing nursing school close to home gave Karla a chance to keep her position on the local handball team, another significant social sphere for her, serving as a metaphor for her present experience at the ICU:

> *The feeling of being in a group then - - in which one masters something - - (.) and at the same time feels (.) the cohesion that in a way (.) one contributes to a very positive (glow) at the same that you are in an arena where you know you have to challenge yourself because you are to deliver in the next game also - - (.) right (.) but you are in an environment in which you feel secure (.) you are in an evolving environment that is built up and in which everybody actually pulls in the same direction and just want to perform".*

The educational path she eventually chose, nursing school, was a surprise in that it was not in any way close to the one she discarded. Instead of entering what traditionally has been, and still is, a male domain, the world of business, she embarked on a traditionally female professional trajectory.

There thus appeared to be a dual interest and pull present in Karla's biographical trajectory: numbers and people, mastering and caring. Growing up in a man's world, "*always enjoyed doing math ... rode the lawn mower, and did all kinds of practical things*", as well as playing handball from age seven, which at the time was predominantly a male sport. A pull between numbers and people that would continue to make a mark on her telling.

Gaining and giving voice, recognition from significant others in the professional context, a sense of mastering, and a feeling of being at home all contributed to Karla's occupational choice and represented what emerged as dominant themes when encountering the death and dying of others. Having the mindset of a doer, once headed in the direction of the business world, one may ask how it was for her to enter such an emotionally charged, relation-intense field. Karla provides two particular incident narratives that described her first ambiguous professional experiences.

Gaining and Giving Voice

Karla brought us back into the sphere of professional care and described the very first day, her first shift, and the thoughts she had following it. She started once more with a broad-brush reporting style. With a few strokes, she created a background image of what colored the very first day: how they were several temporary workers, few regulars, limited training, caring for patients with significant needs, struggling with technical equipment. It made Karla doubt the whole project:

> *...how in the world going to embrace this (.) and that this is not a job for me whatsoever, - (.) thought that 'I shall manage to make it through the summer (.) but the question is if this is the road for me'.*

The panel members very much empathized with Karla the novice and her growing sense of chaos, difficulty, hopelessness, fear of doing something wrong, and fear of violating the dignity of the patient. When revisiting the experience in sub-session two, Karla stressed the sense of insecurity she felt and that she assumed the patient must have been feeling too, her sense of "*not mastering*" the situation. Karla reported that the nursing home experience grew better as the summer went on—proportionally with how "*I mastered my tasks*".

The next PIN, immediately following, took place in the same context. It was an experience no less unsettling than her first shift and, like the latter, also underscored the fundamental importance given to her first professional experiences, and suggested both a willingness to revisit critical incidents and to learn from them. Karla searched for words when describing this first encounter with a dead body, eventually using a Latin term. The Latin, more technical, term for the dead person left not only a sense of reification with the panel, but also the question: How was it that Karla, who encountered death frequently, was searching for the right term for a dead body?

The focus in Karla's telling was on the lack of a sense of mastering the situation: "*Remember I found it very frightening… I just remember the sight (.) a little bit that pattern of breathing (.) felt a little bit (.) felt a little frightened*". When asked in sub-session two what in particular made an impression on her, Karla responded:

> *Coming into that room and watching an old man that actually looked dead… the smooth skin (.) totally emaciated (.3) greyish skin and a particular smell… the characteristic smell that you can sense from (.2) the dying… yes that image sticks.*

She quoted her younger, professional self: "*this is something one has to work with in order to master and be good at in that last phase for those patients*". Karla, according to her own account, had moved as early as that first summer from a focus on "*what I saw in a way (.) the smell and all the senses… (.)*" to a place in which she was "*thinking and reflecting*" on "*these first encounters*".

Related to this dominant theme of "*mastering*" was the emerging realization, while at the nursing home, that her medical field had to be critical care: "*I got a little triggered by incidents a little bit critical*". In sub-session two, when asked if there was a particular incident that had brought this inclination toward critical care to awareness, Karla recounted in an engaged fashion, as if reporting from a sporting event with repeated use of the word "*exciting*", about an elderly patient experiencing a drop in blood pressure. The incident triggered the thought that "*this is a competence one needs to master*". More recently, she had this experience of mastering a critical situation when participating in a bike race and suddenly had to tend to a woman who fell off her bike and was left unconscious. Karla "*acted on instinct*".

Frightened by the Dead, Terrified by the Dying

In sub-session one, Karla moved on to another aspect of the nursing role not as easily mastered. Using the broad-brush approach again, leaving out particulars, she told how during nursing school she did home nursing. This brought her into contact with younger cancer patients. It "*.... did something to me meeting people who were absolutely not ready for it (.) and in my eyes way too young*". This was another early experience, another challenge which made Karla "*reflect*". Quoting herself:

> *'These are groups that are challenging to start to work with' (.) and at the same time it gave a little bit of terror (.) terror (.) not exactly (.) yes (.) terror inside me in a way (.) used a lot of time to mobilize to know how I should relate to them when I came to them (.) considering that you stepped into their homes and a little bit how does one approach the conversation then (.) not least this (.) how direct not direct (.) questions not questions (.) open up for dialogue and what meets you really if you open up for dialogue (.) it was a little bit such factors that I started to buzz with (.) and I remember I spent quite a lot of energy on.*

Karla was ***frightened*** by the sensory impressions encountering the dying elderly man, but what really ***terrorized*** her was having to relate to younger patients, to step into their most private sphere, the prospect of having to engage in a conversation with terminally ill and dying patients.

Was Karla's pull toward critical care due to its demand for action and de-emphasis on talk, the panel members wondered? Why were these encounters with younger patients so terrifying? Was it because they reminded her of her own mortality? Was it the expectation that she should help them in some way that terrified her? Was it the particulars of the context, the blurry boundaries created by a professional stepping into another's home? Was it, as one panel member pointed out, that death is experienced by Karla as something very private and that stepping over the doorstep into somebody's home underscored this? The above may have informed the sense of terror, but Karla herself placed "*the conversation*" center-stage, when fleshing out her concerns in sub-session two:

> *What meets me now... what kind of questions are coming towards me ... how to start the conversations... where do you start... and then actually something can come that you are not prepared for... because you cannot be totally prepared on all questions.*

Karla explained how she, after some time, was able to "*be just present there*" without the need to respond. Yet the shift between past and present tenses may have suggested that the "*stomachache*" lingers into the here and now. How to master the unpredictable encounter with patients and relatives was a challenge of the past and possibly one of the present. Her next move as narrator brought us further into the "*uncomfortable*" terrain already introduced.

Regrets Concerning a Dying Patient in Incredible Pain

The incident started when she was called upon by relatives of a patient who was in "*incredible pain*". "*I come in and see a patient terribly marked by pain*". Karla, not yet graduated, and with only a temporary permit to administer medicine, was instructed to inject morphine by the doctor in charge. She felt very uncomfortable with this, which she voiced hesitantly to the attending physician by phone. Karla regarded her younger professional self as "*in a phase in which one has problems arguing against the attending physician*". Despite the morphine, the pain increased, which made Karla pick up the phone again: "*this is something we cannot handle (.) and the patient definitely must go to a hospital*". Eventually, "*after a little bit of quarrelling*", the patient ended up at the hospital, where she died five hours later in a corridor:

> *THAT was an experience that I remember made a very strong impression on me (.) both a little in regard to being clear distinct (.) know exactly what is our function and profession (.) and concerning being able to argue and be clear and distinct (.) towards those one (.) like i.e., the physicians.*
>
> *How was it for the patient (.) be transported to the hospital and then actually die in the emergency room... that is a little how I think (.) the dignity related to it all (.) is there (.) there is definitely a way we could have solved it totally differently than what we did.*

She concluded:

> *... one of those memories that sticks the most.*

Karla once again placed communication center-stage. Being "*clear and distinct*" seemed to be of core importance, what "*sticks*" from the incidents. What got the panel's attention was the potential sense of guilt-implied in the incident that potentially lingered into the present telling. Karla's injection may have been the last one the patient got, potentially causing her death. The panel members heard Karla being both self-critical, but also critical of the system, possibly annoyed because she let herself be "*pushed around*" as they saw it. The panel also picked up on Karla's mentioning, but not making a point of, her knowing both the relatives and the patient, as "*I came from a small local community*", which implied that she could be recognized later by the family members, adding to the discomfort of the situation.

In sub-session two, when asked whether she could recall the conversation with the physician, Karla responded in a way that seemed to confirm the panel's assumption that the situation had left her with a sense of both guilt and annoyance. She repeated how she had not had the opportunity to stay with the patient to monitor her response to the morphine and how she regretted not being more persistent in questioning the physician's instructions. Self-ironically, she stated: "*I guess I bowed and nodded and said 'okay, yes, I'll go there and deliver those five milligrams*'". Was there a sense of feeling responsible for the patient's death?

At this point, based on the above, a thin line of subjectivity emerged for the panel. In addition to the courage they noted earlier, Karla seemed to them to embody a strong sense of responsibility, which made her liable to feelings of guilt. She appeared as "*a good girl*" who was keen to master and disliked failing. One may say that the "good girl" image suggested by the panel was modified by Karla avoiding the temptation to present merely "*the up-side*" of clinical incidents or her own performance. She did not tie up the loose ends, as illustrated by the following final statement:

Whether it was because I had too much respect (.) towards the one I was speaking to (.) or whether I didn't dare in a way utter my (.1) thoughts about it (.) and manage to argue well enough (.) it is hard to say really.

At this point in her telling, Karla could have diverged in several different directions. She could have elaborated on the emotional impact of the above PIN, entered an argument about systemic weaknesses, or provided another PIN in line with—or totally different from—the above. She could have made the account more messy and chaotic, or even more neatly tied up.

Trying to Master the Most Difficult

In a sentence, Karla changed time and context, moving to her first job as a nurse. Again, having completed her education, one might think that Karla had a sense of the world opening up for her. When she decided to stay and take up a position at the local hospital, it appeared as if she was opting for more of the same, more of the familiar. This of course does not imply that leaving would have been better, but it left the impression that there was no need or desire on Karla's part to distance herself from her place of origin. At age 25, she still lived in close proximity to what had been her childhood environment. Hence, her desire for community as identified above seemed to be reinforced.

During the first years as a nurse, Karla took on a particular role which involved responsibility for teaching the newly employed, as well as contributing to developing the nursing in the unit. Learning about Karla taking steps toward more responsibility as a quite newly employed nurse seemed to underscore the major concern/dominant theme identified, namely the desire to learn and to master. The focus on learning led the panel to suggest that she was a person who took advantage of opportunities, pursued development within the frames provided, and had an ability to adjust to circumstances.

Continuing in an evaluative manner, Karla addressed the "*incredibly*" steep learning "*related to mastering the medical technical equipment (.) and also seeing patients (.) or (.) meeting ill patients (.) very ill patients*

(.) being able to assess very ill patients". She reported a change due to the accumulated experience:

> *After a while now started to build a (.) what shall I say (.) or one's, maybe not tactic but a little bit one's own way to trust oneself for how to handle meeting very ill patients... maybe soon will die (.) that about knowing a little how one shall handle it... because that is maybe what I regard the biggest challenge encountering in a way the dying (.).*

Switching between past and present gave the impression of a process still in progress. Karla pointed out what was different in the ICU context, that it was more about seeing the relatives, as the patients were most often sedated. She elaborated on the change in terms identified as a major concern:

> *One has, as time has passed, been able to retrieve quite some experience with daring in a way to be there, daring to be a little more (.2) direct to put it that way (.) and in a way stand in the somewhat difficult situations (.) and then (.) yes what is difficult with that in a way (.) yes it is that thing about not being vague (.).*

The intensive care nurse on the panel pointed out how non-controversial Karla's focus on communication was, on not being vague, but rather clear and direct. To her, Karla was speaking according to "the book", in line with policy. Still, the two quotes placed relation and communication center-stage. Considering the account as a whole, relation and communication were dominant issues that Karla kept coming back to, underscoring them as principal concerns in her account.

Let us explore another very much related concern, brought up next, namely truth-telling.

To Speak or Not to Speak the Truth—That Is the Question

"*Being able to be present with relatives*" was crucial and carried a certain meaning for Karla:

> *They actually desire (.) often (.) the impression left with me is that they would rather (.) just get the truth as it is (.) of course they want to get hope and that part (.) but most desire to get a direct message.*

The difficulty, as I read her, was delivering those messages of truth, being present with patients and relatives in a way that provided clarity. Karla claimed that health professionals should be "*saying out loud something about what we see*". She continued, "*in 90 to 95% of the cases I am part of, they want us to be concrete and tell it as it is*", but she acknowledged that "*I feel we have a distance to go in regard to be able to be direct with them*". As she made this point, Karla underscored another: "*Why is it always the physician who delivers certain information to the patient*" when it is the nurses that are at the "*bedside*" and have the "*best connection with the relatives and patient*". To Karla, the question "*relates to our credibility as nurses*", sustained by the observation that "*we can often become a little anonymous*".

The above argument was followed in sub-session two by a very pregnant PIN, in which the clear and direct communication she had just argued for was very difficult to attain. It was the story about a young woman, mother of two, who was terminally illwith cancer. Her condition was so serious that when she was opened up in surgery, she was found not eligible for the operation. When she awoke at the unit much earlier than she would have, had she had the operation, the woman figured out the seriousness of the situation. Karla described how she felt trapped by not being in position to say much, as it was the surgeon's call to inform the patient. She was thus left next to an existentially troubled, and grief-stricken, woman, who "*cried and cried and cried*". Karla was thinking about her kids losing their mother, but found herself in no position to address the obvious.

Again, Karla enacted the drama through dialogue, including the one within herself, keeping one eye inward and the other on the patient, considering herself and the other simultaneously:

> *I remember sitting there (.) there was no other alternative (.) no choice to walk out of there (.) in a way I was her support… but I remember (.) answering or not answering her… should I say something or not (.) what is a*

> *natural thing to say - - what can sound totally wrong… didn't have a choice (.) couldn't abandon her then (.) no (.) just had to be there (.4).*

Karla thus added to the complexity of the emerging main concern: relation and communication, not being vague, but telling the truth.

The Dying and Death of a Young Mother—Truth-Telling Revisited

Karla moved on by recounting another particular incident narrative that also described already-identified concerns. The patient, "*an incredibly great girl*", a young woman of the same age as Karla, was infected by a very rare bacterium with a 100% mortality rate. Against all odds, there was a turn for the better around Christmas. The patient was awake and off the respirator, fragile but able to communicate, watching TV, updating her Facebook profile, and participating in the service conducted in the chapel. This turn for the better evoked hope, both in the patient and among her family.

Unfortunately, not long after things got worse. Hence, when Karla was back from holiday, around New Year, "*The decision is made for the patient that there is no more treatment to offer- - and that one choses to terminate treatment*".

> *Two days later I remember I was with the patient as the physician explained to the patient (.) the patient was awake (.2) how one explains that one doesn't have more treatment to offer and that one choses to terminate and that she (.) eventually will be allowed to sleep…*

Karla continued the sentence by explaining what they usually do when situations like this occur. She went from a PIN to a GIN: "*because of course (.) then our focus shifts in a way*". The attention turns, both by the bedside and in the narrating, from the patient to the relatives. The shift reported seemed to be echoed in Karla's manner of speaking as there was a change of pace, as if she was removing herself emotionally from that bedside into a more instrumental mode toward the relatives.

Following a brief pause, Karla again brought her attention back to the focus of the story: "*When the physician explained to the patient that there is nothing more we can do and the patient was acknowledging it to the degree that she was able to take it in*". Karla's voice softened and she spoke more quietly, when shifting to an evaluative manner of speaking and providing what appeared to be the moral of the story, namely that:

> *Even though the patient was very much impacted by the infection (.) I think that it was actually here she was told that there actually was nothing more to offer (.) yes (.) because she was totally preoccupied with 'how am I doing (.) how are my tests (.) what is happening' (.) hence I didn't have any reservations… it was only fair… but of course those images and what one is left with when that is told (.) leaves a strong impression… totally impossible not to be touched by it.*

Having delivered the moral of the story, and been in touch with the impact of having witnessed an act of ultimate truth-telling, Karla again turned to speaking more generally—about how they usually helped the relatives in a situation of the patient's imminent death.

Moving in and out of the patient's room, figuratively speaking, may have indicated that Karla had the need to distance herself from intolerable parts of the situation. In sub-session two, it became evident that she remembered more details from the meeting with professionals (in which termination of treatment for this particular patient was decided) than she did from the actual talk with the patient. From the former, she provided several dialogical enactments, remembering how participants were seated. From the latter, she reported in broader terms, having more difficulty recalling the response of the other, the patient, when told that treatment was to end. This may have been due to the young woman being on a respirator and the fact that they were "*sedating her and she in a way is not present to us*", or it may have been related to this being the part of the incident that was "*totally impossible not to be touched by*".

The red threads identified above—mastering, relating, gaining voice, and telling the truth—run through this particular story. To the panel, Karla appeared to be professional in the most positive meaning of the term. Nonetheless, the fact that Karla was able to share such an emotionally charged story without giving away her own emotions was "*interesting*" to the panel. Did what appeared to be a professional distance in the here and now indicate the same in the there and then? Did the possible desire for professionalism potentially imply too much distancing? If so, how would it inform the rest of the telling? Would there be a need to move further away from the emotionally charged? All these were questions posed by the panel.

The Death of a Young Father—"Why Didn't You Tell Me?"

For the next 35 minutes, Karla devoted the time to "*another case that also was very special*". It took place between three and six months prior to the interview. A transplant patient, father of three, had developed cancer. He lived in another city and arrived at the hospital the night before. There was a critical turn in his condition, and he was rushed into surgery. When arriving at the ICU, he was in very bad condition, in a "*septic phase*" and experiencing "*blood poisoning*".

Karla used a broad-brush approach to tell about the hours of this special shift in reportage style. We learned how the staff discussed among themselves both how to approach the fact that three children were coming and whether it was worthwhile keeping the patient alive. Karla was to be responsible for the relatives that day, and it was decided that they would work to keep the patient alive until the children arrived.

Eventually, earlier than expected into the day shift, the patient had a heart attack and died. Death occurred as Karla was in the middle of a conversation with the family. The narrator could have reached this point in the story way before. Instead, it was postponed due to an elaborate report of the processes that preceded it. Why? Was it because this was the point where conflict entered the narrative? The meeting that had been convened by Karla meant that the patient's wife was "*not allowed*", in Karla's terms, to hold his hand as he died, which was her one desire and had been promised to her upon arrival at the hospital. "*The first thought that struck me*", Karla said when telling how she was pulled out of the meeting with the family was "*oh no, now she was not able to be present*".

After having described how the patient was lying with:

> *…an open gut… it seeps liquid (.) a whole lot of drains (.) perhaps he has received 30 L (.) he looks terrible compared to what he usually does*;

and how this was a dilemma with regard to letting the children see their father, Karla drew a breath and exclaimed:

> *I believe this is perhaps one of the biggest challenges I have experienced as a nurse (.) to handle that group of relatives in that context (.14).*

Just as when she had reached the climactic point in the previous PIN, there was a change of focus followed by an almost abrupt shift in the manner of telling. Without a pause, Karla continued:

> *And then it is a little bit like this 'okay the kids how are we to proceed' and it is obvious when one has resuscitated him with an open gut and then with all the liquids and everything it didn't look good at all in there – right (.) it was just blood all over and yes that is definitely not a nice sight… how are we to adapt to this.*

Karla's evaluative statement, her concern with how the wife might take the fact that her wish had not been fulfilled, was replaced by the pursuit of a more practical question, which she repeated several times in the next few minutes, namely: "*HOW are we to handle this… how are we to handle the wife… all of them*"? Karla voiced the question to Sara, the anesthesiologist on duty—"*definitely one of our best physicians to cooperate with*".

The panel found the repeated use of "*handle*" peculiar, but also that Karla did not elaborate on her own despair. They found her to be action-oriented. The narrating nurse stayed with the situation, but changed focus. Moving on to what happened next fitted with what appeared to be a commitment to a chronological telling. Still, one may ask if this was a way of defending herself against what appeared to be the most challenging part of this highly challenging clinical incident. After having discussed and agreed how to proceed, the three professionals entered the room in which the family, still unaware of the drama that had unfolded, were located. The physician informed them that the patient had had a heart attack and died:

> *And then the wife totally collapses (.) of course and the first thing she says is 'why didn't you tell me' (.) that was the first she said (.) and it was kind of (.) and that sticks (.) it is the kind of thing one has to (.) yes that we had to really work on afterwards (.) both for her part and for our part too (.) for how we should avoid that it remained as a memory for her.*

The panel was struck by the level of detail in Karla's telling at this point—the fact that she could recall exactly what happened: "*It is a professional person reporting... she rationalizes what is difficult... she asks incredibly good questions... sounds like a physician's story... almost a little cold*". As pointed out by the panel, there was a significant difference in character between the detailed, somewhat distanced telling and the subject that was being reported, namely the emotional collapse of this grief-stricken family: "*So the next oldest boy he too totally collapses and screams, hyperventilates, falls apart and we had to carry him to the couch*". As if in disbelief, she continued her narrative about how they all collapsed. None of the three professionals had experienced anything like it, according to Karla. "*But at the same time... it is a natural reaction (.) really it is (.) totally natural reaction (.) really it is (.) totally natural reaction*". To me, it was as if Karla was embracing the naturalness of their emotional reaction as she spoke.

She then took a step back, considering a multitude of experiences in a sentence, and provided a global evaluation: "*Sometimes I think that it is (.) why don't people show more emotion in a way*". Karla then pointed out how the lack of emotion expressed might also be just as natural as some deaths which, unlike in the case of the reported incident, are "*prepared*". In such cases, given the ethical dilemmas related to them, relatives may even feel "*relieved*". In this particular case though she concluded that:

> *It was very very good to see them (.) even if it is different from what one has experienced before it was good to see that they (.) cried like they did (.) really (.) and we sat there for a long time (.) for an hour.*

As Karla was approaching her own emotions though there was (again) a shift in the telling:

> *And then it was really just to break in and and (.) I remember I said 'do you know what (.) now we make him (.) we prepare him (.) and practically prepare in order for you to come in if you want it' (.).*

Once again, we witnessed the action-oriented professional—an impression which was reinforced in the subsequent paragraphs. Karla took charge, not over-ruling the relatives, but neither totally complying with them. Upon getting a hesitant "*no I really don't know*" from the widow in response to the question whether they wanted a chaplain, she responded, "*do you know what (.) I contact him*".

It turned out that the chaplain had visited the patient a few days earlier and could provide consoling information to the family from that talk. Once again, Karla approached another member of the interdisciplinary team, this time the chaplain, with the "how" question:

> *You know what we need now (.) we really need help for how we shall solve this further - - (.) this whole situation.*

Again we recognized the action- and goal-oriented, health professional-looking for her next move in order to "*handle*" the situation, even "*solve it*". She was living with what for her was a general question, felt in various situations, namely "*how shall one grasp the particular needs of those who are there and who don't know me at all*"? One answer this time was a simple memorial service for the family. Karla expressed how pleased she was:

> *That we had taken that decision for them (.) really as we knew they were believers (.) that I think really that it must have been good that a chaplain came in here - - (.) so that felt very good and I experienced them as also experiencing it as good.*

The realization that part of the drama had played out in the very room in which we were having the interview made even Karla's use of general incident narratives (GINs) actually feel experience-near.

Karla eventually came back to "*what still sticks*", the part about the wife not being able to be with her husband at the point at which he died. She underscored how the questions relating to this part of the incident have lingered: "*We have talked a lot about it afterwards that we definitely should or how we should have solved it in another situation*". Even though the family was out of sight, and she had a rational explanation for why it may have been for the best, and she had learned from the physician that "*the family, all things considered, are doing very well*", the situation was obviously not out of Karla's mind. The fact that she spent this amount of time in detailed telling, coming back to "*what sticks*" several times, testified to the opposite, which Karla also explicitly expressed:

> *And it is situations like this that really get burned into the spine to put it that way (.) but, but one senses that one acquires some experience regarding handling relatives (.) when that is what is our focus (.) be direct (.) listen to how they want it (.) be honest about the situation (.) and then use those extra five minutes to see them… sacrifice that little time that makes them feel seen.*

In this global evaluation offered at the very end of the PIN, denoting the moral of the story, Karla was again latching onto the red threads in her account, which were growing increasingly more significant for every new story she told.

The detailed chronological telling of these stories mirrored the former desire to become an economist, making sure that all the small and large numbers were included in the equation. However, although she valued "*direct*" speech, Karla paradoxically conveyed her own experiences in a rather vague manner. The missing number may have been her emotional experience—this was supported by the fact that when Karla was about to become experience-near in her telling, she repeatedly shifted focus and distanced herself emotionally. Throughout, she spoke in terms of "*we*" or "*one*", which underscored the same point. Hence, despite the very clear global evaluation, the underscored importance of direct and honest communication, and the removal of any doubt that this was an encounter that sticks, it remained unclear how or why it stuck with her and what emotion or former experiences it stuck to.

Coming to One's Senses

As Karla was about to end her free-associative telling, the pace slowed and the pauses got longer. What comes last in an account, like what comes first, is particularly interesting in that it can give emphasis to what is most important, or most important for the narrator to convey as important.

Encountering death at the nursing home, Karla was "*busy about the physical and what one saw and sensed*". At this point in her professional development, encountering similar situations, the focus was "*much more on the setting (.) that is how we can make it best possible for the relatives and patients… focus is on a totally different level from when one started*". She then considered what the change implied emotionally. This development has:

> *…nothing to do with one turning cold (.) don't feel that at all (.) but of course we establish a survivor instinct in this setting (.) because if one had taken all situations of this kind at the ICU too close to the heart all the time one would not have survived in this business.*

Thus, Karla navigated carefully between several stereotypical images of what work in acute care meant emotionally to the professional. She distanced herself not only from the cynical health professional, but also from those who get too emotionally involved. Karla situated herself in the position of being just right and 'professional'. At the same time, one may ask whether there was not an emotional distancing in this act of balancing. The lack of expressed emotions, mirrored in the manner of recounting the very emotionally charged clinical situations, may suggest an emotional distance, or that Karla was presenting a processed and thus rehearsed narrative account that she was now about to end:

> *Then I believe I have actually (.1) that (.2) don't have so much (.4) ((takes a deep breath)) so many other (.) viewpoints (.) or so many more (.1) viewpoints (.) or that I need to express now (.) said a lot about concerning what I think about the question or concerning the introduction - - (.) mhm (.3).*

To indicate what she was doing through her telling, Karla repeated "*viewpoints*" twice—a term that gave the impression she had primarily undertaken a rational endeavor, which may also explain the sometimes experience-distant manner of telling. In response to her ending, I repeated part of the SQUIN and invited her once more to consider whether "*there are other events or experiences (.) that you think have been important for you (.23)*". After a long pause, Karla said she didn't think there were, repeating that the ones she just told:

> *… are events that have sat with me and in a way sit well and that have provided me with a lot of experience and that probably have changed me (.2) yes perhaps not changed but built (.1) a (.1) a (.2) what shall I say (.2) or made me in a way into who I am now as a nurse and as a person.*

Karla was reporting change. What changes was she referring to that have made her into a different person and professional?

> *I have built up a significantly greater sense of security for HOW I respond when… that dialogue comes… not avoiding things… ask the questions… am direct… show interest… dare standing in that dialogue and in those difficult answers YOU/ONE can get (.) it is perhaps that which (.) that (.1) that about mirroring one's own self for what comes because that I believe I was very afraid of (.) was much more afraid of that before (.) one avoided the situation because one was afraid of what one would meet… have built up a totally different sense of security.*

Karla raised the question of how to relate to dying patients, the relatives left behind, and the male physicians, at the very beginning of her professional life as a health professional. The question served as a red thread throughout the told story. It informed the narrator's choice of events and experiences, all of which raised questions about how to relate in critical clinical situations. Through the twists and turns of the narrative, it was possible to follow the development of Karla's own voice. Starting out without any experience (the more experienced did the talking), being intimidated by a male physician, to being in charge of following up this family of five in the most critical hours of their lives. At this point, with a firm voice, she made things happen. She was exercising power in a manner that took a certain amount of self-confidence and trust in her own competence.

At the same time, as pointed out above, in the telling of this development and the dialogue about it, the issues of "*not avoiding things*" and being "*direct*" that she reported were not as apparent as in the narrative. Thus, a discrepancy can be identified between the manner of telling and the content. There is little doubt that at this point Karla as nurse was able to "*handle*" challenging encounters. Yet, the same telling left some doubt as to how it was for Karla to stay with and explore the emotions these same situations evoked in her. Where did the "*terror*", reported in the first encounter with death and dying, go?

Despite acknowledging that she was rather new to "*this business*", highlighting the fact that one is never done learning, Karla attributed the change to what she called "*multiple mouthfuls*" of experience. She stressed the importance of reflecting upon experience, which was what she offered the students she was supervising. Having her own experience as a student fresh in her mind, having had "*what one may call models*", she wanted to serve as a model herself to enable them to make up their own minds:

> *One stood in some VERY difficult situations that one feels that one maybe does not have the head totally above water to put it that way (.) actually it is a little bit like drifting on the surface of the water (.) you really have to mobilize for how to handle the situation.*

Some of the panel members wondered whether or not Karla's continuous aspiring toward more responsibility and mastery of critical situations related to a deeply felt sense of insecurity due to the traumatic "loss" of her mother in her second year of life. Through work as an intensive care nurse, she comes close to the personal and emotional at the same time as she "saves" herself behind the technical skills and everything she is good at. Thus, the panel members concluded on a less speculative note, based on what they witnessed in the narrative account, that Karla "*attempts to solve the problems of her life in an incredibly adaptable way*". Karla, for her part, ended her first narrative by voicing with confidence what she regarded as the most difficult aspect of end-of-life care:

But this thing about being present (.) tell concretely what is going on (.) and simply not be avoidant (.) don't be too vague and don't be too avoidant but be direct (.) yes and be present and speak with them loudly about what we are doing and what is going on and simply a little small talk - - (.10). Yes (.) then I think I have said what I wanted.

A Thin Sense of the Situated Subjectivity

To "*master*", "*handle*", and "solve" was placed center-stage in Karla's account. The terms ran through the narrative like red threads. The sense of implied responsibility exposed her to experiences of guilt, which was illustrated by the main story, the incident in which she did it right, but it turned out wrong anyway. Her switch between past and present tenses was perhaps a slip of the tongue, an unintentional way of saying that these difficult situations also take place now and not just in the past. The telling of recent incidents that "*stick*" suggested just that.

Karla constantly took steps to deepen the competence required in the context of her situation, steps that suggested the prospect of more responsibility, more mastering, more dilemmas pertaining to truth-telling, and thus more guilt. This may have related to Karla's action-orientedness, that she, according to her own account, is a doer, and felt "*useless to be at work without doing something*".

This became particularly pressing in professional situations that called for "being", and applying relational and communicative skills rather than "doing" medical work. Hence, this was also what she referred to early on as particularly difficult, what "*terrorized*" her as a young nurse. Karla is still, repeatedly, concerned about the communication with patients and relatives, about not "*not being vague*", but rather a "*clear and direct*" truth-teller.

The pace at which Karla spoke, the clear articulation of words, her mastery of medical terminology, the confidence and manner in which she presented the dialogical enactments, with no hesitation or searching for words, might have camouflaged the fact that her communication was not always "*clear and direct*", but at times rather "*vague*". Illustrative of this was also her extensive use, with important exceptions, of "*one*" or "*you*" when "I" would have been as appropriate.

The relation between the personal and professional in end-of-life care, how to use self, how to relate and communicate, was a concern sustained by challenging clinical incidents at the very beginning of Karla's career as a nurse. It still appeared to be a conflicted area, expressed in particular in the encounters with young mothers and fathers—dying patients that were still awake and in a dire state, resembling that of her own mother.

The unarticulated presence of her childhood trauma could very well have informed her continued devotion to pursue "*mastering*" critical care, as suggested by the panel. That she did not explicitly connect the two was a striking feature of her narrative. The question is whether it dwelt in the shadows of the PINs in her account and in the lack of elaboration of her own emotions in the telling. The above may suggest that she was operating with a dotted demarcation line between the personal and the professional.

To gain and give voice thus became the interpretive principle, the dominant perspective, and the major concern that seemed to inform her telling. This was apparently pivotal regarding which clinical incidents "*stuck*" with her. She made it explicit in the beginning, elaborated on it throughout and underscored it at the very end, letting it thematically frame the account. Thus, it became dots in the thin line of subjectivity, making itself evident during the interview.

7
Dina

Lived Life and Told Story

Setting the Scene

Dina and I met in the hall just outside the palliative unit where she worked as a physician. After initial greetings, we went downstairs to the main entrance. As we stepped outside, we were greeted by the sounds and smells of spring. Life was making a return, at least outside the hospital. Dina took me to the next building and, as we walked to her office, she probed me about my professional background, more so than the previous interviewees had done.

Her particular interest in my background did not strike me until later, when she shared how she sought out male pastors with whom to process her experience of oppressive religiosity. The latter was a theme that ran through her narrative, suggesting that encountering a male who was also a chaplain carried particular meaning for Dina. It seemed equally clear, however, that Dina did not see me as typical of the cast of characters that had inhabited the oppressive religious environment of her childhood. Rather than being a symbolic figure linked to the

K. Moen, *Death at Work*, Studies in the Psychosocial,
https://doi.org/10.1007/978-3-319-90326-2_7

religious oppression of her past, she seemed to link me to the emancipatory process of the present.

The question remained, of course, whether Dina would have told another story at another time to another person. One might ask whether unconsciously I regarded the encounter between us as one that could counter her previous experience with clergy. Did I take this upon myself? Did I take non-verbal signs as proof that I did not represent what she despised? Could this, combined with my sensitivity to her use of terms like “traumatic”, be a reason why I did not push harder for particular incident narratives (PINs) that might complement her dominant narrative and bring in more stories from her long clinical experience? Was it the dynamics playing out between the two of us, or was it rather Dina’s way of expressing exhaustion from encountering so many dying patients, that made her narrative one with so few stories of her encounters at the border between life and death?

Lived Life—In Brief

Dina was born in the mid-1950s. She had two siblings and her childhood and teenage years were spent in a small village in the southern part of Norway. Her mother worked as a homemaker and a kitchen assistant, while her father was an artisan and a social worker. After graduating from high school, she worked at a nursing home while improving her grades in order to get into medical school. During her professional life, she moved both geographically and between different clinical disciplines. Eventually she moved abroad, and for about fifteen years she lived only part time in Norway. Throughout her life she has travelled and spent extended periods in different countries. Dina, mother to a daughter, has been married and divorced. At the time of the interview, after having pursued further education in palliative care, she worked part time as a physician at the palliative care unit.

Told Story—An Overview

Dina’s telling of her lived life was linear and, to a great extent, followed the sequence of events and experiences as they had played out. The account started with early childhood, followed by her teenage years, youth and then early and late adulthood. The narrative ended close to the time of the interview.

Even though the account is largely chronological, it did make circular moves at certain points, most often in relation to actualizations of themes that seemed to have originated in her childhood narrative. Dina's account was only sparsely inhabited, yet, the telling was not without a "*we*". She did not provide any close-up portraits of anyone in her first narrative though; the presence of others was more implicit than explicit. Focus was on Dina's experience, which left a strong sense of "me-ness" throughout her telling. It was a first-person narrative. Dina's lived life could have set the stage for a multitude of other narratives, marked as it was by geographical, professional, and relational movements and turning points, spanning several decades and continents. Setting out from a small community in southern Norway, she traversed the world. She has dedicated her professional life to the well-being of others by engaging in different medical disciplines, and she has facilitated beginnings and endings of life many times.

One might expect such a life to bring forth stories of life-changing encounters at the boundary between life and death. Yet there appeared to be another selective principle for what was included or left out of her narrative. Part of what was left out were her clinical encounters with the terminally ill and dying, making her account the disconfirming case among the four, and leaving me with the pressing question of whether Dina's biographical account could contribute to my central research question.

Detailed Reading of the Narrative

What First Comes to Mind

Dina's very first response to the invitation to tell the story of her life was to go all the way back to her childhood. She started her account with neither demographic nor biographical facts, nor the routines or playfulness of everyday life in the village, but rather with one particular dimension of her childhood. "*What first comes to mind*", she said, "*is my upbringing with Christendom*".

When presented with this sentence, the panel hypothesized that for Dina going to this particular place could be accompanied by feelings of pride, security, shame, or anger. Shame due to "*growing up in the context of something that was inhibiting*", as expressed by one of the panel members. Provided with the full sentence, namely "*What first comes to mind is my upbringing with Christendom and western, black painting, condemning narrow mindedness*", seemingly confirming the panel's darkest anticipation. It fostered an expectation among the panel members of an emotionally charged narrative waiting to unfold.

Dina stated four times within the first few minutes that her religious upbringing and the process by which she broke out of it had been "*very formative*". Giving this part of her life such explanatory power suggested that it was not falling into place as she spoke, but was rather an expression of—a rehearsed narrative about—thoughts she had considered before and with which she was quite familiar. Dina was telling the story of her religious upbringing in terms of oppression and emancipation:

> *From believing that everything was fine as a child, that you are being taken care of by a God, to traumatic experiences with delusions by those surrounding me… that made me not believe in such things anymore… and totally distanced myself from it.*

In sub-session two, triggered by my nudges, Dina added several PINs to this topic, narratives that confirmed that the reported shift from everything being "*fine*" to "*traumatic experiences*" did indeed take place. The first particular incident Dina shared, "*when everything was turned upside down*", and to which her use of "*traumatic*" was related, was about how she came to commit "*the unforgivable sin*" which, in her 11-year-old mind, placed her beyond redemption, apart from her community of origin, significant others and God.

A Threat of Non-Being

One day Dina's sense of "*security*" was totally altered due to her teacher talking about one sin that God did not forgive, that was blaspheming the Holy Spirit. He had hardly finished uttering the words before Dina, in the secrecy of her own mind, did just that, she cursed the Holy Spirit. One thought passed through her head and she immediately understood that her fate was sealed, that she was destined for Hell:

> *In my childish mind I then believed… yes, now you have no one… now I was lost and there was nothing to do about it… RIGHT.*

She went on to talk about how she was existentially shaken by the incident and how she:

> *… became totally neurotic because of it… I remember I lost color vision… I was extremely scared… ehm… and then there was nobody I could talk to about it… I went to talk with my mother… it was not possible to get help, because I have a mom that still believes in Hell ((Dina breathes heavily, before concluding)) and was not able to help me with that.*

Dina was crushed under the weight of the threat not only of eternal punishment, but also social separation: "*It was terrible, everything was ruined… when I die I'll go to hell and everybody else will go to heaven*". Dina continued her first narrative by telling how she left the church when she was 15. In sub-session two, she told a story, a particular incident, that represented a turning point and a contributing factor to her leaving the church. It took place on a bus-ride to visit her uncle and aunt:

> *I was so neurotic (.) I had a lot of neurotic thoughts right (.) thoughts that could be crazy, wrong or sinful… and all that had to with sexuality and stuff like that (.) eh (.) everything wrong (.) I could think - - (.) yes (.) and it bugged me (.) terrible - - (.) because I couldn't manage my thoughts…. so I was thinking 'well, now you are just setting yourself up for hell even more'.*

Dina got to a point at which she realized she could no longer deal with all this. There was a desire to separate herself from the particular religious mind-set of her upbringing:

> *It was so traumatizing (.) I was so sad (.) and so depressed (.) and there was this voice inside me that said it (.) 'I don't want to have anything to do with this'(.) if this is it and this is true and God is like this and people are like this then I don't want to have anything to do with it (.) and then it became light in me (.) it was a decision like that ((snaps her fingers)) … then the colors came back… (.)*

Setting Self Apart

The panel found Dina both "*analytic*" and "*reflexive*", "*a person able to relate to who she is and what she does*". In a sense, when speaking about "*the most formative*", Dina also opened the door on the most painful parts of her life. It was not obvious that a story from a context which would be foreign to most people would be understood. Illustrative of this was how one of the panel members expressed "*shock*" that Dina could have such a negative experience with a Christian upbringing. I have encountered many life-stories resembling Dina's, hence I had no problem appreciating her position. Did she notice?

As she continued, Dina attributed her "*rescue*"—the fact that she "*distanced myself totally from it (.) in order to break out of it*"—to her own inner qualities alone, and that she "*maybe has a personality that was capable of breaking out… and fighting against… and for my own freedom*". She argued the case by listing qualities about herself that were "*always*" there, that distinguished her and set her apart from others:

> *I have always been a human being seeking what is true… I have always been politically engaged… always very questioning… very much a seeker after something other than what I experienced as oppressive… that has formed me very much very… like go in depth, look beyond and find out things… I have always followed that road.*

Dina understood herself as a person refusing to submit to blind faith or external authorities. She was someone fighting for freedom and seeking truth. Following her break with the church, she claimed, "*I came into opposition to everything*". This image of herself as being in opposition to, feeling confined by, and fighting against "*systems*" was a recurring one in her account. At several points, the panel recognized in Dina's telling "*an anxiety of disappearing in the sect*", an urge "*to choose self*" due to "*a fear of becoming nothing*".

In order to truly appreciate the relation between Dina leaving the church and her narrative of herself, one must take account of the religious context she broke out of. That the church was literally located at the center of the community was not peculiar to Dina's village; it is common in villages and cities not only throughout Norway, but also Europe. The village being centered around the church relates to the physical building, but also to the particular place Christianity has had in Norwegian history and culture, and the position the local church has at critical points in the majority of citizens' lives up until today.

Dina withdrew from the evangelical Lutheran state church which, at the time, held a privileged position inscribed in Norwegian law. In 1970, the year Dina withdrew her membership, over 90% of the population were still members. One can thus assume that at this point in Norwegian history, breaking with the church still represented a stigma in a small community. It took courage and determination to go through with it, and it could leave a lasting impression on the one who did. The fact that it also implied estrangement from family of origin underscored what a major decision it was for a 15 year old.

In the narrative unfolding before them, the panel recognized both an "*independent, secure, strong, tough individual who trusts self*", yet also "*a seeker… lonely*". The following statements made in sub-session two, in which Dina alternated between the past tense and present tense, may have captured precisely this impression:

> *It has taken a little time to understand that this can't be true (.2) do you understand - - (.) and still there can be such an anxiety there (.) what if it is there after all (.) uugghh (.)- - right (.) am I really as good as everybody else and do I get to heaven and is there a heaven and stuff like that right- - (.) it is not totally (.) don't have the proofs yet (.) ((laughs)) God (.) do you understand - - (.)*

As more chunks of the account were made available, the panel sensed "*an enormous aggression*" on Dina's part that corresponded to what I wrote in my debrief note just after the interview. At several points in her telling, she expressed distaste with the religious environment in which she grew up by making noises similar to throwing up, as if talking about it was making her physically sick. She thus left the impression that the religious upbringing still very much had an emotional effect on her.

Here and Now, There and Then

Dina had received and signed the same invitation letter as the other interviewees. Like the others, she had heard the Single Question Inducing Narrative (SQUIN) read to her twice before embarking on her narrative. The question why her many encounters from the border between life and death seemed so out of sight became increasingly pressing as her narrative account unfolded.

When asked whether she remembered when she came to the realization that her religious upbringing had been so formative, Dina said that "*it is just a few years ago since I really realized that (.) what (.) had thought about before, but not in the way that I had understood that it has formed something very important*". Having dealt with this so recently might well explain why it was "*the first that comes to mind*". A second hypothesis as to why her experience of a dark and oppressive religious upbringing became the key figure and a red thread in her account was related by the panel to possible interrelational dynamics playing out in the interview: an actualization of the there and then in the here and now. Did she relate to me as a researcher, or was I primarily a male pastor to her? In several passages, Dina in fact related my profession, my maleness, and me to her narrative and the telling of her story. In a not too distant past, talking with a male affiliated to the church would have been very difficult, if not impossible, for Dina:

> *The worst for me was (.) hehe ((laughs!)) (.) you have to know (.) you can be glad that you are here now (.) a male pastor in the Norwegian church (.) that was the enemy - - (.) do you understand - -.*

At one point, Dina made a statement about how she used to hate pastors. Even if I did not fall within the religious category she had grown up in, it felt like an aggressive statement. What first struck me as I later sat down to listen to the recorded interview was her voice—how different it was from the antagonistic and aggressive tone I had heard in the interview. Could the discrepancy between my first and second listening be related to me feeling coerced in the first listening into some hostile interpersonal environment?

The fact that she sought out male pastors with whom to process her own experience of oppressive religiosity, and her later hatred of religion, suggested that in encountering a male minister, his role as pastor could take precedence over other roles he may have, e.g., researcher. The fact that Dina showed particular interest in my professional background, explicitly probing whether I was ordained or not in our initial talk, may have indicated the same.

The fact that I was only able to walk the panel through about half of Dina's first narrative (sub-session one) was partly due to this being my first panel. It may also have related to the point just made, namely that I had a particular interest in lingering over the first part of her account. Whatever the reason, the result was that the panel missed out on the rest of Dina's narrative—her longing to be not only apart, but also a part.

A Need to Be Apart

The years between age 16 and 24 were hardly mentioned in Dina's account. Thus, she hardly talked about fundamental experiences such as leaving home, moving to the city, starting university, or working at a nursing home. Instead, Dina gave attention to topics that many would also regard as significant: living abroad for an extended time, the years in elementary school, choice of education, and career path—in that order. Dina's narrative on these topics did not extend over many lines, but in each she said something about why she regarded these themes as existentially significant in her life.

This was the case when she talked about how her extended visits to other countries provided her with "*another homeland inside me*". What Dina particularly appreciated with France was that it was a culture marked by "*freedom*" and "*openness*" and "*thinkers*". What she particularly appreciated about school was that it provided her with a foundation from which she could be free and make her own decisions. School boosted her self-esteem.

Dina thus related her experience to the dominant themes introduced in "*what first came to mind*", namely freedom and thinking. That her move abroad potentially contributed to estrange her even further from her origins was perhaps illustrated by the indignation expressed by one of the panel members. She questioned how Dina could have moved back and forth between countries when she had a daughter—"*I don't get it*".

The panel grew more and more impatient with Dina not speaking of any persons, or relationships, only countries and cultures. They found the scarcely populated narrative at odds with her professional role in palliative care. Whatever topic Dina covered, she spoke in evaluative terms and left the listener with the sense that whatever she happened to speak about was important and had been formative for her. She had a tendency to focus on inner states rather than detailed recounting of external realities. Focusing on her own inner states—and particularly on the sense of freedom and openness—was also marked when talking about her travels:

> *…enormous sense of freedom there… because it is a large country and very few people and an enormous amount of space… I feel freedom here also (.) particularly when I am in the northern part of Norway (.) because there is so much space (.) but down there I feel it all the time (.) such a strong sense of freedom… it is great (.)*

When asked whether there was a particular episode that encapsulated the feeling of freedom, Dina provided a PIN that underscored what emerged as a dominant theme, namely the need to be apart. It was a trip to a mountainous area in a foreign country in which one could walk for up to ten days without meeting anybody. There were plenty of animals, but no human beings in sight:

> *…an enormous sense of freedom to be out there (.) and not see the end of anything anywhere (.) whatever way you look it is (.) you don't find the end of anything… (.) probably like being on the middle of the ocean when you don't see anything (.) no boundaries in a way (.)*

There seemed to be a craving for open spaces in Dina's life, which she found in culture and nature. The sparsely populated narrative account, yet to introduce any significant faces or voices other than Dina's own, appeared to mirror what emerged as a significant part of Dina's outlook on life, a need to be apart and free.

The longing to be apart was also evident in later years, in regard to her professional life:

> *After having worked as doctor (.) been married (.) had children (.) only been in that system in a way (.) I have had an enormous longing to do other things (.) at times I have done things (.) a little bit with music (.) played the flute a little bit done a lot of dancing (.) all of a sudden I realized that I could paint and stuff like that (.) it just opened (.) just could do it all of a sudden (.) really just like that just (.) things that I thought I never could do.*

Dina labeled work, marriage, and child-rearing as being "*in that system*", as something confining, leaving her with "*an enormous longing*". Perhaps this mirrored a manner of thinking and speaking from the 1970s, and the avant-garde sociopolitical community she was part of in France, in which every "conservative" institution was suspect?

On the other hand, one might ask whether the longing to be apart also related to the character of her present job:

> *IT IS A HEAVY JOB THIS (.) if you work full time (.) then I worked 100 percent (.) and that is too much in this profession (.) just this profession - - with so many dying people (.) then I had (.) then I had noticed 'now I have to take a break'.*

For the first time, Dina referred to the character of her job and did so in rather negative terms. The physician recounted how she had made herself a promise to take "*one year off and do nothing with medicine*". She followed up on the promise and resigned her position in order to travel. At the time of the interview she was back, but with a reduced workload. Did the exhaustion of encountering "*so many dying people*" explain the scarcely populated narrative and the desire to be apart? Was focusing the telling on life outside the clinic a response to a sense of confinement coming from a daily encounter with the death of others? Or, was it the other way around: did the landscapes of palliative care resemble the open spaces and barren land in which one could move around for days without encountering anyone? Moreover, how does end-of-life care answer Dina's quest for a community that not only allowed, but encouraged, truth-telling?

A Need to Be a Part

In her first narrative, Dina moved on from talking about how ending up at medical school happened almost by chance, to tell about her engagement with "*avant-garde*" political groups and how she spent time with people "*who were participating when there was revolution (.)*". She spoke of herself as always having been politically engaged. It is somewhat paradoxical that she didn't address any political-historical events from her time abroad, which occurred during a highly politically charged period in Europe.

Hence, one might ask whether she was attracted more by the social aspect than by the outlet for political engagement in this political social community; at least this seemed to be her emphasis when she recounted how it was all about "*creating social communities (.) in which people could in a way really develop (.) well, get rid of everything from anxiety to oppression*".

Dina talked about a community in which "*the goal was in a way to create a new culture (.) or what do people need to really be free or (.) build real friendships and (.) and love in a way*". In sub-session two, she provided a couple of PINs that illustrated some of the ways in which the members were to "*support each other in order to become better people*".

One of the exercises prescribed for Dina was to be very soberly dressed, old fashioned and wearing no colors for an extended time when attending the university. She also shared the story of a game they played called "*master and slave*":

> *We could come and be awakened in the middle of the night (.) get blindfolded and then they led us into the dark winter night (.) into the woods (.) had to go barefoot (.) eh went swimming (.) only to trust one another - - (.) really it was great fun really.*

Dina summed up the experience by emphasizing how great it was being part of the community:

> *Fantastic, great and one of the most fantastic experiences I have ever had (.) an incredibly exciting time (.) very (.) grew really fond of each other… and then the grief that came with splitting up (.4) I was very sad when it broke in pieces (.) it was sad - - and a grief related to it (.) because it was so beautiful.*

Life in the social community lasted about a year, but it received exclusive attention in Dina's account. What would usually be regarded as significant events and experiences, such as marriage, childbirth, education, her first divorce as well as her first years as a medical doctor—all of which took place during this time—were left almost unmentioned. The same was true for the next six years, between the ages of 34 and 40, when Dina was alternating between France and Norway, taking various jobs as a physician. It was also the case for the following nine years which started with Dina moving in order to undertake her medical specialization. Dina might have wanted to introduce a significant other or a significant clinical encounter into her narrative, but instead she passed over it all without a remark.

It probably wasn't because the life she lived during these years was insignificant, but what she left out suggested a particular focus that informed Dina's account at the time of the interview. What did get attention was Dina's longing for freedom and her desire to be apart, as expressed in her break with the church and her independent oppositional behavior during her teenage years and, on the other hand, a longing for community, a desire to be a part of something. The oscillation between these two desires seemed to inform Dina's narrative; this was reinforced by how she almost exclusively focused this part of her life on a year-long experience of a social political community in France.

The somewhat servile attitude to what sounded like a rather authoritarian social political movement was paradoxical because it immediately seemed to echo the past, what she had wanted to free herself from, as if she was still living according to the script from her strict religious upbringing. This might suggest that alongside the identified thematic thread of being apart was another about wanting to be a part. The following articulation in sub-session two seemed to sum up not only the question of what the community was all about back then, but also what Dina seemed to be about still:

> *What does it take for a human being to grow up in a community without being (.) become un free - - - - (.) YES so I have always sought that road (.) I have done that a lot in France (.) been in communities (.) and on the one (.) on the other side I cannot totally (.) I have never been able to submit really (.) there is a lot of individualism there (.) I really want to be free (.) really free and then not been able not been able to subordinate myself totally in the group either - - (.)*

As if continuing the sentence, Dina moved on to tell how she had been part of many different professional groups. She made the point that despite having difficulties, she had worked on being able to "*submit*" in different professional contexts. She went on, in the manner of a reporter, to talk about how she worked in various cultural contexts. Then it seemed as if she was leaving the former thread of thought and starting to explain how and why she attained broad clinical experience:

> *Everything from surgical, to internal medicine and palliative care (.2) midwifery and stuff like that (.) so have a lot of experience (.) it feels good (.) makes it easy to work now because I have such a foundation in a way.*

Interpreted in line with what immediately went before, it was as if Dina was saying that broad clinical competence provided her with an open space and gave her an opportunity to choose—"*it feels good*".

Death in Life

After a brief pause and a deep breath, in a slightly different tone of voice, Dina introduced what was to become another turning point and shift in perspective, namely the divorce from her second husband:

> *It has impacted me VERY much… EXTREMELY… that feeling of separation (.) brought up a whole lot of things in me that has made me turn my life upside down… my mind opened totally I saw things in a totally different way (.) I was at work, did my things and simultaneously my mind went in high gear to understand what is happening.*

Where there could have been reflections on how the divorce affected other parties, or her work as physician, none were given. Dina talked about how she experienced multiple "*mystical experiences*" during this time. In particular, she recounted one incident—a turning point, an epiphany—similar to the awakening she had had on that bus in her childhood. One day she was passing the cathedral in the city in which she lived and realized that she still believed in:

> *…a terrible, punishing God that sends people to hell and judges people (.) right (.)… and I realized all of a sudden that this was it (.) this was the foundation inside me (.). It was so traumatic to me that I was so radical that I said to myself that I am going to figure this out whatever it takes.*

Through this crisis, Dina became aware that the religious frame and the disturbing images of God from her upbringing were still very much with her. In order "*to figure this out*" Dina pursued "*long conversations*" with both clergy and therapists. Whereas during her younger years, she turned away from the community of faith, now she was turning toward it. This again seemed to reinforce the fact that the selective principle in both her life and telling was the contradictory need to be a part and apart. Her way of engaging this crisis was apparently in accordance with the self-understanding she professed to at the very beginning of her account, namely that she "*likes to go in deep, look beyond and find out things… I have always followed that road*".

Yet, there appeared to be a difference in the depth with which Dina addressed her spiritual awakening in her account, compared to how she had explained her professional choices: the former extensively and in evaluative terms, the latter more in terms of pragmatic arguments, similar to what had triggered her entry into medical school in the first place. Dina cited organizational issues and there being no available job for her in her previous field when explaining her professional move to work with cancer patients. In sub-session two, she added that she "*became very very tired of working nights*". Dina continued in the same pragmatic manner when speaking of another major topic that surfaced after the divorce, namely death.

Death at Work

There was a change in Dina's telling when she engaged the topic of death. She went from the first person to a more general form, from "*I*" to "*you*", from speaking in evaluative terms about values as a matter of life and death for her, to speaking about the value of exploring death as a matter of pragmatics in order to become a good doctor:

> *I am looking at everything in my life (.) turn every stone in a way to find out things (.) then death was the next question (.) look at this thing about death (.) and this I also think is very important as a doctor (.) that you are capable of talking with people (.) that you have a natural relation to death and illness and all this right (.) and not be afraid of it yourself.*

Dina thus talked about death in terms that suggested it was just like any other topic, that she could "*manage it*", so to speak, and "*be done with it*" to use her own words, even though she acknowledged that "*it is a large topic*".

In a similarly distant and pragmatic manner, she went on to tell about how she took up further education in palliative care, moved and got a position as a physician in a palliative care unit in order to live closer to her parents. Invited, again in sub-session two, to focus on her professional life and elaborate on taking additional courses in palliative care, which might have been an opportunity for her to speak about her coming to terms with her own mortality, Dina responded rather briefly and primarily in pragmatic terms: "*We had a need for palliative care for our patients (.) and to get more competence in the field I started on the education*". Full stop.

In contrast, in sub-session two, Dina talked about having many thoughts about death in relation to her divorce. She even bought a book about a Buddhist death-preparation ritual, without finding that it helped her settle the matter:

> *Instead I thought (.) what am I going to do about this (.) I really have to go in deep into this here to look at it and be done with it - - (.) so then I did that – (.) looked at those things (.) listened to it (.)*

This appeared to contrast with her more pragmatic take on death in the professional context. Invited in sub-session two to elaborate on getting a job at the palliative unit, Dina spoke at length, but not about encounters with dying patients at the unit, rather about how she had had "*a vision*", and had known long before it happened that she was going to work there. She then provided more examples of how intuition "*often*" served her in life: "…*also in my profession I have had it with patients (.) that I have had an intuition about what is happening with them*".

Questioned whether she had one such particular patient story to share, Dina provided a narrative about a woman with an extrauterine pregnancy, a condition that can cause severe bleeding:

> *She came in and we had found out about it (.) and then can (.) and it is often (.) sometimes you have to do surgery right away (.) but it is relatively stable here (.) ehm (.) but eh ((stops a little bit)) (.2) and then you can wait until the next day (.)*

Dina continued:

> *And then in there (.) it was an assistant doctor and a head doctor with me (.) and we were in and looked at her and I had this incredibly strong feeling that we should do something - - (.) but leave it to the head doctor right - - (.)*

> *and then we said 'no, we will wait until tomorrow' (.) 10 minutes later huge bleeding (.) right . (.) and this I have experienced ((claps her hands)) very often. (.) and sometimes have I taken steps related to it and done the right things and it has become evident that it was right one may say (.)*

Questioned whether any similar such story surfaced, Dina thought for about eight seconds and responded that she "*cannot think of any right now*", then provided one anyway, which illustrated what she called "*synchronicity*". In this instance, before going on night shift, Dina read about a very particular and peculiar medical condition, and the recently attained knowledge later became instrumental in dealing with an urgent situation.

Dina could have given voice to her own emotions, opinions, relatives, colleagues. Instead it was personal concerns running through her life and narrative which were again placed center-stage: seeking truth (as intuition), speaking one's mind, not submitting to authority figures. They came together in this particular life and death situation, in that Dina was not speaking her mind, but "*but leaves it to the head doctor right*" thus submitting to an authoritative figure.

A Concern with Agency

There is a concern with agency implied in Dina's narrative account, explained toward the end of the interview, when she introduced what was to become the last topic of sub-session one:

> *Yes important for me to follow such (.) I have a part (.) a part of me is very surgically inclined (.) likes it very much and is a little tough and stuff (.) and another is very kind and ((laughs)) (.) I don't know (.) those two together (.) they are my parents (.) they may be likened to my parents (.) my father is one of those tough guys… (.) mom was a little kind (.) maybe a little bit too restrained (.).*

Dina talked about how these inner forces were in play when, in the recent past, she bought a small motorbike and also started kayaking. She related these particular situations to an ongoing struggle between "*the typical masculine and the typical feminine*" within her: "*There are two parts of me that all the time (.) one that wants (.) is very expansive (.) and one that is holding back*". The former is most often the winner: "*but after a while when I think about it I always get it done*".

In sub-session two, Dina repeated and elaborated on both the struggle between the opposing forces within her, but also on the profound effect of being an agent:

> *...am always a little afraid of it (.) because it always implies a change of it (.) you change when you do (.) make decisions and do new things (.) you can tell that you are managing it in a way (.) then all of a sudden you are 'God, you are totally different' (.) oh (.) all of a sudden you see that you are getting a total different emotion in yourself than you have had before - - (.) can be a little scary that too (.) who am I then - - (.).*

After about eighteen minutes of uninterrupted talk, having provided the pragmatic reasons outlined above for pursuing her present position at the palliative care unit, Dina said that she was coming toward the end of her narrative. Upon my question, which she didn't allow me to complete—whether there *were* "*any other events*"—she exclaimed: "*yes, there is one more thing (.) that has also been very important to me (.)*". Then she took a deep breath. What could it be? would she introduce more people, or provide close-ups of the ones already presented? Was she moving from the private sphere to the professional and would perhaps provide narratives related to encounters with the terminally ill and dying?

Credo

Toward the very end of her account, the palliative physician called attention to "*what is most characteristic when I think about myself like this (.)is...*". It was as if here she wanted to introduce something that should linger in my mind, that should not be forgotten, something she would like to be remembered by. She brought me back to the very beginning of her account, to one of her character traits, and repeated that more than anything else

> *… that truth seeking (.1) that is absolutely the most important - - (.) that is what I most identify with- - (.) YES.*

Immediately following this global evaluation, stating *the* most important thing, and before she launched off into a longer argument which explained what she meant by truth, Dina brought up a meta-reflection on our relationship and asked a question that was pressing for her at that particular point of her narrative:

> *I do not know how much you are (.) you are a pastor and stuff (.) I don't know how much you know about these other things (.) a faith in…*

Dina asked a question, but didn't leave any room for my response, instead, without pause, she went on to confess what sounded like a credo, a confession of faith:

> *Actually I believe that our personality is not what we really are (.) he he (.) it is just a construct (.) a tool for something (.) just like an ego or something like it (.) and I believe we have an inspiration inside us that which is what we really are (.2) that one can say comes from God, or it is what we are or (.) it comes from the source that we are coming from (.) something like that (.) that is what I believe in (.) that's what is most important to me and what I try to get into all what I do - - (.).*

After a few lines about the "*so called truths*", "*the double standards*" and the lack of inquiry about whether the claims of truth were "*really true*" in the context in which she was raised, Dina stated:

> *… and always (.) my strongest desire (.) when I was a child and grew up (.) that was to be allowed to say everything I thought about without being judged for it (.) and not judge anyone.*

By asking me the chaplain what I believed, but not allowing me to answer, instead allowing her own voice to be heard, Dina raised and underscored a point: she was not waiting for my approval, but rather allowing herself to speak her mind. This was what may have played out in her many long conversations with other clergy, encounters that have been important in the process of being "*allowed to say everything without being judged for it*".

Three times she stated "*I believe*", resembling the confession in the church she once left. She confessed to being a truth-seeker and made the case that truth is not an external object, something we can point at, but rather something intrinsic, and that we have every reason to speak our minds in courage, because what comes from the inside is "*what we really are*". Hence, Dina was coming full circle as she used the language of religion; "*truth*", "*I believe*", "*judge*", "*inspiration*", but filled it with a different content.

Dina did not elaborate on the philosophical meaning of her credo, but simply stated "*open communication has been incredibly important to me*". She then related her insight to her professional context:

> *And here at the job it has been totally fantastic (.) because here I can use this attribute of mine SO much (.) in being open and direct and of course sensitive - - but still (.) open communication in these situations are so important (.) and it makes things so easy and people feel so secure - - (.) when they are allowed to bring whatever - - (.) YES - - (.) can also let it be (.) many people don't want to (.) that is also part of it (.) but it is so important and it makes things so easy and it lacks in medical professions and particularly among physicians (.) there is an anxiety for ((takes a deep breath)) talking about deep things (.) difficult things (.) diagnosis (.) prognosis (.) tell the truth and stuff (.) there is so much fear around it that it becomes more difficult than it really is (.) can be quite easy (.1) to do it when you are not afraid (.) because (.48)…*

The major concerns identified in the account came together, and Dina finally brought them to the professional context. After having stated again in sub-session two that she used openness and directedness "*all the time*" in her professional practice, I asked Dina for particular encounters in which this had been the case. She paused several times and had difficulty coming up with specific narratives.

Eventually she provided one PIN about having given news to a dying patient about his imminent death without his relatives being present, to which they responded with anger. Dina recounted how she had spoken openly with them about their reaction and it had all worked out well. She then continued by expressing more ambivalence and acknowledged that being a truth-teller was not always that easy. In fact, she was actually "*a little afraid of it*" as the openness and directness at times have served to separate her from people, involuntarily set her apart; "*when I have said things that people don't want to hear (.) then they have just left*" ((speaks in a lower voice)). The structural hypothesis that suggested itself throughout Dina's telling, the desire to be a part and apart, is thus strengthened toward the very end of interview.

A Thin Sense of the Situated Subjectivity

Dina is a disconfirming case in that she almost steered clear of clinical experiences in her narrative. What "*first comes to mind*", when Dina was invited to share the experiences most significant to her, was a process of emancipation from oppressive religiosity. The quest for freedom, and opposition toward any confining structure, ran like a red thread throughout her narrative account, up until the point at which she resigned her position in order to travel. Throughout, often in more subtle ways, she balanced a longing for freedom with a longing for community. This is actualized in "*that feeling of separation*" following her divorce and was also present in the deep appreciation for the community in France and her colleagues at the hospital, both of which aroused her strong sense of belonging.

There may be reasons to ask whether indeed the longing for vast open spaces, the challenge of any confining social structure, and the quest for community, were all informed by what she reported to be an exhausting number of dying patients, encounters with whom were kept at the margins of her narrative account. The fact that the question of how encounters with death have informed her remained such an unaddressed issue in her account, presents a pressing paradox, not least because of what appeared to be one of this narrator's particular inclinations.

Throughout her narrative account, Dina was self-revealing and self-reflective. She related to her inner experiential self and showed awareness of the lingering presence of past and present life experiences. She was also familiar with the presence of contradictory parts of herself, as well as how they might have related to significant relationships. Her telling bore witness to the fact that this was not the first time she had reviewed her life story this way. Thus, the strikingly few references to her clinical work and to the death of others drew attention. The lack of reflection upon how the personal might have related to the professional in her life, and vice versa, suggested that she was operating with a demarcation line between the two.

Dina repeatedly spoke about herself in terms of having "*always*" been a seeker and speaker of truth. In this, she set herself apart, both from those she regarded as hypocrites in her original faith community, as well as current colleagues who were scared of talking about death and dying. A concern for truth-telling was underscored at the very beginning of the account and at the end. It was also this concern that eventually brought her narrative to the bedside of a terminally ill and dying patient. Even though it was a concern that originated outside the clinic, it informed encounters with dying patients and their families within the clinical setting.

8

To Be or Not to Be—An Outline of Existential Concerns

To be, or not to be—that is the question
Act III, Scene 1, Hamlet (William Shakespeare)

Introduction

In the following, I am moving from a separate analysis of four individual cases to a reading across all the cases. The first task is to identify the themes that run across the four star cases; subsequently, these themes are considered individually, in relation to the non-star cases. The second task, outlined in the next chapter, is to relate the identified themes to my research question. This involves linking, underpinning, and challenging my findings with relevant studies and theoretical perspectives that contribute to deepening and developing the relation between dominant themes and the research question driving the study.

A comparison of the "thin sense of situated subjectivities", identified in the previous chapters, serves as point of departure when identifying themes across all cases. Still, a reading across the cases does not imply simple cut-and-paste procedures, or simply adding qualitative data or structural hypotheses. Rather, it involves engaging in a

K. Moen, *Death at Work*, Studies in the Psychosocial,
https://doi.org/10.1007/978-3-319-90326-2_8

different hermeneutic dialogue. The differences that emerge when considering several cases simultaneously facilitate new insights (Bateson, 1972). Reading across the four star cases for common themes requires sensitivity to uniqueness, but also to sameness, similarities and differences, basic shared structure and variations, the whole and the parts (Dahlberg, Dahlberg, & Nyström, 2008, 194).

Findings across the cases do not rest on the assumption that the shared use of terms necessarily implies shared meaning; nor that the interviewees are not addressing similar "realities" even when using different terminology. The fact that all four narrators equally address the identified themes was not a prerequisite for them to be included; on the contrary, unequal "distribution" would be an important part of the findings and central to the discussion. Thus, the following is both artistic and scientific work (Lindseth & Norberg, 2004, 152) as it entails introducing terms and concepts that do not necessarily originate with any of the narrators, but which I imagine capture and encompass the different subjective positions, the thin lines of subjectivity, extrapolated from the individual accounts.

The openness and transparency that marked the analysis of the individual cases, and which is viewed as a navigating post for the whole book, is no less important when reading across all cases. Hence, I will make an effort to stay as close to the narratives as possible, providing the reader with an opportunity to assess the interpretation on his or her own terms.

To Be or Not to Be Fearful of Death

> *Death and life are such a natural process you know everything dies constantly so to me it is a no brainer to be with people and with kids who are going through that.* (Gail)

No Room for Fear?

The interviewees repeatedly witness, in the passing of patients, that death is just a breath away, and that it can strike anyone, regardless of age, at any time. Thus, one likely response to working with death and dying could have been an increased fear of death. However, all interviewees reported to the contrary that their fear of death had subsided following work in end-of-life care.

Eric made the claim that exposure to numerous deaths in the professional context brought an everydayness to it that made the fear subside: "*... this whole process (.) all these hospitals (.) all these deaths and (.) all (.) actually the job (.) made death less prominent (.) or it became so usual*". The other accounts echoed this in different ways. Karla recounted how, unlike in her first "*frightening*" encounters with dying patients when she was overwhelmed by the smells and sights of death, she was now much more at ease with such encounters, managing to focus on other things in the clinical situation. All four reported similar changes.

Even though both Jacob and Dina, the most experienced of the four, acknowledged the toll that working with death and dying took on them, neither spoke in terms of fearing death. On the contrary, Dina stated:

> *... think (it) is very important as a doctor (.) that you are capable of talking with people (.) that you have a natural relation to death and illness and all this right (.) and not be afraid of it yourself.*

Did this imply that the fear of death was regarded as inappropriate to her present professional role? Such an attitude may emerge in the other accounts, insofar as ambiguous feelings and contrasting and conflicting emotions related to death were under-communicated in favor of a more one-sided attitude. The interviewees gave the impression that death, and fear of it, was "*mastered*". In Eric's account, there was emphasis on the good deaths witnessed in "*the calmness of dying patients about what comes after*" and in the "*beauty of palliative care*".

As with the four star cases, in the non-star cases too it was as if fear of death decreased through frequent exposure to the death of others. Anne, an intensive care nurse, stated explicitly: "*this thing about death changed (.) it wasn't as frightening*". Carl, a chaplain, spoke in similar terms when talking about being with dying or dead patients, and stated how "*it is a very big difference (.) at this point I am not afraid at all...*

death is very ordinary… it is a kind of familiarity". Herbert, the palliative care physician, was "*thinking about dying a lot lately*" due to the recent deaths of several colleagues; like Eric, he wondered how he would react when death approached: "*If I wake up with a deadly cancer diagnosis tomorrow, would I be ok with that… I think I probably would*". Admiring the degree of equanimity in the face of death that he witnessed in some of his patients, and also in his father, he wanted to model the same for his own sons. Fiona, an anesthesiologist working in a pediatric ICU, who at a young age had feared death would deprive her of all her loved ones, stated, "*being a physician, doing intensive medicine, is a way of saving my own psyche*" thus suggesting that work with death and dying had a profound positive effect on her.

Thus, as in the four star cases, there was an impression that exposure to the death of others decreased fear of their own death. Did it also increase their indignation and protest against the reality of death? Fiona used to be intensely provoked by relatives who, when encountering the death of loved ones, indignantly asked "*how can this happen to me and mine*". According to her, she had to stop herself answering in return "*how in heaven's name could you not think it could happen to you*?"

No Laments or Protests?

The terror, brutality, randomness, ugliness, and messiness of death, the provocative meaninglessness of it at times, the despair and inconsolable grief it leaves those left behind, was a dimension reported in most of the clinical incidents shared by the interviewees. Another likely response to encounters with death and dying, thus, could be protest, lament, indignation, or other ways of speaking out against the reality of death. Yet, there was little sign of indignation—no revolt or questioning of the gods or fate by the narrators. Even though death was "swirling around" in their everyday professional life, leaving people bereft, none of the accounts problematized the reality of death.

Instead, I heard in the accounts a shared admonition, an expectation that they themselves and other health professionals, would come to terms with death, not primarily in an existential sense, but pragmatically—in order to be able to do the job. Karla repeatedly made use of instrumental terms like "*handle*" and "*master*" when speaking about engaging situations of death and dying; thus, mastering death and dying appeared to be just another item on the list. Jacob spoke of how his years of experience had made it easier for him to handle matters related to death and dying "*purely professionally*". Similarly, Dina related to death as a thing she intentionally set out to control: "*I have to go deeply into this in order to be done with it*". She addressed death as a matter of pragmatics, not merely because it had existential importance, but more for pragmatic reasons, namely to become "*a good doctor*". The palliative physician thus talked about death in terms that did not make it qualitatively different from other challenges faced in the clinic; in her own words, she could "*manage it*", so to speak, and "*be done with it*".

Gail, a female chaplain working mainly with terminally ill and dying children, shared a similar take on death—namely that it rained down on the just and unjust alike. According to her, she had experienced sudden disasters at the farm during her upbringing—"*we got hailed out (.) we didn't get enough rain (.) cows got sick (.) your dog and cats die*". Like Fiona, she considered the question "why" to be a dead-end road, as "*shit happens to all of us*". According to Leah, the youngest of the interviewees and a nurse in palliative care, death was "*neither fair nor unfair*". Yet, in contrast to Fiona's statement above, the young nurse was "*wondering why [they] don't get more dramatic reactions from relatives… more despair (.) more anxiety (.) more aggression*".

Both Anne and Bente, another intensive care nurse, stated in almost exactly the same words, that "*it is not always death that is the worst*", which seemed to mirror a shared understanding among the interviewees. "*Death is a relief*", more often than not, "*in the context we are in*", according to Leah. Yet, like Karla and Fiona, Anne also opposed the thought of a child losing her mother and a mother losing a child. She expressed clearly what the star cases also conveyed, namely that it was not possible to find meaning in death: "*I find it brutal and things like this one cannot understand or say that there is any meaning to* it".

Gail, like Fiona, had been exposed to much death and dying growing up. She claimed it made her come to terms with the reality of death early on: "*death was not a scary thing for me (.) ever*". Like most of the interviewees, she "*didn't know anything about hospitals - (.) I was never hospitalized (.) never had any major illnesses (.) never had any minor illnesses either*". More than the exposure to relatives passing, she attributed her familiarity with death and mortality to growing up on a farm:

> *I witnessed a lot of death and dying, a lot of suffering (.) a lot of changes (.) (you know) when you are working outside in the environment you are at the mercy of mother nature and (.3) if you get a wet year you get great crops great animals - (.) you get a dry year you see that a lot of things die (.) so I was constantly in that rhythm of life and death (.2).... everything dies constantly - (.) so to me it is a no brainer and to be with people and with kids who are going through that (.9).*

Instead of being filled with indignation, or opposing the very idea of the death of a child, Gail found those times "*most rewarding*" when she was allowed to convey to patients and relatives what farm life had taught her, namely that:

> *'Death is natural (.) I mean this is a horrible thing for your family (.1) but this is a part of what we all must face' in whatever words I use at the time, whatever fits for that family.*

She acknowledged the grief, but did not raise her fists in anger toward the sky.

She did express indignation though, echoing Bente, Fiona, and Jacob, toward what she repeatedly witnessed, namely how medical treatment deprived patients of their death. It postponed inevitable death and prolonged suffering by "*doing things to the patients, not for them*". Herbert gave voice to the same paradox:

> *We are supposed to be helping people and we often make things worse for them ((whispers the last part)) (.) so (.4) America is not getting it right.*

Whereas for Herbert this grim reality compelled him to make the patients' experience better, Gail's overall experience in health care left her with little faith in hospitals' contribution to healing. It also left an impact on her notions about her own future death:

> *If you ask me 'what would you want for your death if you had this or that disease', I'll be like 'I am not having anything to do with transplants or (.2) you know (.2) anything like that' (.) it is like 'nope (.) just give me some good pain meds and I ((laughs)) I'll deal with it that way'.*

Fiona's narrative seemed in a poignant way to resemble what was evident in the star cases, namely a paradoxical concern with mastering death. Death had terrorized Fiona and those close to her from the age of only two when it took her father away. Powerless, she subsequently watched death take her grandmother, grandfather, and aunt. At one point, she thought it would do away with all those dear to her. Instead of fleeing, guided by the repulsion she, like Eric, eventually felt toward sickness and death, paradoxically, she was the one that took on the most difficult cases within her profession—"*the small people*". Where everybody else backed down, she decided to stand in, seemingly motivated by a desire to face and master the most difficult.

No Changed Outlook on Life?

Corresponding to the decrease in fear of death was the lack of evidence in the star cases that encounters with dying patients raised questions pertaining to the interviewees' own mortality. The lack of a heightened sense of vulnerability or risk related to living was both surprising and interesting. One could imagine that exposure to so many deaths would leave a strong sense of the constant vulnerability of their own lives.

Indeed, Dina did report extensively on engaging more actively with life, pushing her own limits, engaging in new activities, and pursuing authenticity in relationships. She did not relate her changed priorities to encounters with the death of others though, but rather as a gain coming out of her very painful divorce. None of the four interviewees spoke of changed priorities due to an enhanced sense of their own mortality. That is not to say that they did not articulate deep concerns, but the concerns raised related primarily to the interviewees as social and moral beings, rather than as mortal beings. The former were triggered by experiences and situations outside the clinic rather than encounters with death and dying within it.

How did the non-star interviewees convey how encounters with suffering and death had changed their outlook on life? Leah attributed the insight that "*one is not immortal anymore*" to getting older. She had "*never related it to a particular encounter*", merely to growing up. Like Dina, Iris, a chaplain quite new to the clinic, placed most of her narrative outside the patients' room: "*so there are three areas I would point out that bring me to today*". Encountering the death of another in the professional context was not on the list, but "*relationships, wonderful church experience and my love for learning being nurtured*" were. Again like Dina, attention was given to the unhealthy dynamics of her "*chaotically enmeshed*" family of origin and the process of breaking away and eventually reconciling herself to it, more than to her experience with clinical encounters.

Gail related her value statements and lifestyle choices primarily to her upbringing at the farm; it was as if she had made "*a commitment to live simply so that [I] can simply live*", which implied "*healthy living, little spending, buying of organic food, no TV, no longer being constantly angry at politics (it didn't help my work life)*" and thus living a predominantly withdrawn life. She did relate the latter to her work in end-of-life care: "*I listen to some people how they do their lives on the weekend I am like (.) I cannot do that and be a hospital chaplain (.) not with what I see and do*".

She very much related her decision to leave her profession and take early retirement to the realization of her mortality: "*I do not want to die in the city… I do not want to die in my job*". She attributed this realization to her upbringing, not to encounters with the death of others. Still, having witnessed too many professionals pass away soon after retirement, she and her partner made the decision "*to quit our jobs… make a different kind of life*". It is "*the rat race… the demands in US hospitals right now… you do more with less*", that, according to her, pushed her toward early retirement.

Carl, whose narrative, more than the others, may be termed a systematic thematic reflection, stated that encounters with people in general, not only the dying, changed his "*theology and thinking*". One insight appeared to be informed by encounters with dying patients though. It was about how we as human beings share the same conditions, regardless of faith—"*there is no difference*". He did not find any significant difference in dealing with death and grief between those claiming a particular faith and those that do not. To Carl, the chaplain "*personality traits*" rather than faith were decisive for a peaceful death.

Herbert, up until his thirties, had been a very active Presbyterian and head of a church; now, he regarded himself as a Buddhist. He confessed having "*personally come to a deep and abiding faith in myself that (.2) … WHEN WE DIE WE ARE DONE*". Like Dina, Herbert attributed the major change of outlook in his life to his divorce, and like his Norwegian colleague, he described the process, which involved therapy, as an emancipation. In almost exactly the same terms as his female counterpart, he stated: "*it is like everything opened up*", and he too, despite being inclined to seek security, took up new activities pushing out the boundaries of his comfort zone, for example, by learning to fly airplanes. Hence, as with the star cases, it seemed to be incidents outside the clinic, more than encounters with death inside it, that served as awareness-raising experiences for the interviewees.

For Herbert, the turning point came at around age forty: "*I lived rather blindly up until forty (.) just working at being a good doctor*". Carl, having just turned sixty, like Herbert, pointed to turning forty as "*the most difficult turn*", giving him a depressing sense "*that everything pretty much was over*". He found though to his surprise that "*the intensity in life experience didn't decrease… it was an enormous relief*". Hence, the fundamental shift in his outlook on life happened prior to him entering end-of-life care. The experience was echoed in clinical encounters though: "*I believe that encounters with dying and death in a way confirm this interpretation of experience*".

Iris reported a turning point in her early twenties, due to "*everything falling apart*" and having no sense of "*how to put my feet firmly on the ground*". It was an awareness experience in which she came to the realization that "*you cannot control life*". She recounted how during her low point she had a death wish, how she:

> *… would drive a car down the road as fast as it would go just to see if I might die… I could have easily died (.) it was really stupid (.) and I was hurting and mad (.) it was the way my insides just screamed.*

The fact that one cannot control life—an expression of mortality—was repeated and placed center-stage in a couple of her clinical incident narratives. Throughout her telling, she contrasted this insight with paradoxical statements about doing just that, taking control of life:

> *I have always had people around me who say to me 'you are so lucky' (.1) 'you get everything you want' (.) 'why do things always work out for you' (.1) I laugh at that (.) I think that is hysterical (.2) I have worked very hard for everything that I have.*

When talking about her father almost dying due to serious illness, yet beating the odds several times, she mentioned "*his will to live*". This was a somewhat paradoxical statement when considering how Iris encountered, on a daily basis, how randomly brutal death struck patients and relatives regardless of their will: "*she did what she was supposed to do (.2) but all this bad stuff kept happening to her*".

Summary

What the above seems to suggest is that the interviewees shared and reported a common decrease in fear of their own death due to encounters with the death of others. Implicit in this seemed to be an understanding that one should not be fearful, but rather accept death's reality; as if it was not fitting for end-of-life care professionals to fear, lament over, or protest against death.

This does not reflect the attitude toward dying and death depicted in the *Ars moriendi* (Ariès, 1976, 34) or *Speculum mortis* (ibid., 51) prevalent in the Middle Ages and later. Still, it is possible to recognize strands of the cultural realities in which the professionals are situated. Across the accounts, one can identify "the secular age" (Taylor, 2007) in the problematizing of certain traditional Christian beliefs, and in the lack of reference to beliefs about death or the afterlife.

It is also possible to identify the merging of Eastern and Western ideas in the accounts. The latter seemed to inform an emphasis on the "here and now" and a de-emphasis of the hereafter. This is no less evident among the chaplains, who underscored the importance of the individual's experience rather than dogmatism and "correct beliefs".

There is a sense of mortality conveyed across the cases. More often than not, however, this was related to situations outside the clinic, not least in encounters with the fragility of life in early years, sickness and loss of family members through death or divorce. At the same time, there was nothing in the narratives that revealed a heightened sense of risk to one's own life as a result of witnessing the sometimes sudden, brutal, and random occurrences of death. There were no reports of a radical change of priorities, due to being repeatedly exposed to the fact that there may be no tomorrow.

To Be or Not to Be a Truth-Teller

> *Remember one of the days before he died he took me by the hand and kind of… felt that 'we are going to overcome this'… and… deep inside I knew already at that point that he is not going to make it. (Jacob)*

Speaking the truth was a primary concern, not only in the four star cases but across them all. It was placed at the center of the accounts of the interviewees' encounters with the dying and their relatives. Dina and Karla both began and ended their narrative accounts with the importance of truth-telling, as if wanting to make sure that if everything else was forgotten, this should be remembered. Jacob also gave substantial place in his narrative to questions pertaining to speaking the truth. All three unanimously adhered to "*speaking the truth and nothing but the truth*". Yet, on taking a closer look, the theme was more conflicted, ambiguous, paradoxical, and tension-filled. Having or gaining a voice was a prerequisite for speaking up. The process of having/gaining a voice was emphasized by Dina and Karla and downplayed by the other two.

Gaining a Voice

Dina's account could be read as a narrative about gaining a voice. From the very start, according to her, her longing for freedom concerned a sense of being silenced "*and always (.) my strongest desire (.) when*

I was a child and grew up (.) that was to be allowed to say everything I thought without being judged for it (.)" This desire led to a break with the church and potentially to her leaving the country. Throughout her account, more so than the others, she spoke in terms of "*I*", as if practicing her hard-won right of speech. **Karla**'s account was similarly very much about gaining a voice. The concern announced itself as a dominant theme early on, as in Dina's account, and it ran throughout her account. Her emancipation took place within the hierarchical structure of her professional context. When entering the hierarchy of health care as a novice, she had a feeling of not having a voice:

> *... whether it was because I had too much respect (.) towards the one I was speaking to (.) or whether I didn't dare in a way utter my (.1) thoughts about it (.) and manage to argue well enough (.) it is hard to say really.*

She also needed to gain a voice in relation to patients and relatives. Karla was "*frightened*" by the sensory impression of her first dying patient, but she was "*terrorized*" by having to relate to and communicate with awake and alert cancer patients. We can follow Karla, in her narrative, from being painfully timid early in her career to having gained more of a voice, in relation to both other members of the interdisciplinary team and patients and relatives. The voice she had gained came through as she self-quoted extensively. What emerged as a moral of her story, what she was aiming for throughout her career, repeating its importance several times in her account, was to be "*direct... not vague... not avoidant... clear*".

For both Dina and Karla, gaining a voice was a concern of both the past and the present. Dina's response to my question about whether there were any other thoughts before we ended the interview revealed that she might not have come full circle in regard to trusting her own voice, relating this dominant theme to another, discussed below, namely guilt:

> *I just have to watch out so that I don't start to critique myself (.) or (.) having said something wrong or (.) been unfair against someone or something (.) it is when I say that my father is in such and such way (.) think 'O God, you have*

to say that he is nice also' - - (.) ((breaths out as if frustrated)) do you understand. . (.) it is what they call bad conscience.

Gaining a voice was not a concern expressed to the same degree in Jacob's and Eric's accounts, suggesting that there was perhaps a gender issue here. Jacob's prevailing concern was almost the opposite, as described below, namely having, or being "accused" of having, too much of a say in life and death decisions. There was not as much intimidation to trace in the men's narratives. Considering the non-star cases though, the gender distinction was not important.

Several of Anne's clinical PINS were related to the issue of gaining a voice, primarily in relation to physicians. Over the years, there had been a change from situations in which "*nobody knows you and you sense that they didn't always care about what you said*" to "*the advantage of getting older (.) you gain some kind of authority*". Leah, who was in the earlier stage of her career, echoed Anne's experience: Despite "*always [having] had a tendency to make people listen to me*", she experienced "*[not being] recognized for what I said*". Anne recounted how she used to be stressed about how to relate, and what to say, to relatives. Leah also mentioned the experience of not being recognized, that "*[they] didn't want to talk to me (.) didn't have enough to offer*". Though she was 25 years younger, like Anne she found it "*wonderful to get older*" as "*people might listen more to somebody who it is obvious has been around a little longer*".

Gaining a voice, being honest and direct, was a significant and dominant theme in Bente's account too. The intensive care nurse spoke in terms of "*always*" having been "*self-confident… stood for the choices I have made… I speak my mind… it can be difficult at times but I believe it is for the best in the long term*". Yet, it was evident in her story that when she was younger her professional life had been characterized by a lack of voice and a sense of timidity toward authorities, particularly older male physicians. Fiona, a physician at a pediatric ICU, more explicitly regretted not speaking up to colleagues in a situation which resulted in a death and to which her input might have made a difference: "*I didn't contribute to the conversation*".

Gaining a voice was also a dominant theme in Carl's account. He reported feeling intimidated, fearful, and lacking a voice when encountering bereaved people early in his professional career as a parish pastor, "*not knowing what to say or do*". Recognition from others mitigated this sense of intimidation. Yet, it was not colleagues who helped Carl find his voice; it was grateful relatives, who recognized his contribution in the midst of their loss. When sharing his experiences, his colleagues were not able to acknowledge him, but repeatedly made emotionally charged forays into "*questions of theology or politics*". Like Dina, Carl was thus left with a desire for a space in which he could speak his mind and heart; he reported having found this in his present collegial community.

Gaining a voice related not only to the ability to be outspoken, but also to be authentic. It was placed center-stage in several accounts and was an important aspect both of their current professional situatedness and of past choices of educational institutions and clinical fields. Gail spoke of how she left the Presbyterian Church she grew up in and was ordained in another church in the name of authenticity. Coming toward the end of her career, a lingering sense of not being 'at home' as an ordained minister might have been apparent as she said, "*I will be glad just to be me*". Herbert and Leah gave voice to how palliative care promoted authenticity; how "*when illness, death, knock on the door it is seldom welcome, but often implies… more real conversations*"; and moving beyond "*all the external [issues] and what most people are busy with as long as they are healthy*", how it invites "*removing the doctor façade… not playing the doctor role*". Thus, I related this dominant theme to another major concern across the cases, discussed below, namely to be a part or apart.

Giving Voice

While the concern of gaining a voice shows up differently among the star cases, the related one of giving voice to truth was shared more equally. Of particular concern was giving voice to truth about the imminence of death in encounters with dying patients and their families. Among the four interviewees, there was unanimous agreement about the appropriateness of "*saying out loud something about what we see*", as

Karla put it. All four shared particular incident narratives that pertained to truth-telling. Yet, as already indicated, after looking more closely, the issue that had initially seemed crystal clear was messier and murkier than it first appeared.

Dina considered herself a notorious truth-seeker, which she regarded as her most "*characteristic*" trait, one she related to being a truth-teller. She used this *ability* to be "*open and direct…a lot* in her work", even though, at times, it was like "*breaking through a wall in order for people to understand stuff*". Dina related the urgency she felt to speak the truth to an upbringing with too many lies and double standards: "*Never going to tell another lie in my life*". Compared to Dina's urgent and almost compulsive need for truth-telling, Jacob voiced a more ambiguous relation to telling the truth to patients.

The fact that he, as the treating physician, had privileged information about the imminence of death seemed to represent more of a dilemma to him than Dina, who was in the same privileged position. Initially, he stated the importance of "*not hiding*" information: "*I believe one profits from being honest with the relatives and telling the facts*". Further into his account, though, he appeared to contradict himself as he made the case that "*personally I don't think it is right that one should inform a terminally ill patient that 'now you are going to die' (.) I think that is totally wrong*".

When asked, he could not recall one instance in which he had informed a patient about imminent death, but he provided several illustrations about how he had intentionally done the opposite, saying that it was going to be fine when he knew differently. The issue for Jacob, as I understood him, was not about withholding information altogether, but rather the importance of posing the moral question of how far into the process of dying would it be appropriate to remind the patient of what had already been made known to him or her.

Karla was also torn about truth-telling, which could be part of the reason why the theme lingered throughout her account. She kept coming back to it and it seemed to inform her choice of particular incidents. She argued that "*90-95% wish that we could be concrete and tell it as it is*". On the one hand, she used a long PIN to advocate for telling a dying patient that death was imminent; on the other, when asked whether there were times in which she considered it not appropriate to speak about what she saw, she admitted, "*yes absolutely*".

Eric included several situations in which truth-telling played a part. A couple of these related to himself, or someone close to him, being on the receiving end of the truth-telling. In one of them, the truth had quite detrimental consequences for the person addressed. In another, Eric recounted how he got very negative feedback from having been direct. As in Dina's case, Eric's attitude toward truth-telling may thus have been informed by negative experiences outside the clinic.

Eric stated that the truth about the imminence of death should be addressed at the right time and on the initiative of the patient. When talking about his encounters with dying patients and their relatives, he described the meetings as "*conversations*", "*dialogues*", and "*sharing*". A dying woman he was caring for at the time of the interview did not want to talk about her death and instead allowed herself "*hope*". Referring to another encounter with a young female patient, he "*got a sense that being direct with her was the right thing*". In other words, it was not a given. In this, he adhered to a recognizable therapeutic and pastoral discourse, in which the role of the helper is to listen rather than deliver a message. Downplaying the topic in his account could thus relate to his professional formation and/or painful experiences of truth-telling outside the clinic.

Anne stressed the importance of speaking the truth—"*I have emphasized that one should be honest*". She continued: The "*art*" is all about "*preparing them, yet not being brutal*". The only PIN she provided though was about how she spoke the uncomfortable truth to her own dying father about his imminent death, despite the fact that he would have preferred her not to. She underscored the value of "*daring to say things as they are, don't wrap it in too much*". Yet, as is evident below, part of her wanted to conceal her own thirty-year-old mistake, committed as an inexperienced young nurse. Thus, she was conflicted in relation to openness and transparency.

Fiona, working primarily with children, talked about how at times she becomes the truth-teller, a messenger between the parents and their dying child. In one instance, the parents did not want to be by the bed when the medical equipment was turned off, "*but can you please tell him that we love him*". Fiona returned to the bedside to fulfill what she had just promised. The many health professionals present turned very quiet ("*in a not uncomfortable way*"), when she gave voice to a last message of love to the little boy about to lose the struggle for his life.

Speaking Out or Holding Back?

For Carl, Herbert, Leah, Gail, Iris, and Eric, there seemed to be no urgent need "*to tell the truth and nothing but the truth*". It was more about tuning into the truth of the other, allowing them to give voice to their own experience, and reach their truths in their time.

Gail talked about how she had worked with a family really "*guarding the gates*" around their eleven-year-old son who was dying from cancer. The frustrating instructions from them were clear and persistent: "*Do not tell him he is dying*". According to Gail, for his part the boy asked that very question—"*Am I dying*"—at every opportunity. Despite it being "*agonizingly painful*" and "*upsetting*", leaving her "*powerless*", Gail believed that it was "*not for me to set the agenda*".

> *As chaplains we walk with people (.) we are present with people (.) and it it's kind of like you know (.) watching your crops grow… not wanting to fix things… social work tends to get into that… I don't need to take a rope and lead you… that is a sweet deal.*

Like Jacob, Herbert gave voice to the dilemmas of being the treating physician with privileged knowledge about imminent death: "*I am all the time with people who are dying (.) they may or may not know it at the time but I know it (.2) and (.4) I don't want their death to be sort of unattended by themselves*". Thus, he regarded himself as "*the messenger of bad news*", which he didn't approach with a sense of dread, but rather found "*rewarding*" as patients and relatives were often grateful for the honesty.

Herbert spoke about facilitating "*considerations of the dark side*" of what patients bring up, like having limited time to reconcile with family members: "*as a doctor you come with this authority (.) you get to say stuff like that and not get kicked out*". He also stressed the importance of "*not coming with an agenda*", but "*being open to suffering as opposed to fixing it*". As the experienced physician elaborated on this topic, it was hard not to contrast the values expressed with those inherent in the very first memory he had shared in his narrative: How he had been deprived, at age five, of any opportunity to express grief when told by his father that his grandfather had died.

It may have informed his present sensitivity, and so holding back at times left him with a sense of guilt and self-reflective questioning. Reflecting on an encounter with a young man who passed away just a couple of days prior to the interview, he questioned himself: "*Did I fulfill my role (.) was I honest enough (.) did I short-change him in any way?*" "Short-changing" by giving too much information and thus depriving someone of hope was the other side of insisting on conveying medical truths, according to Leah. A relative once asked her whether she was going to take the patient's blood pressure: "*My gut-feeling was 'why in the world should I… what does it help*'"? Yet, she did not know how to convey this without depriving the other of his hope.

Iris was sensitive to the significance of language, both how it can facilitate expressing deep experience, but also how it can get in the way of expressing oneself. In the latter case, "*when people need something different or something more (.) that is when you have that conversation*". Holding back one's own truths though—which appeared to be a shared value among the chaplains—seemed to come with a price. All four reported an uneasiness that came with being identified with beliefs they did not adhere to. Thus, they reported a loss of voice.

Gail experienced certain families leaving her out: "*if I am not talking about triumphalism, whatever (.) God is gonna fix this… I don't do that (.) I cannot do that*". Similarly, Carl faced a loss of voice when encountering patients and relatives with a strong belief in the power of prayer. In contrast to the mother who, according to Carl, was shouting to him over her dying son's bed: "*prayer helps, right*", Carl was informed by his own skeptical realist inclinations and years of facing the ultimate power of death: "*I don't see that people get well when they are dying (.2) if they do it is because we were wrong about them dying*". Yet, seemingly more pragmatic than Gail, he responded affirmatively to the desperate woman: "*it always helps to pray*". Downplaying his own convictions was necessary, but at the same time it was at odds with the concern that ran through his account, namely "*to be one's self*".

Despite his claim that he himself "*never had a crisis of faith*", it seemed that having patients' and their relatives' beliefs projected upon him, challenged his sense of authenticity. All the chaplains conveyed in a similar fashion how, in encounters with patients and relatives, they downplayed essential parts of themselves that related to truth-telling, a dominant theme addressed below.

At the point in the interview when Carl stated that the "*Christian answers aren't necessarily helpful (.) because they are not*", it was as if the insights just shared had exhausted him: "*now I feel a little tired in the head*". Perhaps it was the discrepancy he felt between the meanings projected upon his role as a leader of a particular faith—"*people do have an image of my theology*"—and what appeared to be his own more relativist and skeptical position. According to him, in his mind, he posed the silent question to patients and relatives: "*do you really believe that*"? On the other hand, perhaps it was rather the realization that "*you are not protected… one can never be safe… it doesn't necessarily help to pray*", and thus being "*theologically challenged about God's way of being God*", that drained the chaplain? In any case, it mirrored what was expounded more in Carl's account than the others, namely that "*the hospital experience and encounters with this manifold life challenges one's thinking*". It also raised what was particular to chaplaincy as compared to the other professions in end-of-life care, namely that one can be called upon and challenged about one's personal convictions.

Summary

It is the physician's task to provide patients and relatives with their medical status, speak the truth about their current medical situation. Yet, truth-telling, as outlined above, was a dilemma felt across the accounts. Its importance was recognized regardless of actual responsibility for delivering medical news and updates, and also regardless of professional discipline, gender, or cultural context. Still, the chaplains appeared more accepting of the other's truths, even when that meant defending oneself against medical truths and imminent death.

Whether and when to speak the truth about the other's imminent death was the most pressing moral issue, particularly when the dying patient was awake and able to hold the professional accountable by his/her glance. It was presented as a "Catch-22" situation in that the professional could short-change the patient and the relatives with either too little or too much information, too early or too late, resulting in deaths going unattended, on the one hand, or risking depriving patients and relatives of hope, on the other.

The concern with truth-telling was conveyed as a multilayered stressor, in that the professionals both witnessed the short-changing of truth either by other professionals (physicians) or by family. The dilemma they felt was enhanced by not being in a position to deliver the messages themselves. When the professionals stressed the importance of truth-telling, it seemed to align partly with a discourse, outlined in the previous sub-chapter, suggesting that the dying individual should face up to death. Additionally, this dilemma seemed more related to the professional's need to be authentic. This originated in life experiences outside the clinic, but seemed to have been enhanced in encounters at the border between life and death.

Herbert's concern about not short-changing patients and relatives seemed to have a negative counterpart in his own experience of having been short-changed by his own father at the death of his grandfather. Dina's and Bente's claim to "*always having been a truth-teller*" could serve to illustrate the same; the former related her urge to speak the truth to having had a religious upbringing that left her with a sense of having to cover up. Whatever the origin, the matter of truth-telling for the professional represented a sense of individual responsibility and raised questions pertaining to authenticity and guilt.

Gaining a voice, speaking up, and holding back—in relation to patients, relatives, and colleagues—were major concerns identified across the narrative accounts, to the degree that they served as selective principles in the narrators' accounts. Gaining a voice in relation to patients and families was a concern across cases, whereas gaining a voice in a collegial community appeared to be more of a gender issue. Gaining a voice was primarily dealt with as a matter of the past. Still, all three concerns appeared as prevailing matters of pressing concern in unfolding patient relations at the border between life and death.

To Be or Not to Be Guilty

> *... did one make a mistake (.) could one have done something different... would he have died anyway (.)*
> ***((sighs))** never get an answer* (Jacob)

Guilt, or the prospect of it, was a dominant theme in all four star cases. In various ways, encounters with dying patients and their relatives gave the professionals a sense of responsibility and raised the related concern about moral trespassing. This was related in part to particular situations implying concrete choices that have unforeseen effects, but also in part to situations seemingly unrelated to what the professional has or has not done. Let us begin with an analysis of situations in which choices have unforeseen outcomes.

The action-oriented situations of the interviewees' routines, described in the multiple PINs they provided, made the actors prone to making mistakes or in some cases, question whether they did or not. Karla, Jacob, and Eric all gave this significance by recounting experiences of having made choices that had unintentional and unforeseen effects that left them with a sense of guilt. Karla placed the question "*what could we have done differently*" explicitly center-stage throughout her account. Often she omitted the question mark and instead stated positively that they could have done something different.

Mistakes come with the game, according to Jacob, the experienced anesthesiologist, "*nothing is 100% certain in this world*". Still, this kind of intellectualization and self-reassurance did not dispel the sense of responsibility and guilt, which was a dominant theme in his account, and in those of the other interviewees.

A Sense of Extreme Visibility

It was the unpredictability and randomness of life and death saturating their occupational routines that seemed to leave our professionals with a sense of guilt—more so than making measurable mistakes. When it was not evident how to proceed, when consensus was not obtainable due to the urgency of the situation, when "*you are pressured to make decisions you had rather not*", or keeping patients alive and "*prolong[ing] that death process in a way... that is an enormous strain*", according to Jacob. He was left with similar feelings by the demands to prioritize, when one is "*playing 'musical chairs'...and then you are to prioritize who is most sick*".

The one incident that stuck in particular with Karla, and to which she devoted the greater part of her narrative account, was about taking responsibility for the family of the father of three children, summoning them to a meeting, which, as we remember, had the unforeseen result that the wife was not next to her husband when he died, and in desperation she had exclaimed: "*why didn't you tell me*".

This incident resembled several in Jacob's account, in which he didn't make any particular professional errors, but happened to be the one who took the final steps allowing the inevitable, namely death, to come. Spoken accusations such as "*if you had not turned off the respirator he might have survived*", or those acted out, like the desperate son who jumped onto his father's bed and continued CPR furious that Jacob had stopped, are illustrative of situations in which unreasonable blame is attributed to the professional.

Eric referred to a situation when he was asked to give a blessing as the medical equipment was turned off. The patient, somewhat unexpectedly, did not die for another six hours. During this time, the relatives started to ask about the ethical legitimacy of the decision to end treatment. The decision was not Eric's, but he had given his blessing. When asked what his sense of discomfort was related to, Eric responded: "*I was feeling responsible, because I had given my permission for it to happen*".

Jacob repeatedly raised the question "*who am I*" to appraise whether a life is worth living or not? He repeatedly claimed the "*impossibility*" of the situation, of having to make life and death decisions. This suggested that being engaged in end-of-life care implied a strong sense of conflicted responsibility that went beyond possible violations of concrete moral and/or legal codes in their respective professions. It came with the territory.

Accusations are also perceived in the stereotypical images of professionals who do their work dispassionately; this too might have enhanced the sense of being scrutinized and induced feelings of guilt:

> *Physicians are easily accused of having lack of time and when they sit and talk with patients they look into their computer or ((laughs)) turn pages in the prescription book.*

Jacob took care in his account to show how he was not like that; how, on the contrary, he engaged patients and relatives in talk. Both Karla and Jacob felt they had to comment on and defend themselves against such perceived accusations:

> *It is not that we are cynical or (.) that everything just bounces off us (.) we have to behave professionally (.2) and do what we have to do without mixing in too much emotions and feelings (.6).* (Jacob)

> *Has nothing to do with one not (.) that one becomes cold (.) I don't feel that at all (.) but of course we establish a small survival instinct (.) because if one had taken all situations one is part of at the ICU too close to heart all the time one would most likely not survive.* (Karla)

One could identify an unspoken, yet implied, defensive argument claiming that working in this kind of occupational environment leads to cynicism and emotional detachment on the part of the professional. In a constructed statement from the two sub-sessions, Eric addressed a similar perception of the outside world, considering what "*I think maybe other people may think*":

> *I relate to death in a different way (.) in that sense I have lost the grip… to understand how others may have it… that has struck me lately … people can comment and say things (.) about working at the hospital (.) it has to be painful (.) and difficult (.) meeting so much death… and then I can say yes it is in a way (.) but it is not that hard and difficult (.) and then people are wondering… I get a hunch 'it cannot be right (.) one cannot speak like that'.*

Dina's account contrasted with the other three in that she didn't convey a sense of guilt related to work in the clinic. Yet, at the same time, it was her narrative account, as well as her own life story, that was most colored by the issue of guilt—more so than those of the others. Her emancipation story was very much about freeing herself from the sense of guilt and shame which, according to her, was imposed on her by the religious environment in which she grew up.

Unlike the other interviewees, she did not relate her feelings of guilt to patients or relatives, colleagues or authorities, but rather to the scrutinizing stare of a higher being. Toward the very end of her narrative, when all things were considered, and her way to emancipation and freedom made clearer, the fear of judgment and a sense of guilt seemed to linger nonetheless.

An Internal Court of Justice

Considering the above, the "courtroom" is a suitable metaphor for understanding not only Jacob's account, but also those of Karla, Eric, and Dina. Different contexts, different courts, different proceedings, but an internalized ongoing "trial" nonetheless; an ongoing conflicted sense of responsibility; and the feeling one needed to defend oneself. The narrators alternated between raising charges against themselves, on the one hand, and defending themselves, on the other. They both questioned the legitimacy of their accusers and answered perceived "accusations" voiced by patients and relatives, their colleagues, and their respective professional codes.

It made sense to extend the notion of the internal court of justice to the non-star cases. They did not discuss guilt or the prospect of it any more explicit than the star cases, nor did they turn the interview into a confession of past clinical transgressions. Yet, behind claims such as "*I have no regrets about how I have worked with people*" (Gail), it was repeatedly possible to identify responsibility, guilt, and defense as implicit dominant themes.

As was evident in the star cases, the accounts contained guilt related to having made particular choices and actions as health professionals. Anne told a very poignant story, which served to illustrate this and what was also true for several of the interviewees, namely that they were living with "stories that haunt them" (Rashotte, 2005):

> *When I worked at the unit (.) there was a man who was dying and we had someone attending to him at all times... I remember I got in there and he had such a frantic anxiety in the eyes (.) horrible anxiety (.2) and so I was*

> *afraid, really, and then I ran out to grab a drink and when I came back he was dead (.) that I struggled with (.)... in hindsight I could say almost that I ran out to grab the drink to get out of there (.) it was like vicarious (.) right (.) - and that I struggled with for a while (.) I remember I had to sleep with the light on afterwards. I was a completely novice nurse (.).*

The thirty-year-old story related to unprocessed shame and guilt which were evident as she spoke:

> *I hope this is anonymous (.) because this is not something I tell people (.) it doesn't sound like a very good deed right (.) I had a very bad feeling that I had not done my job and had failed really.*

Herbert, early in his career, was sued for malpractice. It was "*devastating*" as his "*identity as a doctor was called into question*". He then gave voice to the guilt he experienced having "*failed to help*" a young cancer patient with "*horrible symptoms*". The patient's caregiver was very angry with him, and the whole situation left him "*feeling very inadequate... that failure to help really stuck with me*". Leah, who was at the other end of her career as an end-of-life professional, gave witness to similar incidents and testified, "*that feeling when you make mistakes is so terrible that you pretty much do anything to avoid it*". The sense of being "*extremely visible... and leaving deep tracks in people's lives*" was persistent. She reported having had "*a continuous sense that I would make a wrong step... that it would leave a deep mark on them*". She said that minimizing the number of those who were not happy, "*those that felt we made it worse*", was one motivation to go on doing end-of-life care. Yet, early on, she had sick leaves because she was "*afraid if something happened and I couldn't deal with it*".

Several of the interviewees referred to haunting looks exchanged with patients or relatives. Fiona, like Jacob, spoke in general about the situations that "*stick*" being those in which the patient was awake. "*When they lock the glance they see your soul*", was Fiona's interpretation. In particular, she mentioned a fifteen-year-old boy who "*kept his eyes on mine for a long time before he fell asleep*". He was never to wake up again due to complications during surgery. "*The autopsy showed that we could have saved him had we read the picture a little better*". "*Sticking*" also referred to those situations in which she could have pushed more, as well as those "*in which I feel we pushed it a little far… leaving grotesque images… patients bleeding out of their eyes*".

Bente, an intensive care nurse working in similar clinical "*terrain*" was "*haunted*" by an encounter that occurred when she was newly trained and worked at a post-surgery unit. One day, she received an older patient:

> *He was full of cancer hence they closed him up again… came to post-operative unit on a respirator… the head physician came and said to me 'now you go and get stesolid and morphine… and he was awake this patient but one cannot speak while on a respirator (.) then he asked me to give him the medicine (.) then he took off the respirator and then he died… one may say that it was euthanasia… it was those eyes (.5) … I remember that tears were running (.4) and I remember the anesthesiologist said to me 'just give everything you have in the needle.*

As she continued, it was as if the intensive care nurse with close to thirty years of experience had forgotten what she had just recounted, taking a defensive position: "*if I had done something that killed a patient I don't know how I could have managed (.) but I have never been in so grave situations that I have really felt that it was my fault*"—apparently contradicting what she just claimed to be the case (euthanasia). She came to terms with the intolerable in the situation by claiming she had no choice: "*I cannot turn the time back (.) and if I had not done what I was asked I would have been charged for misconduct (.) I didn't have a choice*".

Considering the above, and in light of concerns about "*the reputation one gets through the media*", as well as accusations from other members of the interdisciplinary team—"*why didn't you terminate treatment earlier*"—it took the form of an internal court of justice. As with the star cases, the "accusations" were only partly related to actual transgressions. Like Jacob, Anne, the intensive care nurse, claimed the impossibility of making life and death decisions—"*he came off the respirator, but he didn't wake up (.5) and then what (.) you cannot kill him… some survive that possibly shouldn't*".

The Pain of Unwanted Care

Gail added to the picture by telling how "*the hardest part*" was powerlessly witnessing the process of treatment when it was obvious that there was going to be no good outcome. What Herbert called "*the unwanted care… the prolongation of death*", "*the overtreatment*" which "*spin our wheels for a week*". He told several stories about how colleagues, oncologists, simply did not recognize that patients were dying: "*The night he died the oncologist put up a note that said 'continue high dose of steroids'*".

Thus, in all accounts there was a conflicted sense of responsibility, often related to that which was beyond what they, or anybody, could be held responsible for—i.e., death. Still, it left them with the sense of "*falling short of giving the best care*". Leah, the youngest of the interviewees, spoke about this when stating that end-of-life care workers "*put more on themselves than is reasonable (.) one thinks that one is responsible for life and death*". According to the nurse, this was stressed by people outside the clinic, who made admiring statements about "*one having life in one's hands… doing such an important job… such a big responsibility*". She has learned to arm herself with the thought that "*it is not our fault that they are sick (.) it is not our fault that it doesn't always go as planned*".

Despite her attempt to hold the accusing voices at bay, her patients and the inadequacy she felt when confronted with the death of others haunted Leah in her dreams—"*most often there is nothing I can do in these situations*". She would wake up in tears, sad "*that I lost him*".

Guilty of Surviving and Forgetting

As if the above was not enough, survival guilt was added to the picture. Anne stated:

> *So it makes me aware of how lucky one is (.) how privileged having healthy children (.) at the same time one can be embarrassed when you come home and get irritated about the mess (.) right (.) in a way you live in the reality in which you live anyway (.) and you walk around irritated about the same things that others get irritated over (.) but when you look at the big picture I*

believe I have the capacity to think that one actually is lucky (.) but it is not always apparent in the everyday.

Bente, in very similar terms, talked about how grateful she was for her family, but also regrettably about:

… not always being kind at home… I am not nice even if I have done a lot of thinking (.) I am so unwise… but one needs some free spaces too (.) I am so angry at times that I could have cracked (.) but never at work.

A similar "survival-guilt" was recognizable in Gail's final exchange with the parents who had just lost their three-year old. The bone marrow transplant was not successful. "*He [the father] said 'I hope you have a good life in North Carolina' and I said 'yeah, away from the suffering*". For the first, and only, time during the interview, Gail was emotionally overwhelmed, seemingly by the realization "*that they have to deal with that the rest of their lives*". All choked up, she was unable to speak for a long time. It was at a similar point in his account that Herbert, the palliative care physician, also had tears in his eyes. He shared a heart-breaking story, one that had particularly got under his skin, about two young mothers, both dying on Christmas Eve. Herbert eventually went home to celebrate, but the bereaved children's uncomfortable questions lingered in his mind—"*does she have to die at Christmas?*"

A conflicted sense of guilt was also apparent when Bente was talking about not being able to remember patients even if it "*had been an extraordinarily tough situation… then I think it is probably good… but I am put off by it at times*". Similarly, Gail recounted how "*I don't even dream about my patients (.) it doesn't come up (.) it is very odd (.) as much crap as we see in guts and gore and horrible situations (.) it doesn't come out in my dreams at all (.2) which is nice ((laughs))*". Herbert admitted "*that most deaths don't do too much to me… it happens once in a while… so I wonder sometimes if I am really particularly compassionate or not and (.) I don't know ((whispers)) (.10)*".

In other accounts, like in that of Iris the chaplain, guilt was even more subtle and implicit; part of the absent presence, but no less identifiable in the narrative account. Iris, like Dina, placed much of her emotionally charged narrative outside the clinic. Guilt was very much part of the picture, even if primarily implicit, poignantly yet subtly expressed in the following sentence: "*I had the role of caring for my brothers and sisters as well as my parents… I was twelve years old*" and "*I felt like I had let them down because I couldn't handle it (.) because I always handled everything*".

One heard the same sense of heightened sensitivity to the needs of others when Iris talked about encounters with patients and relatives, and when supervising students in the clinic: "*At the end of the day you never know if everybody is okay (.) if everybody's stuff has been taken care of (.) and tended to in a way that works for them*". The narrator herself did not relate the sense of responsibility experienced in her upbringing to what she experiences in her professional role. She identified her lifelong desire to learn as the primary driving force, thus seemingly leaving guilt out of the equation.

Summary

It has been established that a conflicted sense of responsibility and guilt ran across the cases. "Conflicted" in the sense that it did not come as a confession, an unambiguous admission of guilt; rather, it was a matter of feeling questioned, a dynamic involving defense. This process is what I call guilt, and it appeared to be a thread woven into the narrative accounts of each interviewee, regardless of gender, profession, or clinical field.

It was as if the interviewees were in a continuous "hearing", like when people in power are summoned and systematically questioned about their dispositions. Questions were posed and accusations made by various voices from different viewpoints. The "accused" oscillated between pleading guilty and claiming innocence.

Unlike the two previous themes of fear and having a voice, guilt was less the subject of meta-reflection by the professionals. Although what seemed to trigger guilt, from traceable mistakes to stereotypical images of their own profession, was made explicit, the narrators seemed unable to address the experience of guilt with a corresponding explicitness. In contrast to the way they talked about mortality and truth-telling, the narrators conveyed guilt more implicitly and not in terms of a recognizable discourse, as if there was shame related to it, or a lack of words to articulate it. Hence, guilt appeared to be something that the professionals carried individually and thus something that individualized them.

Dina was the disconfirming case. She differed in that she dealt explicitly with guilt and made it a major concern in her narrative, but also in that she addressed it in terms of a particular religious discourse. Dina's contrasting case contributed to making what was identified across the cases visible: That the narrating subject conveyed a sense of being scrutinized, or being on trial, or even of being summoned by a higher being. Jacob's and Anne's questioning of the legitimacy of making life and death decisions might lead one to identify a sense of being accountable to a higher being; or at least an acknowledgment that certain tasks are too large for any human, even those set apart for end-of-life work.

To Be or Not to Be a Part or Apart

> *My reality and what I go through daily is (.) it is a reality and a dimension that they don't know or that they don't relate to.* (Eric)

In different ways, all the cases oscillated thematically between being a part and being apart—belonging and separation. For several, this seemed to serve as a selective principle in the telling, informing what they told and what they left out. The oscillating movements between finding a home and leaving home informed both the lived lives and the told stories, as well as life inside and outside the clinic. This came as no surprise, one might say, having invited the narrators to tell the story of their lives. Yet, I found concerns relating to being a part and being apart implicitly and paradoxically present in the accounts, and not necessarily part of what the narrators explicitly conveyed.

Set Apart by End-of-Life Care

Implicit in all the accounts, though more explicit in some, was how the professional became part of the lives of the patient and his/her family, and vice versa. Gail stated how she loved to visit people and how she expected to miss it when she would retire in a few months. Herbert said:

> *There is a real joy for me in sitting down with strangers and connecting… fills my vessels back up… it is just wonderful and I come alive doing that (.) connecting with people… having those relationships.*

He "*really gets attached*". Hence, "*for me when death comes it is often an anticlimax (.) what's been important is all this stuff leading up to it*". In this way, he voiced a sense of personal loss. Yet, this was an engagement that left a sense of guilt with Herbert: "*I worry sometimes about it, do I go there because I need it?*"

The interviewees' identification with, and relation to, patients and relatives very much added a dimension to the ambiguous experience of being apart and a part. The professionals not only participated in the treatment, but also became part of the existential dramas playing out in the lives of the patients in the units. Hence, they were not only becoming inhabitants in the others' lives and narratives, but the latter were inhabiting theirs. Eric referred to a sense of loss: "*The loss of no longer being allowed to be in it (.) that conversation (.) or that process then - - (.) - - to it in a way becomes silent*" which illustrated the mutuality and intersubjectivity at play.

Bente recounted how "*the one who has received the patient at the unit becomes special and the one who is there when the patient dies becomes special*". This sense of being set apart in a heroic manner mirrored their role in the clinic and resembled important strands in their accounts, not least those of Dina, Jacob, Eric, Gail, and Bente. Dina's experience of emancipation from oppressive religion took focus in her account and left the clinical experiences more in the shade. Still, what set her apart in her original context, namely "*always having been a truth-teller*", was what at times set her and the others apart from their colleagues.

Bente spoke as if she were participating in a war: "*I have always been where there is a fire (.) right (.) I have always been in the saddest situations… I have been in touch with most of what it is possible to be in touch with*". Thus, she set herself apart from most. Like Dina, she regarded herself as a truth-teller, "*not having hidden agendas*", advocating for dying patients. This also set her apart from other professionals in end-of-life care. Repeatedly, she stated that working at an ICU is not for the faint-hearted:

> *Had it not been that I have thick skin (.) because that I have (.) I can take a lot (.) and I can forget (.) then I would never have been in an ICU (.) one cannot be a 'leaf of parsley'* [refers to being fragile] *working in a place like this.*

Leah was feeling unfulfilled in other—less challenging—clinical areas, where she "*found nothing that was important enough*"; she felt inclined to "*the most difficult*" *areas* and had a sense of being set apart for this particular work: "*when I feel that somebody else could have done it then I don't see the point of going there*". Gail pointed out how having no children of her own was key to her perseverance among the terminally ill and dying at the children's ICU. It set her apart for this kind of work, and she attributed colleagues' burnout to having young families.

Anne turned the argument upside-down: "*some say that it is much harder to work with children after having had children themselves (.) I find the opposite to be true (.) I am a little different from others, I believe*". Gail elaborated on her feeling apart in that she could tolerate witnessing human suffering:

> *I am not like dreading it,* but – *you're (gonna think) I am crazy here - (.) I cannot stand to see animals suffer (.) so if I (.2) if there is an animal in pain it is like (.) that is really difficult for me (.) I wouldn't (.) I wouldn't ever be a vet.*

A Social Anomaly

As was evident in Jacob's account, being set apart for the good and difficult work in end-of-life care comes with a price. Eric and Jacob in particular expressed a sense of being anomalous because of their work with the death of others. Jacob conveyed the experience more implicitly than Eric; the sense of being set apart was articulated clearly in Eric's account. He related the sense of apartness to what for most would be considered anything but natural, i.e., death, which for him has become just that "natural". The chaplain provided us with a glimpse into his understanding of how working with death and dying informed other people's perceptions of him. According to Eric, "*others commented fiercely*" about how impressed they were that he could remain in this work. A response that made Eric understand that "*my reality and what I go through daily(.) it is a reality and a dimension that they don't know or, yes, or that they don't relate to*".

Carl, like Eric, shared a PIN that illustrated how his familiarity with death at the same time worked to estrange him, even to those close to him. One time he took it upon himself to facilitate a gathering around the open coffin of a family member and "*was told afterwards that it was a little too much… it wasn't totally okay… they were in the same situation as me when I was young*". Gail expressed a similar sense of being apart by being at ease with the death of others: "*I want to say I enjoy being with people during the death process… that's a weird thing (.) you can't say that to anybody who is not a chaplain*". Leah added: "*many find it strange that I can work as I do*". On the other hand, several times, almost apologetically, Carl came back to how he has lived without experiencing significant losses in his personal life, and how sharing this fact in his professional context came with awkwardness. Hence, there seemed to be the feeling of stigma related to both over-exposure and under-exposure to death.

Gail made a similar point, that working with death and dying left her at times with a sense of being apart, even from those closest to her:

> *When people ask me 'how do you work with dying children (.) I just don't (.) that is so awful' (.) in fact my mother won't talk about it with me (.) she absolutely will not talk about it - - (.) ah it is taboo with her (.) it is really hard to say even to my boss 'I am exhausted - - (.) ((whispers)) I don't think I can come to work after this' ((laughs as she speaks as if to tone down the seriousness of what she is saying))* ….

Fiona also talked about feeling estranged due to encounters with death outside the clinic. She talked about the continuous presence of death and dying in her home, mainly related to her mom being the "*health department for the whole family*". This lingering presence of death and dying in her home of origin made someone comment, "*Gee, you are really growing up in a hospice*". With all the annoying "*poor you's*" added due to the loss of her father at age two, she felt feelings projected upon her that did not correspond with how she felt inside. The other side of this estrangement was the strengthened sense of being a part of her small family. She said how it was herself, her brother and her mother, "*it was us against the world*". Thus, being a part and apart was a theme in her narrative account that resembled how it was dealt with in relation to clinical contexts in the other accounts. This suggested that involvement with death and dying, whether outside or inside the clinic, both come with the risk of feeling estranged from other human beings, and a sense of affinity toward those sharing similar experiences.

Similarly, Jacob expressed ambiguous feelings related to being set apart by his professional role. In both his and Karla's accounts, as in Eric's, the implicit gaze of the other(s) was identifiable. Affirming and admirable gazes are mixed with critical and scrutinizing ones. On the one hand, Jacob was set apart to do, in his own terms, "*unimaginable things*" as he could "*keep our patients alive indefinitely… if we decide for it… there are no limits for that…*". On the other hand, he realized that he was up against "*the impossible*"—making life and death decisions in regard to fellow human beings, "*prolonging*" the death process or "*allowing*" the patient to die. Hence, he was set apart not only for the good, but also for the difficult and painful. Jacob was the one that called the shots; he was set apart to make the final decisions.

Jacob's account could thus be read as a trial in which numerous nameless people who inhabited the close-to-thirty particular incidents he recounted were summoned partly by the prosecutor and partly by the defense. The account could be read as a narrative that systematically added pieces to a picture of being singled out to answer for decisions made and actions taken in the complex, unpredictable, and rugged terrain at the border between life and death. The physician took the stand in the courtroom and claimed the impossibility of being in charge of such a place: "*what do you do*?"

A Sense of Imprisonment

Gail told how, as a child, she had watched the dogs digging under the fence that surrounded their farmhouse, and how she was doing the same to free herself from what she experienced as her mother's "*over mothering*", her "*overprotectiveness*". She used this metaphor to explain leaving the professional life for an early retirement: "*I think I am gonna feel I have dug under a fence and gotten out once I go back to North Carolina*". She thus conveyed a prevailing sense of imprisonment.

"*The death and dying is not driving me away… I want to stress that health care politics really sealed the deal for me*". She elaborated on the lack of regard for the workers and the increased demand to do more with less, "*prove that our work makes a difference*", leaving her with a love-hate relationship to her job: "*I think I like it, but I hate it… the politics and the corporate crap I hate (.) I love the people part*". Herbert echoed this when he said he was finding the hospital to be "*a system to treat sickness not to treat people*". These are expressions of a sense of occupational hazard, as if the speakers were set apart for risk.

Leah was open about the darker, more conflicted side of her involvement with patients and relatives; how at times she dreaded meeting them in town, and how she felt her personal space was being invaded. She admitted that at times she had sunk into her car seat at the parking lot when spotting one of "her" families approaching, taking cover and hiding:

> *…because I couldn't stand meeting them… for some time it felt as if they were stalking me (.2) they were everywhere.*

The experience of being fenced-in was a significant red thread in Dina's account as well. The quest for freedom was less subtle, more explicit, than in the other accounts, but voiced in terms that perhaps captured a major sentiment in several of them: "*What does it take for a human being to grow up in a community without becoming unfree… I have ALWAYS sought that road*".

Being a Part

Dina's longing for freedom, her desire to be apart, was expressed throughout her account: In her de-conversion, her break with the church and her independent and oppositional behavior during teenage years were all complemented by a longing for community, a desire to be a part, an "*enormous longing to belong to something…*". Thus, the palliative physician once again gave expression to what was the existential experience of the other interviewees in the context of their professional work in end-of-life care. This probably accounted for the following sentence, in which she named the gift of being a part of her present clinical community—"*we are friends here (.) a group of friends… you can say what you believe and think… it is fantastic*". Her strong identification with the professional group mirrored a similar "we-ness" expressed in the other accounts.

Unlike Dina, Karla's biography played out in every way close to her home of origin. The prospect of staying part of her original context seemed to have informed her decision to pursue nursing school instead of business school. Karla's biographical and professional trajectories didn't stand out in any significant way from what may be regarded as mainstream—nothing suggested a need to set herself apart. Yet, she continued to pursue training in critical care, moving toward this expertise, setting herself apart for the good and for the challenges of end-of-life care.

Using handball as metaphor, she made a profound point about how, for her, mastering something was related to feeling secure in a group. In various ways, all the narrators echoed Karla's emphasis on belonging to a team. Thus, thematically they balanced the strong sense of being apart by also giving attention to being a part; "we-ness" complemented the "apartness". In different ways, they all explicitly stated, and gave significance to, the fact that their present professional context provided them with a sense of being a part. Among the star cases, Karla in particular attributed her decision to remain in the field to the recognition of others, but the importance of recognition by specific individuals in order to feel "at home" in the clinical context was evident in all. Hence, the other side of working with death and dying, setting them apart, was the experience of strong affiliation with others working in end-of-life care, a "we-ness" countering the apartness.

In similar vein, Gail found her primary support among people with similar experiences—others set apart for this kind of work—her colleagues:

> *As chaplains I think we have a very wonderful way of being with each other as a team (.2) that helps with (.1) staying in the saddle (.) staying on the job (.) Sue and I have a very cohesive great friendship and working relationship so that she gets what I do and I get what she does (.) so we have each other (.1) to sound off (.) you know (.) shut the door (.) scream yell swear (.) whenever we need to tell jokes and be obnoxious (.) and I think that is just a huge reason why I was able to stay in pediatric chaplaincy so long.*

In several accounts, the collegial community took on characteristics resembling those of "home" and "family". One dimension of this is how most if not all the interviewees, in one way or another, described the profound effect of good mentors on the early part of their professional careers; how it was decisive for their choice to pursue their profession in the first place: "*I still count her as the reason I chose nursing*" (Leah).

Iris, who gave a lot of attention in her account to her mentors—"wise people"—both in church and in the clinic, speaks of them in almost idealized terms: "*I wanted to be near her all the time (.) whatever she had I wanted some of it too*". Considering her "*chaotically enmeshed family of origin*", it is hard not to relate the idealization of figures in the professional context to a need for a supportive "family". Yet the narrator herself did not make such a link. Carl had an uncle who provided him with support and wisdom. Yet that could only partly compensate for the lack of support and understanding he felt among his colleagues: "*didn't get any response (.) no help (.) no recognition (.) except from my uncle*".

This is in stark contrast to Carl's present collegial community, that met "*as we meet the patients*", and in which Carl finally felt at home as he could share "*the experiences (.) the insecurities and the dilemmas*". Yet, this is not the case across the board. Herbert, when sued for malpractice, "*learned to get my satisfaction from patients—not from other doctors*". Leah made a promise related to her professional context that "*I will never again be in a situation in which somebody can tell that I am afraid or insecure or stressed*".

Recognition was a shared factor that moved the pendulum from feeling estranged to feeling at home, from apart to a part. The interviewees reported how recognition by more experienced colleagues brought them to visibility, from having no voice to being listened to. Herbert recounted how he used the first twenty years of his career "*trying to define myself and gain the respect of my peers (.) because honestly palliative medicine is a little bit of hand waving… a bit fussy yet… always a challenge to feel equal to the pulmonologist, the oncologist*". Hence, the professional context could serve to estrange the interviewees, set them apart, from both colleagues and people outside the clinic.

Several of the interviewees thus kept coming back to the quality of the relationship with colleagues in the interdisciplinary team. In their accounts, some dwelt more on collegial relationships than relationships with patients, relatives, and their own families of origin. They delivered extended dialogical enactments from both good and challenging feedback situations with colleagues. The good thing about having friends among colleagues was that "*confidentiality is not a problem*" and one could "*talk with them about anything… complain, cry, be angry and in despair*". Thus, they found space among other professionals in end-of-life care in which they could be "at home" with their professional experiences. However, according to Bente, even when with friends among the professionals working beside her she had to be very conscientious about "*who to talk with… where one absolutely shouldn't vent frustration*".

Nonetheless, particular relationships within that context also answered the fundamental need to be seen and recognized. From early on, Herbert pointed to the team as being among the most rewarding aspects of his job. Bente said, "*when you are new then you are just a number that may disappear again… after a while I got a lot of recognition for the assessments I made and that I dared ask questions (.) that I dared do things*". She also underscored how being recognized continued to be important: "*one needs a little praise even if one has worked for 28 years*".

Summary

Being a part and apart was a dominant concern in the narrative accounts. The sense of apartness was voiced partly in positive terms, pointing out what the interviewees positively brought and gained from working at the border between life and death.

The sense of playing a part in the very last phase of the patient's life was conveyed as a significant and valuable part of end-of-life care across all the accounts. It implied being present at very intimate moments, and when the relationship ended, it might have left a sense of separation, loss, and grief. Yet, becoming a part of the lives of dying patients and their families also came with conflicting emotions; a sense of being invaded, involuntarily sucked in, left with limited personal space, or left with a sense of guilt related to an implied prohibition against "feeding off" somebody's unfortunate situation, or having a personal gain. Hence, being apart might have represented links between the professional's own profound needs and encounters with death and dying.

It was as if the professionals' sense of having forged a natural relation to death also left them in a more ambiguous, partly offensive, position in the eyes of others; that end-of-life care turned them into social anomalies, even to those close to them. It was as if end-of-life care marked them, distinguishing them from others who did not work with death and dying. In their narrative accounts, the interviewees related to this as if it questioned them being at ease with death and dying, having forged a natural relation to death, in a world in which death is "forbidden" and anything but natural.

On the other hand, the interviewees had a sense of being a part. They are part of a community of colleagues also engaged in end-of-life care. Several of them reported how the early phase of their work with death and dying was marked by insecurity and being overwhelmed, much like being in the liminal phase of a "rite de passage" (Von Gennep, 1960). Several identified recognition of their competence by an older and more experienced professional as marking the end of their feelings of in-between-ness, and a prerequisite for entering and staying in the field; that made them part of a community.

To Be or Not to Be Personal in the Professional

A Pressing Question

Thus far, the discussion showed that regardless of gender, profession, clinical field, and length of experience, professionals working with the death of others lived with several, partly overlapping, existential concerns. Hence, in encounters with the terminally ill and dying, there was something personal and existential at stake for the professional as well. The final dominant theme that was identified and discussed pertained to whether and how the professionals actively related to the personal in the professional.

The willingness of all the interviewees to participate in the study and share their stories, remaining in their chairs even after several hours of narrating, suggested an attitude of openness and transparency; a willingness to engage the personal in the professional, and an interest in linking experiences inside and outside the clinic in order to understand the impact of working with death and dying.

Yet, when reading and re-reading the transcribed interviews, it became evident how the interviewees related the professional and the personal in varying degrees, which suggested a more conflicted relation between the two.

A Demarcation Line

There are many instances of bridging life inside and outside the clinic in all the accounts. For example, when Dina argued that her need to turn every stone in her life, also her own mortality, a desire that originated with her divorce was relevant to her professional work. Likewise, when Jacob related the question of "*what is a dignified life*"—very much linked to his professional role—to his mother's recent surgery and rehabilitation; or when Karla talked about how her evolving sense of feeling more secure in her professional role was also evident when communicating with her own family members in crisis.

Eric and Dina, in particular, made explicit links between significant relationships and events of the past and present emotional states and perspectives. They displayed a familiarity with their own narratives and used ways of including and relating to experiences outside the clinic that differed from those used by Karla and Jacob. This suggested a self-reflective capacity in Eric and Dina. Not that Karla and Jacob's accounts were devoid of this capacity, but the other two referred explicitly to having sought out spaces in which they processed parts of their life stories.

What was of particular interest, however, was not the degree of linking primarily between life outside or inside the clinic, but rather relating the realization of what was specific for the individual in professional encounters.

Herbert offered an illustration of this. He marked his narration with long pauses and a quiet, at times almost inaudible, way of speaking. Several times he linked the personal in the professional. He linked the insight that "*part of my nature is conflict-avoidant and [I] like to see everyone on the same page*" with how he "*loves to see people work together*". Another such link was made when stating "*I have a remarkable need for security in my life but I love ideas that kind of (.2) throw out old thinking (.) and the hospice was certainly one of them*". Thus, he related his engagement in pioneering hospice work with inherent paradoxical personality traits, connecting the personal and the professional.

Dina's narrative certainly suggested that she worked intentionally to link past experiences and her present outlook on life. Yet, speaking in terms of "*always*"—"*always... a truth-seeker*", "*always... seeking freedom*"—did not necessarily carry the promise of relating actively to herself. The urgent need to gain an understanding of the relation between painful past experiences and present perspectives also seemed limited to her personal life. How working with death and dying informed her was not articulated as much, but rather located more on the boundary of her narrative in vague terms of "*an enormous desire to do other things... having to take a break*" due to the character of the job.

The small number of clinical encounters in Dina's account might have suggested that her interest in considering clinical experiences self-reflectively was not as pressing as being self-reflective about experiences outside the clinic. In this, she seemed to be drawing a demarcation line between the personal and the professional, like Jacob. Jacob apologized both for bringing in his world and for offering me an account of "*loose ends*". What was missing, and thus perhaps contributed to a sense of incoherence, was the kind of self-reflectiveness that links events, experience, and present perspective. Jacob admitted that physicians are not good at debriefing, but also claimed an understanding of professionalism in end-of-life care that left little space for the emotions it might evoke in the professional. Did the apparent lack of emotional processing mirror a lack of emphasis on this in the professional training of physicians; did it come with the territory of intensive care?

The selective principle of telling for Karla, the ICU nurse, seemed to challenge such a notion. Her narrative was informed by clinical situations that:

> *... are events that have sat with me and in a way sit well and that have provided me with a lot of experience and that probably have changed me (.2) yes perhaps not changed but built (.1) a (.1) a (.2) what shall I say (.2) or made me in a way into who I am now as a nurse and as a person.*

Different from the notion of what "*sticks*"—repeatedly used by Karla to denote why certain experiences are shared—"*sits*" suggested an even more processed relation; that the events and experiences found a dwelling place in her perhaps, or she in them; and that she had the sense that she could work through and integrate them. Her firm voice, consistent pace, the inclusion of dialogues and a coherent, and "just right" emotionally distant way of telling may suggest the latter.

Nonetheless, often when Karla was about to become experience-near in her telling, she shifted focus and thus distanced herself emotionally. Throughout she spoke in the impersonal terms of "*we*" or "*one*". This also occurred at points in the narrative calling for reference to her emotional experience. Thus, leaving no doubt that these were encounters that "*stuck*", it remained unclear how or why they stuck with her, and what emotion or former experiences they stuck to. She didn't hide the fact that they made a deep impression on her, yet she didn't reflect on how in any depth at all.

Paradoxical Blind Spots

Iris, more than any of the other interviewees, underscored the importance of the personal in the professional when working with people:

> *In order to grow professionally and develop skill (.) my skills for chaplaincy (.2) I have to also grow personally (.) they can't be separate or disconnected and when you do chaplaincy (.2) whatever situations or conversations affect the chaplain deeply (.) most deeply (.) I believe that there is a personal connection (.) a deeper personal connection (.5) in my opinion (.4) we must find a way to process that with somebody else.*

In contrast to Jacob, Iris did not apologize for bringing in her world. On the contrary, she explicitly adhered to a discourse of relating the personal and the professional. In the unfolding of her narrative though, despite professing the value of it, it was not always easy to identify how she linked the personal and the professional in her own account. There were instances in her narrative in which Iris explained how her experiences outside the clinic informed those at the patient's bedside, yet there were not as many reports about learning from encounters with patients and relatives. A closer reading of her account suggested that even she, the self-professed defender of the personal in the professional, operated with a demarcation line between the two.

In the very first sentences of her account, Iris pointed out how she "*learned deep caring*" in her "*chaotic and enmeshed*" family of origin. It has taken her "*many many years to sort that through and figure it out*". This suggested that Iris had an active relation to herself and the relation between life inside and outside the clinic. However, when challenged to share particular incidents in which she was cared for, Iris struggled. What came up instead were stories in which she cared for somebody else—"*well, isn't that interesting*". Hence, when exploring under the surface of her self-report there was a painful realization of a potential discrepancy between the narrative self and the experiential self.

More than any of the others, Iris pointed out that "*whatever situations or conversations that affect the chaplain deeply, I believe there is a deeper personal connection*". Despite making a point of how people pursue helping professions to facilitate their own healing, and even providing a PINin which she pointed out such a connection in the narrative of one of her students, Iris did not provide similar links between her own personal and professional life. Claims to the opposite notwithstanding, it was as if Iris, as with the other interviewees, operated with a thin, invisible, but significant, dotted demarcation line between the personal and the professional.

Carl reported that becoming a chaplain had been an emancipatory experience, a homecoming to a collegial space in which he did not have to hold back his own self, but was allowed to share "*how life is right now*" without feeling "*theologically or in any other way*" evaluated. This was just what he tried to achieve in his encounters with patients and relatives.

Paradoxically though, his account did not provide thick descriptions of his own experiences. He claimed, "*my biography is of great importance*", yet in his account he very much limited "*person*" to "*theology and thinking*". Carl was the most explicit theologian among the interviewees, and his account was marked by reason and argument, not emotional experience, unlike Iris, the female chaplain. Thus, even when explicit adherence to a discourse suggested the opposite, the demarcation line was maintained.

Anne provided a particular incident narrative that illustrated what seemed to be a paradoxical blind spot. When she was eight or nine years old, Anne—who was now working at an ICU for children—had a near-death experience. This triggered frequent anxiety attacks in the years that followed: "*[I] felt that I disappeared*". Like Eric, she invented techniques in order to ground herself in the present. Still, in her use of the present tense it was as if the experience still triggered anxiety: "*I suddenly wake up from a sense of suffocating… but even if I have that sense of suffocating I do not get scared (.) it is really strange*".

Relating her personal trauma to her professional life, Anne stated "*I have never considered what it did to me... don't have a sense that this has had significance for my choice of occupation... all one does and all one experiences I guess have significance*". Hence, the impression was left of a paradox unaccounted for by the narrator, similar to Karla, namely between one's own personal trauma and the pursuit of work in critical care.

Fiona, working in an ICU, very much centered her account on questions pertaining to her "*choice of occupation*". Hence, throughout she related the personal and the professional. She talked about how she had grown up with "*a steady flow of illness and death in the family*", including the death of her own father when she was a toddler, and subsequently deaths of her grandparents and aunt. They had all stayed in her home during their terminal phase. As an eight- or nine-year old, it had left her "*afraid that all around me would die*". The presence of death combined with growing up with a partially absent mother who, due to her work as a nurse, served as "*the health department for the entire family*", initially triggered avoidant feelings against health care and "*not something I wanted by any means... Sick people were the worst I could think of (.) they were everywhere and took too much time*".

As a coping strategy in relation to her fear of those around her dying, Fiona stated that she "*wanted to fix most things*". This desire seemed to linger and inform her choice of pursuing critical and intensive care, as both involved "*special and difficult patients that I wanted to master*".

Ending up at children's ICU was "*a coincidence*" according to Fiona. But was she not perhaps overlooking her persistent desire to master the most difficult:

> *... discovered that doing child anesthesia stressed people considerably... one was afraid of not mastering it and felt uncomfortable with small patients... so then I thought after a while that either you opt out... or you try to master it somehow.*

Like Eric, Karla, and Anne, Fiona ending up in end-of-life care was something of a paradox that was not made explicit in her own account. Like Eric and Karla, without explicitly linking her desire to master critical situations and people in vulnerable positions, the physician provided clues that made her choice of vocation more comprehensible to the reader—but perhaps not to the narrator herself.

Herbert ending up in palliative care was similarly paradoxical. He talked about his anger related to how his family of origin revolved around his mother's continuous complaints about her pain and sickness. According to Herbert, she was "*too absorbed in her pain*". The anger was particularly about how this limited the life of his father. Hence, one may assume that Herbert had had enough pain already. Yet, in his early clinical assignments as a medical student, he was particularly drawn toward "*pain patients*".

A related paradox, not mentioned in his account, was related to him, like Dina, growing up "*short-changed*", dealing with pain, emotions, and intimacy in a "*stoic*" manner: "*to me personally it felt awkward to say something consoling, encouraging… in our family we just didn't know how to react to that stuff*". In his present marriage, he still found it hard to be emotionally transparent. Yet, in his professional life he explicitly treasured the intimacy by the deathbed, as it was "*those interactions with patients where we 'touch' each other that really get to me (.) that is what fills me up*".

It Is Not My Pain

Fiona, like the other narrators, provided fewer links, when turning things around and considering the impact of the professional on the personal, she pondered whether working with death and dying "*has changed me as a person*". In addition to providing few PINs from the professional context, she included general statements about how death "*comes with the territory*", "*not primarily my pain*", and how "our loss is not meeting the aims of what we are trying to achieve", seemingly disconnecting the personal and the professional. She admitted that end-of-life care was having an impact, but related it, like Dina and Jacob, to the amount of "*life spent at work*" and not to encounters with death *per se.*

In this, she echoed Gail, who also claimed "*I don't get overly involved in people (.) they aren't my children (.) they aren't my relatives (.) they aren't my family*". She spoke about how younger health professionals struggled to keep good boundaries, telling *patients and their relatives too much about their own personal life as if they were friends or family*. The result is that, after having tended to the third or fourth death, they often decided to leave end-of-life care. Gail did not seem to see how her own experience might have resembled that of the burned-out young nurses:

> *The more I know the family and the patient the more difficult it is to kind of keep that (.3) that from creeping in (.) the (.) all those emotions (.) all that suffering (.) all that sadness (.) that is difficult to keep from creeping in so that you're (.2) you are not emotionally exhausted for days and days and days - - (.) so that is a HUGE challenge (.) how do we do that and how do you stay sane ((laughs)) and balanced (.) and calm.*

Gail talked about how her father had taught her to be tough. Watching her parent's response to recurring "*wiped out fields*" due to natural disasters, taught her not to cry, and to follow her parents' example, despite major difficulties. "*Does it help anybody to lose their center*", she asked rhetorically. Her supervisor confronted her with the need to learn to cry. He held her "*feet to the fire*" by making her engage emotionally with experiences she had had in the clinic. It took years, according to Gail, and "*I still don't like to cry*". This was perhaps why she seemed to be in the paradoxical situation of maintaining in her own mind good professional boundaries—"*I am HUGE on boundaries*"—and yet, like burned-out nurses, experiencing being "*exhausted*" and "*ready to be done*" with chaplaincy.

Instead of pondering why the encounters seemed to have the same draining effect on her as on those younger inexperienced nurses, she maintained the notion of the latter having a poorer demarcation line between the personal and professional. She attributed this in part to them having children of their own. Thus, she avoided critically reflecting upon the high degree of involvement, similar to that of the parent's care, implicit in her tending to seriously ill and dying children on the unit several times a day for weeks; she did not reflect upon what was in it for her standing intimately alongside grief-stricken families. She rather maintained the idea of a demarcation line, "*I don't get overly involved with people (.) they aren't my children*".

Summary

One can identify to varying degrees in the narrative accounts a discourse that encourages the professional to actively link the personal and the professional. Such thinking seemed more explicitly present in the accounts of those working in palliative care and/or chaplaincy. Even if several of the narrators were hesitant about bringing in "*my own world*", it was still possible to find some measure of such linking across the cases.

Still, the majority of links were made in terms of how the biographical-historical had informed the professional, and not the other way around; not with how emotionally charged clinical encounters with dying and death had left their traces. What was less evident than expected, though not totally missing, was the kind of self-reflectiveness that linked critical professional incidents and present-life perspectives.

What captured the eye of this researcher was a thin dotted demarcation line between the personal and the professional running through and across all accounts, not least those that underscored the importance of linking the two. The thin line was particularly visible when the interviewees chose not to address how critical clinical incidents had informed them emotionally. It was also evident when the narrators made a division between life inside the clinic and that outside, as if the two were not related. Finally, the thin line became visible in some of the paradoxes identified above—links between the personal and the professional which are visible to the observer, but unmentioned by the narrator.

Is this kind of linking too much to expect from a first-person narrative? Does it suggest an understanding of professionalism that leaves little space for the emotions end-of-life care might evoke in the professional? Does it mirror a lack of emphasis and training in self-reflection in the respective courses, or does it come with the territory of end-of-life care? These and other questions will be pursued in the next chapter.

Final Remarks

Through a gestalt analysis of four cases, and a thematic reading across all the cases, we have identified five, partly overlapping, existential concerns. Through the four star cases, I intentionally gave sufficient space to look at how the individual made sense of his/her "world" before suggesting how the professionals (in the plural) made sense of theirs. I made a point of not looking across cases before looking sufficiently into each of them. This was to ensure that the idiosyncrasy, the subjective, the tensions and paradoxes inherent in the various ways the participants made their own being an issue were not lost in the process. For the same reason, I explored potential discrepancies between reported self-understandings and implicit, interpreted self-understandings. I sought to balance the general conclusions reached by including disconfirming cases (Booth, Carroll, Ilott, Low, & Cooper, 2013). The move from data to conclusions should thus be sufficiently accounted for, hopefully leaving the reader able to identify idiosyncrasies, contradictions, and paradoxes.

"Concern" rather than "theme" better captures the existentially and emotionally charged, ambiguous, contradictory and dynamic "forces" informing the lived lives and the told stories of the interviewees. It should be obvious that it is not merely an intellectual report or positioning on the part of the narrator; rather, as is evident in the discussions of each concern, more often than not, the narrator expresses an ambiguous relation to fear of death, speaking the truth, guilt, being apart or a part, and thus the personal in the professional.

Considering the whole chapter, it appears as if the end-of-life care professionals are concerned not merely or primarily with the threat of physical non-being. The threats to one's being as a social and moral person, encountered at the border between life and death, appear to be just as pressing. The existential concerns identified in the narrative accounts are present regardless of the age, gender, ethnicity, profession and clinical field of the narrator; although these social distinctions may indeed influence to what degree and in what manner the concerns make themselves evident. Focus in the next chapter will be on trying to understand how these concerns may, or may not, relate to what is specific to end-of-life care, i.e., death.

References

Ariès, P. (1976). *Western attitudes toward death: From the Middle Ages to the present*. London: Marion Boyars.

Bateson, G. (1972). *Steps to an ecology of mind*. Chicago and London: The University of Chicago Press.

Booth, A., Carroll, C., Ilott, I., Low, L. L., & Cooper, K. (2013). Desperately seeking dissonance: Identifying the disconfirming case in qualitative evidence synthesis. *Qualitative Health Research, 23*(1), 126–141. https://doi.org/10.1177/1049732312466295.

Dahlberg, K., Dahlberg, H., & Nyström, M. (2008). *Reflective lifeworld research* (2nd ed.). Lund: Studentlitteratur.

Lindseth, A., & Norberg, A. (2004). A phenomenological hermeneutical method for researching lived experience. *Scandinavian Journal of Caring Sciences, 18*(2), 145–153. https://doi.org/10.1111/j.1471-6712.2004.00258.x.

Rashotte, J. (2005). Dwelling with stories that haunt us: Building a meaningful nursing practice. *Nursing Inquiry, 12*(1), 34–42. https://doi.org/10.1111/j.1440-1800.2005.00248.x.

Taylor, C. (2007). *A secular age*. Cambridge, MA: Belknap Press of Harvard University Press.

Von Gennep, A. (1960). *Rites of passage*. London: Routledge & Kegan Paul Ltd.

9
An Existential-Psychosocial Reading

A Death blow is a Life blow to Some
Who till they died, did not alive become—
Who had they lived, had died but when
They died, Vitality begun.

Emily Dickenson

Introduction

In order to come to terms with how the death of others may inform the concerns outlined in the previous chapter, I will engage in an in-depth dialogue between the interpretive framework outlined in Chapters 2 and 3, i.e., the existential-psychosocial reading of the narrative subject, and the concerns outlined in Chapter 8. The aim is to present lines of thought that establish credible relations between the major concerns identified and the reality of death encountered in end-of-life care. In the following, key aspects of the fundamental ontology of Martin Heidegger, as well as particular aspects of psychoanalytic theory, will enable a simultaneous consideration of the research question—how encountering the death of others may, or may not, inform the self-understanding of health professionals working in end-of-life care—and the findings outlined in the previous chapters.

K. Moen, *Death at Work*, Studies in the Psychosocial,
https://doi.org/10.1007/978-3-319-90326-2_9

"The care structure", central to Heidegger's conceptual universe and elaborated below, resembles the understanding of the relation between the individual and his/her social context intrinsic to psychoanalytic object-relational thinking. Central to both is the mutual constituency of that which is inside the individual and that which is, or has been, between him/her and significant other(s)—individuals, organizations, and cultures. Within both frames of thought, the individual subject struggles to navigate the relation to her/his "world(s)" of significance in an idiomatic way: through introjections and projections (Bion, 1962; Klein & Segal, 1998), oscillating between more or less authentic states of self (Winnicott, 1960), forgetfulness or mindfulness of being (Heidegger, 2002).

Talking about two perspectives may leave the impression of them being two easily accessible unambiguous monolithic theoretical bodies, which of course is not the case. Heidegger is subject to interpretations; different scholars outline his philosophy in various ways, several of which contribute to this discussion (Benktson, 1976; Cerbone, 2008; Dreyfus & Wrathall, 2007; Fløistad, 1968). Similarly, the human condition is addressed in different ways in different psychoanalytic theories. Thus, the following will be a dialogue between different, partly opposing, classical Freudian, and object-relational voices.

Heidegger's fundamental ontology and psychoanalytic theory both overlap and complement one another. The former Heidegger's fundamental ontology engages with mandatory basic conditions and constitutes a delineating of being, not least being-toward-death. Relational psychoanalytic theories, on the other hand, offer a conceptual framework that explains how the individual may relate to and digest experiences at the borders of language. The discussion will extrapolate both the similarities and the peculiarities of each theoretical perspective. In order to underscore that it is a merging of perspectives, I call my application of them an existential-psychosocial reading.

Heidegger states, "It is one thing to report narratively about beings and another to grasp beings in their being. For the latter task not only are most of the words lacking but above all the grammar" (Heidegger, 2010, 36). Hence, the German philosopher took it upon himself to invent a language that captures the fundamental ontology of being. The result was a conceptual universe, not very accessible and in part not easily translatable. To most readers, getting a grip on the Heideggarian set of terms implies moving into foreign and almost inaccessible terrain and is a process that requires the same kind of faith as that of the farmer waiting to see the seed grow and mature. Efforts have been made to make the philosophy of Heidegger (Dahlstrom, 2013) and psychoanalytic concepts (Auchincloss & Samberg, 2012; Hinshelwood, 1991) more accessible. I do not include a glossary of terms of either tradition, as the meanings of concepts are made evident in how they are applied in the discussion.

Being on the road, as opposed to being an observer by the roadside, is what marks all true thinking (Benktson, 1976, 12). This is not about taking any thinker or thought system at face value, but engaging oneself with the tradition and with thinkers. It is not about applying a set of fixed philosophical ideas, but engaging oneself philosophically and critically with those provided by certain traditions. Hence, even if the aim of the following is to bring it all together, it is not a matter of leaving no question marks. It is rather an attempt to present possible ways of understanding how the identified concerns relate to one another and to the research question: not an edifice waiting to be unveiled, but one way of organizing the pile of bricks. At the outset of this endeavor, I want to adopt the words of Ana-Maria Rizutto, an Argentinian psychoanalyst, whose object-relational thinking is outlined below:

> The richness and depths of human experience, the complexity of psychic phenomena, the convolutions of the private world of man, the limitations of human communication, our ability to repress and distort, our inexhaustible capacity to hope and idealize, make any study of this sort hopelessly complex. It is therefore only with modesty and humility than one dares to talk in theoretical terms. (Rizzuto, 1979, 11)

Interpretation is central to any hermeneutic phenomenological endeavor. Theory serves as a necessary interpretive means. Yet, it should be stressed that any theory "exists to assist in the understanding of complex reality: it is not the reality itself… never completely true, only partly true to what we say and see" (ibid., 11).

First Concern—Fear of Death

Decrease in Fear of Death

The interviewees repeatedly witnessed, in the passing of dying patients, that death is just a breath away and that it can take anyone, regardless of age, out of this life in an instant. The terror, brutality, randomness, ugliness, and messiness of death, the provocative meaninglessness of it at times, the despair and inconsolable grief it brings to those left behind, can be identified in many of the clinical incidents shared by the interviewees.

Hence, one possible, perhaps even expected, response to encounters with death and dying could be protest, lament, indignation, or in some way speaking out against the wild reality of death. Yet, there was little indignation to trace, no revolt or questioning the gods or fate by the narrators, nor any evidence of trembling fear. Thus, even though death swirls around their everyday professional lives, leaving people devastated in its wake, none of the accounts problematized the reality of death as such. What the interviewees did report unambiguously, however, was a decrease in their fear of death due to encounters with death and dying.

A Matter of Defensiveness?

The amount of exposure to suffering and death on the part of end-of-life care professionals resembles extraordinary situations, like those of soldiers in war. Hence, one may ask whether the defensive attitude toward death represents a shrinking of consciousness, the kind of numbing and emotional withdrawal witnessed in the face of potential destruction, in order to halt the awareness of a threat, which appears to have been the collective response to other such potential threats, e.g., atomic warfare (May, 1950, 11)?

Sanford Gifford, psychiatrist and former teacher at Harvard Medical School, in his paper "Some Psychoanalytic Theories about Death" (Gifford, 1969) reviewed empirical psychoanalytic case studies of terminally ill patients, systematic investigations of attitudes toward death, and testimonies of survivors from death camps and civilian bombings during the Second World War. He found that soldiers, perpetrators, and victims alike, in the face of the possibility of death, displayed an "irrational belief in their own immortality". Gifford took this to mean that there is an "inability to believe in one's own death even under the most extreme circumstances" (ibid., 649).

The author pointed out how an emotional deflection took place in people facing death, even when lining up at sites of killing or digging their own graves. He suggested that "there is a strong impression that mass behavior resembles the behavior of individual patients with fatal illnesses, as in the disbelief in rumors about extermination camps" (ibid., 647). He elaborated: "the tendency to stop asking questions recalls cancer patients [Abrams, 1966] who cease questioning at a certain phase of their illness" (Gifford, 1969, 649). That terminally ill patients, approaching death, "cease questioning" was also reported in the narrative accounts of the present study. Whether to tell, or engage in a "conspiracy of silence", became an ethical dilemma for the professionals, a concern addressed in a later sub-chapter.

The question in focus here is the quiet acceptance of death among the health professionals, reported as a decrease in the fear of death. In Gifford's text, survivors of extermination camps suggested that it was possible to gain "freedom from fear of death through constant habituation" (ibid., 52). There were reports of a naturalness and familiarity with death due to exposure to it, resembling the reports by the interviewees in the present study. Gifford related the thwarting of curiosity, the "conspiracy of silence", the mastery over conscious fears of death, to death being beyond experience, so to speak.

According to Gifford, this position was "based on the familiar observation that no one can imagine his own death without including himself as a spectator" (ibid., 639). There is no prototype of death in actual experience, according to the author. A decreased fear of death due to exposure to it does not alter this understanding, as "a supreme sense of mastery over fear may intensify primitive beliefs in immortality" (ibid., 52). Having undertaken a selective historical review of systematic investigations of attitudes to death, he concluded that:

> There is no clear evidence from recent experiences with mass death – in thermonuclear war, civilian bombing, or the German extermination camps – that would require any revisions in Freud's concept of 1915, that in the unconscious everyone is immortal. (ibid., 952–953)

Investigations of attitudes to death among other health professionals will be considered below. Gifford's position resembles Freud's argument that there is no unconscious representation of death, conveyed in *Thoughts for the Times on War and Death* from 1915 (Strachey, 1957, 275ff). Below, I will explore the position that death is not "at hand" when engaging Heidegger's existential interpretation of death. For now, let us further explore the attitudes of those who participated in the present study.

Several of the narrators related actively to their own mortality. This was particularly evident in the accounts of Herbert, Dina, and Eric, who called attention to their own deaths. Others were not as vocal, appearing more to avoid the topic of their own mortality, which raised the question whether working with terminally ill and dying patients necessarily implied developing "a personal philosophy of death and dying", as suggested in another study (Iranmanesh, Ghazanfari, Sävenstedt, & Häggström, 2011, 208).

On the other hand, several of the interviewees stated positively that death "is not always the worst", and "it can be a relief", and for some, death has been considered a possible escape at difficult points in their own lives. Adding to the picture was the evident indignation when relatives posed questions like "*why me*?" when death struck, as explained in Fiona's response—"*who do you think you are?*" There seemed to be an implicit recognition of the inevitability of death.

In order to explore this "positive" attitude toward death further, I will examine Freud's major idea about death which is included in Gifford's discussion, namely the "death instinct", and see whether it can illumine positive statements and expressions of indignation when its inevitability is questioned. In *Civilization and its Discontents* (Freud & Strachey, 1962), Freud undertook a cultural analysis in which the interpretive principle is the antithesis between "eros" and "a death instinct". His claim was that both the pursuit of genital love and opposition to it by destructive aggressive tendencies are intrinsic to the human being, to the degree that it may explain the developments of culture, its established institutions and norms.

The idea that there should be an instinct inherent in all organic life to "reinstate... antecedent inorganic life" has been controversial ever since it was introduced, and was regarded as speculative even within Freud's immediate psychoanalytic circle. Nonetheless, eleven years after first proposing the idea, Freud stated that what he first put forward only tentatively "in the course of time has won such a hold over me that I can no longer think in any other way" (ibid., 99). This time, he appeared to be arguing less biologically and more emotionally:

> Perhaps we have adopted the belief because there is some comfort in it. If we are to die ourselves, and first to lose in death those who are dearest to us, it is easier to submit to a remorseless law of nature, to the sublime Ananke (Necessity), than to a chance, which might perhaps have been escaped. It may be, however, that this belief in the internal necessity of dying is only another of those illusions which we have created "um die schwere des Daseins zu ertragen" ["to bear the burden of existence" – Schiller). (Freud cited in Gifford, 1969, 663)

Decades later Gifford showed how Freud's "biological theory of death" was criticized and challenged, but not necessarily discarded. It is beyond the scope of this endeavor to decide the matter. However, the potential power and comfort in a notion, conscious or unconscious, of the inevitability of death, as suggested by Freud, should not be underestimated. Still, it cannot be concluded whether it also informs the decrease in fear of death reported across the narrative accounts of the present study.

It is worth noting though that more relationally oriented psychoanalytic theorists later found the dual instinct theory fruitful and corresponding to what can be observed in human behavior, oscillating as it does from the very beginning between destruction and creation, love and hate, life and death (Gifford, 1969, 653ff).

This is also true of Melanie Klein. The notion of a death instinct was central to the development of her conceptual universe, which also included the notion of "splitting" (Klein & Segal, 1998, xi). Klein identified the latter as a defensive strategy on the part of the infant to manage unbearable anxiety triggered by birth trauma, death instinct, and frustrating experiences of unmet desires. Thus, according to Klein, splitting is an earliest defensive strategy against both psychic reality and external reality and "forms the basis for the most severe psychosis" (ibid., 262). This way of organizing reality in internal "good" and external "bad" continues throughout life and is accompanied by an oscillation between the "paranoid schizoid" and the "depressive" positions.

The "depressive position" is not synonymous with "depression" as in the clinical term. It denotes a state of reflection and integration, "a mourning—the ability to acknowledge that our lost and loved objects are gone and to sustain our feelings for them over time"; it implies a "capacity for ambivalence" (Froggett, 2002, 39; Klein, 1959). When applied as a lens through which to view the accounts of the present study, Klein's binary conceptualizing makes it possible to identify such pendulums in the narrative subjectivities. This is particularly evident at those polarizing points in the accounts, when the other(s) is characterized in terms of black and white, and at those integrated points when the narrator owns the complexity of his/her own experience.

Is the decrease of fear of death to be interpreted as a "splitting" of one's own mortality, and a projection of it into the other, so that death becomes something that happens to others? Alternatively, does it speak of an integration of anxiety, an owning of one's own mortality? The reflective articulation of their own mortality by several of the interviewees suggests the latter; underscoring fear of death as something dealt with, handled and thus belonging to the past, may suggest the former.

As outlined above, both the "death instinct" and "splitting" are concepts that facilitate psychosocial thinking about the reported decrease in fear of death, the positive statements about death, and the indignation at the question of its inevitability. Both serve as imaginative theoretic edifices (Gifford, 1969, 664). In the following paragraphs, I will explore other ways to illuminate the attitude of death conveyed by the narrators.

A Matter of Acceptance?

Absence of fear of death ("negative thoughts and feelings about the state of death and process of dying") does not necessarily reflect denial of death, according to Wong & Reker (Neimeyer, 1994). They relate this to there being a variety of possible attitudes toward death, even if historically the focus has been on one, namely "fear of death". The authors themselves proposed four additional attitudes, namely: "neutral acceptance" (death is a natural part of life), "approach acceptance" (belief in an afterlife), "escape acceptance" (escape from painful experience), and "avoidance" (avoid thinking or talking about death) (ibid., 127). These accepting attitudes seem to resemble some of the interviewees' statements about death outlined above.

Based on the above-mentioned five possible attitudes, Wong & Reker developed the "Death Attitude Profile", a questionnaire later used in many studies (Black, 2007; Gama, Barbosa, & Vieira, 2012; Matsui & Braun, 2010; Peters et al., 2013; Zyga, Malliarou, Lavdaniti, Athanasopoulou, & Sarafis, 2011), some relating to professionals, others to students, most relating to the professional field of nursing. Frommelt's attitude toward care of the dying (Frommelt, 2003) and the Collett-Lester "Fear of Death Scale" (Lester & Abdel-Khalek, 2003) are other tools used to survey death attitudes among end-of-life care professionals (Mastroianni et al., 2015) and students (Edo-Gual, Monforte-Royo, Aradilla-Herrero, & Tomás-Sábado, 2015; Thiemann, Quince, Benson, Wood, & Barclay, 2015). The tools have also been used in combination in order to examine relationships between nurses' attitudes toward death and their care of the dying (Braun, Gordon, & Uziely, 2010; Matsui & Braun, 2010).

The accepting attitude toward death identified in the narrative accounts of the present study both align and contrast with findings from studies which used the above questionnaires and which were more quantitative in their approach. Most significant is perhaps the finding that acceptance seems to come with experience. In their initial study, Wong & Reker had three age-differentiated groups (young, middle-aged, and old), with 100 participants who each responded to the 32 items in the questionnaire. One significant finding was not only that individuals often carry a "mixed bag" of the attitudes identified, but also that "neutral acceptance" seems to come with age and experience. Both correspond with findings in the present study—not least the latter—specifically, in terms of how the interviewees reported that through experience they gained a neutral relation to death. Still, the notion that neutral acceptance comes with experience contrasts with findings in other studies (Black, 2007), in which fear of death is more dominant among the older participants in the study.

Several studies identify differences between the attitudes to death of palliative care nurses and those of nurses in other clinical fields like hematology (Gama et al., 2012) and emergency (Peters et al., 2013). It is possible to identify similar differences in the present study, namely in how the interviewees working in intensive care spoke differently about death from those in palliative care. However, as argued below, the picture is not black and white. The centrality of attitude to death in care of the dying is thus underscored (Black, 2007; Matsui & Braun, 2010; Michal, Dalya, & Beatrice, 2010); further, such findings call for investigations into how culture may inform attitudes to death (Michal et al., 2010).

In line with an existential-psychosocial reading, I will move from identifying attitudes toward death within the individual, to exploring how these might be shared entities in the cultural contexts in which the professional is situated.

A Matter of "Feeling Rules"?

Carey Candrian, collected data from both an emergency department and a hospice over a period of 22 months in order to critically analyze implicit discourses (Candrian, 2014). Using ethnographic methods, she identified how providers of end-of-life care reduced complexity, "the disorderly nature of these things" and "tame[d] the wildness and overwhelming emotional struggles of this type of work" by "linguistic practices". Her findings resemble "the tame" attitude toward death and "the comfortableness" with which the professionals reported relating to it in the narrative accounts of the present study.

According to Candrian the "taming" is both enabling and disabling. The suppressing power of the implicit rules, "without which death would be wild and out of control", enables the professional to stay in a very "conflicted" and "ambiguous" field. At the same time it "precludes change", because "it prevents different types of discussions from ever taking place, and different types of questions from ever being asked" (ibid., 66), "standardizing what should be said, and not said. Further yet, even specific smells, sounds, colors, spaces, and feelings around end of life are becoming tamed and standardized" (ibid., 67).

Candrian's interviewees, like mine, report what will be discussed below, namely how this familiarity with death works to estrange them from family and friends outside the professional realm. The pressing question addressed at this point though is whether the unanimous report of a decrease in fear of death is a loyal response to an invisible rule of language. Does it point toward an implicit and shared expectation that applies to working with death and dying across geographical borders and empirical fields, regardless of gender, years of experience, and profession? Let's explore "the suppressing power of implicit rules" through first-hand experience of their presence.

During the course of the present study, I participated in a "visual matrix" (Froggett, Manley, & Roy, 2015), central to which was a free-associative sharing of images reflecting the topic of transition from life to death. Quite a few images appeared to me during the session. Most related to my own previous professional experiences in a funeral home and at various hospitals. They included images and memories related to the bodily aspect of death, such as the smell of a decomposing body which had been dead for three weeks at a cabin one summer; a tiny hand sticking out of a white sheet, which was the just-bereaved parents' only point of access to their child's body, due to the child's head being too damaged; and the warm body of a grandfather, minutes after a fatal heart attack, surrounded by his confused and grief-stricken wife and grandchildren.

What I became aware of as these images emerged was an inner censorship. I hesitated sharing them, even in the safe context of a friendly collegial community. I somehow had the feeling that they were inappropriate, and that they were at odds with the images that surfaced for the other participants. When talking about it afterward, we wondered whether the sense of inappropriateness related to the fact that all the sharing that far into the matrix had been of beautiful, "Victorian" images of death; tranquilizing images of beautiful gardens, graveyards, and oceans, leaving no space for the smelliness and ugliness of death.

Hence, one may ask whether what Candrian identified among her interviewees—which seemed to be mirrored in the present study—was an expression of discursive structures, culturally shared "feeling rules" (Hochschild, 2003) related to encountering death. Is the dotted line between the personal and the professional which runs across the narrative accounts, identified as a concern on its own and addressed below, an expression of the same? Moreover, what about the apparently shared notion that encounters with death are to be "handled"? Does it all suggest that there is in fact a shared (Cartesian) understanding implying that rational human beings should "master" nature, death, and emotions? The case can be made that such notions are intrinsic both to modern Western medicine and New Public Management, and that they are significant discursive structures, dominant narrative constructs, in the contexts within which the narrators are situated. As will be elaborated in the next sub-chapter, these are narrative "plots" that outweigh other possible discursive structures, limiting the space not only for the experiencing and vulnerable professional (Froggett, 2002, 112), but also those she/he is there to care for (Frank, 2013).

What is the cost to the individual? Adapting to the norms does not dispel the feelings, on the contrary. That was my experience with the visual matrix. Yet, when I shared the contrasting experiences, the "improper" images, they were welcomed. In various ways, the narrators conveyed the necessity of withholding feelings in order to sustain professionalism. This was particularly evident in the narrative accounts of those working in intensive care in which it was possible to identify less expressive language.

Karla was not in any way without warmth in her telling, but her narration was "efficient" and appeared informed by a medical technical language not conducive to conveying emotions. Jacob was less technical, but emphasized that professionalism implied a withholding of his own emotions. Fiona and Anna, both situated in pediatric ICUs, were both more expressive about their feelings. They also included significant parts of their childhood and life outside the clinic in their narrative accounts, thus leaving the picture more nuanced.

It is thus suggested that the narrators were engaged in partly overlapping discourses, and that each individual "finds itself always already in a symbolically structured world" (Dreyfus & Wrathall, 2007, 270) and takes for granted ways of speaking that also imply rules regarding feelings. How these may have inhibited the narrators from conveying fear of death is harder to account for. Complicating the picture is the fact that whatever feeling rules were at play, they did not prohibit any of the narrators from expressing feelings in general. This is underscored by the fact that part of gaining a voice implied rebelling against oppressive, religious, cultural, and professional discourses, and related to their implicit feeling rules as well. In addition, in the interviews they demonstrated a willingness and ability to express and articulate a variety of feelings evoked by working with dying and death.

However, what remains as somewhat at odds is the unanimous report of a decrease in fear by the interviewees in regard to what for many is quite anxiety provoking. As outlined in this sub-chapter, discourse, as identifiable linguistic practices with implicit feeling rules, is one possible way to understand this. Yet, the case is also made that rules don't dispel the experience. One may ask, what is particular to the experience of death and mortality that might explain the "rules" and cultural measures undertaken to tame it? This is the question pursued in what follows, when I return to psychoanalytic theory and existential philosophy to explore the experiential burden of human beings in order to shed further light on the reported decrease in fear of death.

A Matter of the Experiential Burden?

What distinguishes human beings from other living beings is the paradoxical situation of being both animal and symbolic, both hopelessly in nature and self-consciously out of it, determined and free. Becker calls this existential paradox "individuality within finitude" and explores how we come to terms with this impossible situation:

> Everything that man does in his symbolic world is an attempt to deny and overcome his grotesque fate. He literally drives himself into a blind obliviousness with social games, psychological tricks, personal preoccupations so far removed from the reality of his situation that they are forms of madness – agreed madness, shared madness, disguised and dignified madness, but madness all the same. (Becker, 1973, 27)

The tragic existential situation calls for the child to adapt, to shield itself against the full realization of its terrifying paradoxical situation, what Freud called "the great necessities of fate, against which there is no remedy" (Becker, 1973, 53), as a "god-worm", a "god who shits" (ibid., 58).

One may ask whether the fear of death is inherent in existence, a matter of nature, a universal response to the "worm at the core" (Kiser, 2015), or unevenly distributed according to the development of the individual human being? These are at least two possible positions, which if not entirely clear-cut can be seen as accentuations that can be extrapolated from the psychoanalytic literature in regard to coming to terms with fear of death. Perhaps, they are also mirrored in the various degrees to which the narrators addressed their own finitude. Possibly.

In the one case, fear of death is related to the utter dependency of the child on his mother, and thus the grave anxiety that is provoked by "object loss", by being abandoned, and possibly annihilated. A good mothering, a sufficient nurturing, will, according to such an argument, relieve fears and anxieties. The other school of thought, which Becker calls the "morbidly-minded" argument, does not necessarily ignore the above arguments, but locates more centrally the idea that fear of death is natural, biological and universal, an arming for self-preservation, and present in all living beings. I will elaborate on the former position below, but give more space to the psycho-physical understanding of the subject.

Becker acknowledges that developmental processes may inform the level of "inner sustainment" of individuals and hence contribute to a less anxious presence in life as it fortifies the feeling of indestructibility. Still, he warns about making too much of it:

> Even the unusually favored Freud suffered his whole life from phobias and from death anxiety… I don't believe that the complex symbol of death is ever absent, no matter how much vitality and inner

> sustainment... a very favorable upbringing only serves all the better to hide the fear of death. (Becker, 1973, 22–23)

Becker relates the fact that most people grow up without a pressing conscious realization of the terror of death due to the reality of repression. Repression serves a purpose and makes life manageable, a "strange power of living in the moment and ignoring and forgetting" (ibid., 23), making possible the forward momentum of activity without which people would suffer psychotic breaks. Hence, according to the "morbidly-minded" school, described by Becker, it is neither the parents nor other relations that fundamentally bother the child, it is life itself.

Solomon, Greenberg, and Pyszczynski (Baumeister, 1986, 189–207), who developed terror management theory (TMT) based on Becker's existential analysis, claim that death anxiety as an interpretive principle for understanding individual and collective human behavior is "generally consistent" with a diversity of theorists, such as Cooley, Mead, Horney, Sullivan, and Kohut (Snyder & Forsyth, 1991, 24). Underscoring its applicability is the fact that TMT is applied in numerous studies (Bassett, 2007; Dunne, Gallagher, & Matthews, 2015; Hui, Chan, Lau, Cheung, & Mok, 2014; Taylor, 2012), related to existential care (Lewis, 2014) and end-of-life care (Stevens, 2009), yet more difficult to identify when related to the experience of end-of-life care professionals.

The decrease in fear of death unanimously reported by the subjects of my study does not seem to comply with the "morbidly-minded" position which makes the case that the reality of death always informs life, even when not actualized as a threat of imminent death. The latter claims that death anxiety is intrinsic to life and that no one can opt out. Thus, the identified decrease in fear of death remains a paradox. In order to shed light on this from another perspective, I will use Martin Heidegger's fundamental ontology and existential interpretation of death.

A Matter of Death Not Being "at Hand"?

What is the possibility of experiencing death and hence grasping a total sense of one's being? Heidegger claimed the obvious that "such an experience is at any time not available for Dasein regarding itself". Thus, he echoed the claim made by Epicure, "where death is, I am not and where I am, death is not" (Yalom, 2008, 177). Heidegger added:

> The death of others, then, is all the more penetrating. In this way, an end of Dasein becomes 'objectively' accessible. Dasein can attain an experience of death all the more because it is essentially being-with with others. (Heidegger, 2002, 229)

The other's death is experienced by most, as was the case for the participants in this study. Yet, according to Heidegger, experiencing it does not necessarily contribute to a sense of death's inevitability or to a sense of finitude.

What of the other's death can be experienced, according to Heidegger? Not death as the end of Dasein, not "the real having-come-to-an-end". "We do not experience the dying of others in a genuine sense; we are at best always just 'near by'" (ibid., 230). Death reveals itself as a loss, but more as a loss experienced by those left behind, according to Heidegger, than the actual loss of life, which we cannot experience as we are always present. "No one can take the other's dying away from him" and thus "insofar as it 'is', death is always essentially my own" (Heidegger, 2010, 231).

"Dying, which is essentially and irreplaceably mine, is distorted into a publicly occurring event which the they encounters", according to Heidegger (ibid., 265ff). "One also dies at the end, but for now one is not affected [unbetroffen]" (ibid., 243). Thus, paradoxically, the death of others encountered in end-of-life care may keep death at arm's length as it will:

> …allay any sense of death being my possibility here and now. In other words, experiencing the deaths of others contributes to Dasein's tendency to evade or cover over its own finitude. This is so primarily because the deaths of others are experienced as terminating events, something that happens at the end, and to end, a person's life. Such experiences contribute to a purely futural way of thinking about death, as something that will happen somewhere off in the distance, thereby encouraging the thought that 'one also dies at the end, but for now one is not involved'…

> In other words, 'Dying, which is essentially and irreplaceably mine, is distorted into a publicly occurring event which 'das Man encounters'. Calculative thinking of this kind is thus not a way of living one's own death, projecting it ahead of oneself as one's 'own most possibility'. (Cerbone, 2008, 87–88)

It is not as if death is not spoken about: "Everydayness acknowledges something like a certainty of death. Nobody doubts that one dies" (Heidegger, 2010, 245). It holds the reality of death to be true, but it is a kind of truth that misses the mark, concerning the meaning of truth as uncovering Dasein.

Open and direct talk about death, a displayed sense of certainty about the reality of it, a sense of familiarity and naturalness to it, a lack of fear regarding it, as reported by the interviewees, is thus not necessarily an indicator of somebody authentically relating to the reality of death, if we follow Heidegger. On the contrary, it could actually imply the opposite, namely that the narrators related to it in terms of das Man—at arm's length, not yet something he or she was involved in, perhaps complying with linguistic practices in order to keep the unpleasant and ambiguous at bay, as suggested by Candrian. If this is so, it corresponds with the claims made by Heidegger that "the 'they' provides a constant tranquilization about death". This is as much for the dying as it is "for those comforting him" as "the they does not permit the courage to have anxiety about death… What is 'proper' according to the silent decree of the they is the indifferent calm as to the 'fact' that one dies" (ibid., 243–244).

I cannot experience my own death, nor the death of my neighbor. The latter is my neighbor's "most own possibility", implying that it is his and his alone. In regard to my own death, "the possibility of the impossibility of being", it is non-congruent with existence: "In Dasein there is inevitably *(undurchstreichbar)* a constant 'lack of wholeness' which finds its end in death" (ibid., 233). When it eventually does attain this "wholeness", it becomes "the absolute loss of being-in-the-world" (ibid., 228). Thus, death as termination of life is always beyond reach, not at hand as "Dasein is never authentically related to its end" (ibid., 249). Still, paradoxically, Heidegger did not marginalize the importance of human mortality; on the contrary, as elaborated below, he placed it center-stage and gave death—"that which makes impossible all our possibilities"—an unparalleled position among the basic conditions (Yalom, 1998, 187).

Concluding Remarks

In the above, I have tried to come to terms with what appears to be a paradoxical response to encounters with dying patients, namely a decrease in the fear of death. As shown in the literature, fear is not the only possible attitude toward death. However, the fact that the decrease in fear is so unanimously conveyed in my material calls for further exploration. Hence, I have undertaken an existential-psychosocial interpretation, mirroring the understanding of the narrative subject outlined in Chapter 2. This involved engaging sociological, fundamental ontological, and psychoanalytical perspectives, in order to shed light on how the reality and mystery of death may relate to the concern in focus.

The case has been made that attitudes toward death are psychosocially constituted and discursively appropriated. Unspoken discourses, culturally embedded feeling rules, may inform and suppress both the individual professional's experience and the sense of freedom to express those experiences, at the boundary between life and death.

Through an existential investigation of the essential condition of mortality, the case has been made for an expansion of the notion of death. The existential reading undertaken places the threat of non-being in life, and not merely as a terminating event at the end of it, from being limited to a future terminating event, to understanding it as a threat of non-being intrinsic to life, a "worm at the core" (Kiser, 2015). According to this line of thought, human beings respond to the former in the same way as they do to any threatening future event, as something that can be handled and mastered. It is suggested that one effect of encountering the death of others is the confirmation that one's own death lies in the future.

Hence, according to the above argument, the reported decrease in fear of death as a future terminating event does not exhaustively address how encounters with dying patients may inform the self-understanding of the professionals. It is argued that death-in-life is accompanied by a profound object-less anxiety, perhaps resembling the "nameless dread" mentioned by (Bion, 1984). Hence, in the remaining discussion I assume that, as opposed to fear of a particular controllable object (like one's future death), covert and overt anxiety are to be placed center-stage as we continue to pursue the question how encountering the death of others may, or may not, inform the self-understanding of health professionals situated in end-of-life care.

Second Concern—Angst

Implicitly and explicitly the interviewees reported an oscillation between a sense of being apart and a part that comes with working with death and dying. On the one hand, they expressed a sense of feeling estranged from people outside their clinical field due to the "familiarity" and "natural relation to" death they had attained. On the other hand, there was a strong sense of being a part, both of the life and death of patients and their relatives, but also of a collegial community. I will discuss the former before addressing the latter.

A Matter of Stigmatization?

The experience of feeling estranged does not quite seem to fit sociologist Erving Goffman's discussion on stigma, yet the case will be made that the experiences reported by the interviewees in part resemble key features of stigmatization as he outlined it. Goffman understood stigma as "discrimination" and "failure to accord respect and regard" due to "abominations of the body", "blemishes of individual character" or "the tribal stigma of race, nation and religion" (Goffman, 1968, 15).

Even though none of the narrators reported being socially excluded, their narratives bore witness to the notion that working with the death of others brings "a heightened self-consciousness and other-consciousness" (ibid., 30). The need to defend oneself against an assumed, or experienced, questioning about how one can stay in this kind of work suggests that "sensitizing" toward people outside the clinic is related to an experience of "facing an unaccepting world" (ibid., 31).

Considering the marginalization of death in Western society, and how it is hidden and institutionalized, it makes sense that there is something strange, perhaps even repulsive and "tainted" (Kessler, Heron, & Dopson, 2012), about professional end-of-life care. The professionals themselves become living reminders of the culturally dominant "restitution narrative" (Frank, 2013) which doesn't always correspond with reality—eventually we are all going to die.

The interviewees' identification of their "natural" relation to death was uttered in a society in which death is "forbidden", if we follow the argument by the French historian Phillipe Ariès (Ariès, 1976, 85). It is thus regarded as anything but natural, potentially even a provocation. Is that perhaps the context for feeling estranged? Staying with the notion of stigma, and considering all that is said this far about the individual and cultural defense against the reality of death, the end-of-life care professional represents a "discredited attribute" of life. As such, she/he may be regarded as a social anomaly (Douglas & Douglas, 2013).

Working with death and dying thus represents the professional's relation to society at large. As pointed out in Chapter 6, a close working relation to death serves to leave the professional end-of-life care worker in an ambiguous relational situation, which also implies positively being set apart for something good. This is evident in reports of being the object of gratitude and awe among patients, relatives, and people outside the clinic which, however, can also be part of a stigmatization. Goffman introduced the notion of "wise persons":

> … persons who are normal but whose special situation has made them intimately privy to the secret life of the stigmatized individual and sympathetic with it… wise persons are the marginal men before whom the individual with a fault need feel no shame nor exert self-control, knowing that in spite of his failing he will be seen as an ordinary other. (Goffman, 1968, 41)

This resembles the traits of an anomaly, described by the British social-anthropologist Mary Douglas in her work *Purity and Danger*. In the animal kingdom, the anomaly fails categorization due to having attributes from different species. Douglas explains how the anomaly becomes untouchable, unclean, not to be eaten. Similarly, in human society, people failing categorization may become social anomalies. One may ask if positioning the self in between the dead and the living has such an effect.

Let us expand the perspective and move from a sociological interpretation to a fundamental ontological exploration of the entanglement of the individual and society, in order to attain an in-depth understanding of being a part and apart.

A Matter of "Familiarity" with "Forbidden" Death?

Part of Heidegger's fundamental ontology, as pointed out in the previous sub-chapter, is an existential interpretation of death:

> The full existential and ontological concept of death can now be defined as follows: as the end of Dasein, death is the ownmost, nonrelational, certain, and as such, indefinite and insuperable possibility of Dasein. As the end of Dasein, death is in the being [sein] of this being [Seienden] toward its end. (Heidegger, 2010, 248)

If death is stripped of its physicality by Heidegger, or if being toward the possibility of non-being is also about relating to death as a future terminating event, is debated by commentators of *Being and Time*. What is essential for this argument is that death relates to life and more particularly to the entanglement of Dasein and the world (the referential totality):

> What is characteristic about authentic, existentially projected being-toward-death can thus be summarized as follows: anticipation reveals to Dasein its lostness in the they-self, and brings it face to face with the possibility to be itself, primarily unsupported by concern that takes care, but to be itself in passionate, anxious freedom toward death, which is free of the illusions of the they, factical, and certain of itself. (ibid., 255)

According to Heidegger, the "world" is often subject to "a familiarity" and a taking-for-grantedness, which implies that Dasein misses or passes over the phenomenon. In "breakdown situations", the "world", and how Dasein relates to it, may "announce itself" (Cerbone, 2008, 44–45). Such a situation would imply a questioning of the "world(s)" in which one is a part, a confrontation with the possibility of non-compliance with that world, and thus possibly also a sense of meaninglessness and the prospect of a dissolving of self, a threat of non-being.

This is an existential reading of death, placing it within life, as an intrinsic part of it, and not merely as an end to it.

Was such an existential threat of non-being implied in the concern about to be or not be a part or apart, identified across the cases of the present study?

Against such a notion, it could be argued that the health professionals rather had a sense of becoming, not dissolving, in encounters at the bedside. Not that the encounters were void of pain or conflict or ambivalence, but there was a clear demonstration of the professional's capacities, not the opposite. There was a unanimous voicing of the meaningfulness of the encounters; they provided "coherence" (Antonovsky, 1987), not a fundamental questioning of the "referential totality". It "*fills my vessels back up*", according to Herbert. Hence, the reported sense of apartness seems not to have been related to encounters with the death of others per se.

Nonetheless, the familiarity with death reported by the interviewees was accompanied by a sense of apartness. This may be due to the notion that the "natural" relation to it is contrasting, and implicitly questioning, the taken-for-granted "forbidden" death of Western society, a significant part of the "referential totality" of the interviewees. I suggest that it is not encounters with the reality of death *per se* that fundamentally alter the individual's sense of being-in-the-world; rather, it is how death is interpreted in the "world(s)" in which the professional is entangled.

Below, I will probe more deeply into an existential reading of death and show how it elucidates the entanglement of self and world and facilitates an existential-psychosocial reading of the concern in focus. It is a fruitful perspective that elucidates what is at stake, namely a threat of non-being, being apart as a social person—death to "being-in-the-world" as Dasein knows it. I will explore situations included in the narrative accounts in which "the world" seems to "announce itself" to the narrator, situations which perhaps call the subject to disentangle self and thereby provide him or her with an enhanced sense of being apart.

A Matter of Angst?

In Heideggarian terms, Dasein is *"befintlich"*, attuned, in *"grundstimmung"*, moods—"[a]ttunement is an existential, fundamental way in which Dasein is its there" (Heidegger, 2010, 135), "it comes neither from 'without' nor from 'within', but rises from being-in-the-world itself as a mode of that being" (ibid., 133).

> All moods are in some way disclosive or revelatory of 'being-in-the-world' as a whole. That is, whatever mood I find myself in thereby conditions or determines how everything shows up to me and is thereby constitutive of anything's showing up at all. (Cerbone, 2008, 89)

Heidegger works to identify an "attunement in Dasein in which it is disclosed to itself in a distinctive way?" (Heidegger, 2010, 176), which discloses the entanglement with "the world". Angst, or anxiety, is such a mood as it "discloses Dasein in its thrownness" and "reaveals something like a flight of Dasein from itself as an authentic potentiality for being itself" (ibid., 133). This in contrast to "falling prey"—a forgetful state of being, in which Dasein turns away from itself (ibid., 180). According to May, "life fear is the anxiety at every new possibility of autonomous activity", whereas "death fear is anxiety at 'going backward', losing individuality, being swallowed up in the whole" (May, 1950, 151).

Anxiety then, on the one hand, is a disclosing of the entanglement through a collapse of the familiar, a crowding-in upon the individual a sense that his/her "world" takes on "utter insignificance… complete unimportance" (Heidegger, 2010, 180). On the other hand, anxiety implies an anxiety provoking confrontation with the ultimate threat, namely what Heidegger called "existential solipsism", "individualizing":

> In anxiety, the things at hand in the surrounding world sink away, and so do inner worldly beings in general. The "world" can offer nothing more, nor can the Dasein-with of others. Thus, anxiety takes away from Dasein the possibility of understanding itself, falling prey, in terms of the "world" and the public way of being interpreted. It throws Dasein back upon that for which it is anxious, its authentic potentiality-for-being-in-the-world. Anxiety individuates Dasein to its ownmost being-in-the-world which, as understanding, projects itself essentially upon possibilities. (ibid., 181–182)

"Mood", used in the particular Heideggarian way, resembles "thematic field" used in BNIM to denote the "selective principle"—the characteristic way in which the individual is disposed to receive and organize experience; that which informs which stories surface in a narrative account; that which structures and patterns not only the telling, but also the living in the world (Wengraf, 2001). The "two tract" model in which both the "living of the lived life" and the "telling of the told story" are analyzed separately allows for an explication of the multitude of possible paths both the lived life and the told story could have taken. Thus, the idiosyncrasy of life and narrative is explained, and a "structural hypothesis" is formed as a "thin sense of the situated subjectivity" at the point of the interview—a "thematic field", "*grundstimmung*"—responds to the question "why was this life told this way?"

Thus, it is possible to identify explicit and implicit individuating processes, attempts to disentangle self from "worlds", in the narrative accounts. Across the accounts, self was being made visible through the questioning of "referential totalities" in which one is entangled—those of parents, faith communities, professional codes, and society at large. At times, it appears as a realization of having "fallen prey".

There were several situations in which the interviewees seemingly found themselves in a state of angst in the Heideggarian sense. These were situations in which "'the world' announces itself" to them, confronting them with possibilities and opening up different ways of making own being an issue. Dina's break with the community of faith and her divorce seemed to be two such "breakdown" situations—the latter possibly informing her the most at the point of the interview:

> *... ehm (.) it has impacted me VERY much... EXTREMELY... that feeling of separation (.) brought up a whole lot of things in me that has made me turn my life upside down... my mind opened totally, I saw things in a totally different way (.).*

Herbert, Iris, Eric, Carl, and Gail, in particular, spoke in similar terms about experiences in life which made "the world" and the possibility of non-being "announce itself", thus possibly enabling a changed self-understanding. Important for this discussion is that "worlds" "announced" themselves due to experiences outside the clinic, not as a result of encounters with the terminally ill and dying. Still, the professional's experiences of threat of non-being may have resembled those of terminally ill and dying patients. Dina stated, when outlining the impact of the divorce:

> *I am looking at everything in my life (.) turn every stone in a way to find out of things (.) then death was the next question (.) look at this thing about death.*

The palliative physician reported how the divorce made her look at her life and "turn every stone", how "the enormous pain" made her entertain the thought of death. Thus, the divorce seems to have brought about an altered sense of being for Dina. The "worlds" announced themselves to her in an individualizing experience, not only the relation to her ex-husband, but to God and the social context in which she grew up.

In Dina's case, as in Herbert's, it appeared as if a shift had occurred: from "das Man" to Dasein, from "forgetfulness" to "mindfulness" of being, a shift from servility to agency:

> *... all of a sudden I realized that I could paint and stuff like that (.) it just opened (.) just could do it all of a sudden (.) really just like that just (.) things that I thought I never could do.*

This suggests that it was the threat of non-being that comes with disentangling oneself from the "world" of significant others that carried most angst for the interviewees, and thus, most fundamentally informed their self-understanding. Encountering the death of "strangers" did not seem to have the same impact. This is perhaps, as suggested in the previous sub-chapter, related to death as a terminating event not being "at hand", a phenomenon for which there is no internal representation, and thus which cannot be experienced.

The case has been made that any attempt on the part of the individual to disentangle self from the "world" is accompanied by existential angst and a sense of homelessness. Remaining within an existential-psychosocial interpretive frame, keeping an eye not only on death but also on the mutual constituency of the psychic and the social, I will examine below how existential angst is at the heart, not only of the individual, but also of the culture in which she/he is situated.

I will explore how heroism is a defensive measure which may inform and enhance the health professional's sense of apartness. Two claims made by Ernest Becker form the point of departure: that the terror of death is constitutive for "heroism" (Becker, 1973, 5) and that cultural differences in the world are very much differences in regard to established social "hero systems" (ibid., 7).

A Matter of Terror Management?

Being apart, as conveyed in the narrative accounts, is not merely a matter of being set apart, but also of setting self apart. In various ways, the interviewees portrayed their work in qualitative terms that distinguished them from others: Truth-tellers (Dina, Bente), repeatedly put themselves in the line of fire (Bente), staying when others left (Eric, Herbert), choosing patients that others did not (Herbert, Leah), inclined to pursue the most difficult work (Fiona, Leah, Herbert) and subject to the awe and gratitude (Jacob, Karla) of others. Thus, I interpret being set apart from others for "the most difficult", even though in subtle ways, as part of the self-understanding of the narrators. None of them were speaking of themselves in terms of being wise or heroes. Yet they spoke in ways that resembled heroism, indicating a return to the argumentative lines of Ernst Becker and terror management theory which, as will become apparent, enables a psychosocial consideration of the concern in focus and how it relates to death.

According to Becker, one of the central concepts to understanding man's drive toward heroism is the psychoanalytic concept of narcissism. It "seems to come from his animal nature", according to Becker, who links the human hero system with the self-preservation one finds in all living things, including plants and animals. The organism's narcissism feeds on symbolism and can therefore "expand into dimensions of worlds and times without moving a physical limb; it can take eternity into itself even as it gaspingly dies" (Becker, 1973, 3).

The deep instinctual absorption of self and the feeling of being immortal is thus "physiochemical" (ibid., 2). This is most visible in childhood, according to Becker:

> Sibling rivalry is a critical problem that reflects the basic human condition: it is not that children are vicious, selfish, or domineering. It is that they so openly express man's tragic destiny: he must desperately justify himself as an object of primary value in the universe; he must stand out, be a hero, make the biggest possible contribution to world life, show that he counts more than anything or anyone else. (ibid., 4)

Human beings are thus engaged in a life-long pursuit of standing out, of setting themselves apart, making something of lasting value. This is constitutive for the human animal, separating him from other species, a pursuit to "earn a feeling of primary value, of cosmic specialness, of ultimate usefulness to creation" (ibid., 5). Becker relates heroism to what distinguishes the human animal from other animals, namely the "the experiential burden".

In order to act and move ahead, the human animal "cannot keep gaping with our heart in our mouth, greedily sucking up with our eyes everything great and powerful that strikes us" (ibid., 50), rather the human animal builds defenses that:

> … allow him to feel a basic sense of self-worth, of meaningfulness, of power. They allow him to feel that he controls his life and his death, that he really lives and acts as a willful and free individual, that he has a

> unique and self-fashioned identity, that he is somebody, not just a trembling accident. (ibid., 55)

This is evident from early on in the child's style of life, his character, "his way of using the power of others, the support of the things and the ideas of this culture, to banish from his awareness the actual fact of his natural impotence" (ibid., 54). Hence, according to Becker, in this sense "human character is a vital lie" that serves to keep us ignorant of the fact that "we always rely on something that transcends us"; that our "courage to be" (Tillich, 2000) does not come from our own center, because at the very center is the threat of non-being.

The metapsychological notion of narcissism as a response to the threat of non-being, central to Becker's argument, is one possible axiomatic ground for the interpretation of heroism. I would, like Taylor (1992), be very hesitant in making the former grounds for moral evaluation of the individual (Lasch, 1991). There are no grounds for stating that any of the interviewees in the present study are engaged in end-of-life care solely for the purpose of self-fulfillment. Recognizing that self-perseverance highlights the importance of undertaking an existential-psychosocial analysis of the concern in focus (to be or not to be a part or apart), I will stay with heroism and explore below how it may be a fruitful interpretive principle for understanding health care, which is the immediate context of the narrative accounts in focus.

A Matter of Being Immersed in a Hero System?

According to Becker, cultural differences in the world are very much differences in regard to established social hero systems as "society itself is a codified hero system, which means that society everywhere is a living myth of the significance of human life, a defiant creation of meaning" (Becker, 1973, 7). This relies on, and resembles, Otto Rank's argument in *The Myth of the Birth of the Hero* (Rank, 1932). Every cultural hero system, including that of the modern West, according to Becker, is religious in nature:

> Civilized society is a hopeful belief and protest that science, money and goods make man count for than any other animal. In this sense everything man does is religious and heroic, and yet in danger of being fictitious and fallible. (Becker, 1973, 5)

According to the American cultural anthropologist, “what characterizes modern man is the failure of all traditional immortality ideologies” (ibid., 190). This would appear to be reflected in the material of the present study, as noted, in the seeming lack of shared beliefs about the meaning of either life, death, or the hereafter.

Relying on the above analysis, we may ask whether, in a time of the decline of meta-narratives, religious, and political ideologies, health care has become a significant hero system in the Western world. According to Becker, the dethroning of God and soul implies that the human being is “thrown back hopelessly on his own resources, on himself and those few around him” (ibid., 190). In a secular age (Taylor, 2007), following the de-mythologizing of the world, the psychologizing of the human being, and the emerging of health as an ultimate concern, the case can be made that health professionals have taken over roles traditionally held by clergy—as experts on life, authorities in general, providers of hope.

Such an analysis resonates with how the interviewees voiced the multilayered pain that goes with playing the part of “hero” in such a cultural defense system. This includes the thin line between being a “god”—“doing unimaginable things”—and becoming the scapegoat, the recipient of accusations; the short distance between being a hero and ending up in a courtroom, real or imagined—the latter due to the constant scrutiny of authorities, employers, colleagues, and relatives. Finally, the moral distress that comes with undertaking or witnessing useless, over-optimistic treatment, “the unwanted care”, and the prolonging of suffering and death that follow. Becker appropriately asks, “how can a human being be a god-like ‘everything’ to another”? (Becker, 1973, 166). Thus, the other side of making human beings and human endeavors “religious”—entities in which ultimate hope is placed—is that everything human is finite and decaying, hence the necessary ambiguity toward the hero, and perhaps to those in end-of-life care.

The fact that being a health professional entails having larger-than-life expectations projected onto one seems to be apparent in the indignation expressed by panel members toward vulnerabilities, inconsistencies, and contradictions inherent in the lives and narratives of the professionals. This underscores the sense, also conveyed in the interviewees' narrative accounts, that as end-of-life care professionals, they have to be larger-than-life and less paradoxical than others. Becker points out the dilemmas that come with sticking "out of nature so much that you yourself have to create your own heroic justification" (ibid., 172). This is the situation of the artist whose work asks him accusingly: "what right do you have to play God?" Does this question resemble the one heard in the narrators' accounts, repeatedly in Jacob's, when posing the question "*who am I*" to assess whether a life is worth living or not?

The relevance of heroism as interpretive principle is underscored in the explicit concern voiced by the interviewees regarding the threat of "annihilation". The threat is not primarily represented at the bedside; it relates more to the structural conditions in which one is working. Several of the interviewees (Bente, Jacob, Gail) said they experienced the increased demands of their employer who "*wants more money out of every buck*", as a threat to their own lives—more so than the demands of encountering death and dying on a daily basis: "*the death and dying is not driving me away… I want to stress that health care politics really sealed the deal for me*" (Gail).

Gail was retiring early because she did not want "*to die in my job*". It was "*the rat race*", the expectation of having to do more for less, which left her disillusioned. The work itself was "*exhausting*", but meaningful. The lack of organizational recognition and validation made her question whether it was any good for her. Jacob suffered "soldier's heart", pain not identified with heart failure, a few months prior to the interview. He linked suffering stress-related chest pains to the amount of work and the impact of ongoing organizational changes—it is "*killing you*".

A Matter of a Subordination of Professional Concerns to Managerial Imperatives

New Public Management (NPM) is an umbrella expression for different principles and methods for organizing and managing public services. It takes the market as a model, assuming that public services aligning with the rationale of the market will provide better quality and more efficiency. It is historically related, in particular, to the political orientation and times of Margaret Thatcher and Ronald Reagan. Since the early 1990s, New Public Management has served as the dominant model for the organization of public services in Norway, as in many other countries. It is performance-based, outcome/results-oriented, and it is marked by financing and reporting systems.

In the Norwegian context, tensions both between individual professionals and professional affiliations and New Public Management are regularly reported in the media. Frequently, we read stories about the merging of hospitals, re-organization for better efficiency at hospitals, budget crises, and health professionals on strike, due to new regulations and instructions. V. B. Wyller and a group of physicians at the University Hospital of Oslo are one such critical voice in the literature. Based on the experience of the largest hospital merger in Norway ever, they are voicing concern that New Public Management is in fundamental tension with both the professional subject and the health care professions.

Under the heading "Reclaim the Profession", they argue how NPM is an expanding system of monitoring and reporting that signals a fundamental distrust in the health workers, a demand for loyalty that turns autonomous professionals into disciplined officials; clinical services deteriorate in quality, since priority is given to "profitable" rather than "unprofitable" patients, and moral language is displaced by financial cost–benefit analyses.

The concerns raised are also voiced in the emerging field of psychosocial studies, concerned with the professional in relation-intense welfare professions (Clarke Hahn, & Hoggett, 2008; Froggett, 2002).

There is a questioning of the implicit understandings of the subject in the various ideological underpinnings of the social welfare system, particularly the lack of recognition for the other as an experiencing subject and thus the potential reductionism applied to the "professional" subject (Clarke et al., 2008, 70). There is a concern that the cost reduction gained has a high prize in terms of the health of the employees, a pointing out how technocratic managerialism does not go well with relationship practice.

New Public Management (NPM) has influenced welfare professions over the last decades (Hood, 1991) and is experienced by many as a discursive structure which to a large degree has suppressed any other. The interviewees experienced this as a subordination of professional concerns to managerial imperatives. In Gail's terms, it implied "a mathematical reason" that does not have the means to take account of matters of the heart; perhaps, one may suggest, because it is itself anxiety driven. From the above argument and the interviewees' reported experiences, the case can be made that NPM is taking the form of a hero system, in that it offers—not least by its focus on what is quantifiable—a system of significance and a sense of control, including a set of rewards related to a certain kind of loyalty to particular standards.

A notion of health care as a system marked by the mere "heroic" pursuit of budgets in balance is challenged in that one-third of Medicare expenditures in the USA are spent on end-of-life, and most on life-sustaining care. This suggests that the obligation felt by treating physicians to keep going at any cost, even where the treatment is painful and the benefits highly uncertain and speculative, is not uncommon (Zhang et al., 2009). Such a priority was witnessed and fundamentally questioned by the interviewees, and in particular by Herbert and Jacob.

In reference to the individual physician or health professional pursuing treatment in spite of the inevitability of imminent death, one might ask: "How conscious is he of what he is doing to earn his feeling of heroism" (Becker, 1973, 5)? It may be as important to consider the organization in which the individual is situated and ask the very same question: How conscious is it of what it is demanding of its employees in order to earn heroism?

Being a Part

In the last paragraphs of this sub-chapter, the focus will be on the reverse aspect of being apart, namely being a part. In various ways, the narrators described a shift from not feeling at home to being at home in end-of-life care. The transition was related to experiences of acceptance and recognition from significant others within the clinic.

The significance of acceptance and recognition was evident, too, in the telling of "negative" stories in which these elements were missing and replaced by a lack of affirmation by the other. This was witnessed in stories of encounters with colleagues, patients, and relatives, and corresponds with other studies that explain how recognition and positive mentoring serve to prevent burnout and compassion fatigue, but also enhance professional development (Benner, 1984; Kalicińska, Chylińska, & Wilczek-Różyczka, 2012; McMullen, 2007; Powell, 2013; Skovholt & Trotter-Mathison, 2011).

Axel Honneth, German Professor of Social Philosophy (Honneth, 1995), places the struggle for recognition at the very center of his philosophy. To be or not to be a social and moral person depends on seemingly insignificant physical movements and gestures, or the lack thereof. The human being does not live by bread alone, but by movements of eyebrows, offering of hands, smiles—small gestures that in some contexts mean nothing, while in others separate the living from the living dead.

"The making visible of a person" can, literally in the blink of an eye, be replaced by marginalizing, silencing, and making invisible (Honneth & Margalit, 2001). By our gestures and facial expressions of recognition, we concede to the other person a moral authority over us. Simple gestures not only make the other visible, but also concede moral authority in that we have to treat the other according to the worth that we have just assigned him or her. One's becoming or dissolving within a professional context, as in other social contexts, depends on recognizing gestures from significant others. Being deprived of this recognition, one may face "death" as a social and moral person.

In order to feel recognized, at home and a part, having a professional task-oriented relationship is not sufficient. The latter needs to carry certain relational qualities. In the last part of the next sub-chapter, relying heavily on object-relational psychoanalytic thinking, I will explore "thirdness" as one such quality. I will investigate how it may play a part when the anxiety, the professional's sense of uncanniness, finds a home and thus leaves him or her with a sense of being a part.

Concluding Remarks

The above existential-psychosocial analysis suggests that the sense of being apart, conveyed across the narrative accounts, relates to the fundamental ontological situation of the human being as always being a part, always entangled with "world(s)". Angst is the condition of the human being when this every day being "fallen prey" is questioned, when the world "announces" itself and she/he realizes the entanglement. The contrasting "familiar" death of the professionals with the "forbidden" death of society may be interpreted as one such "announcement" of the individual's entanglement with his/her world.

One urgent question pursued was whether encountering the reality of death has the effect of "the world" "announcing" itself. A close reading of the narrative accounts suggests that it is rather encounters with situations in life outside the clinic that reveal the entanglement to the professionals, and thus the possibility of individuation, authenticity. and mindfulness of being. The interviewees reported an enhanced sense of mortality, and a different outlook on life, not due to encountering death as terminating event, but when encountering threats of non-being. Existential angst is the mood in which the individual is attuned, when faced with the possibility of non-being, which indicates that it was not encounters with deaths of others that "untangled" the worlds of the narrators.

The case is also made that a sense of moral conflict in regard to hero systems inherent in the health care system makes "the world announce" itself to the professional. She/he becomes mindful of her own being. Both New Public Management and experiences of over-treatment are referred to in the narratives as having such an effect. Both represent dominant discourses, which raised "strong evaluations" (Taylor, 1989) in the narrators. On the one hand, over-treatment represents a discourse that appeals to the very strong value of doing whatever possible for the patients, of "doing good". On the other, futile treatment is at odds with the ethical principle of "not doing harm" (Beauchamp & Childress, 2013).

The above analysis suggests that working at the boundary between life and death does something to how the individual understands self. However, just as central as encountering the reality of physical death is how the reality of death is perceived by the culture, both at large and within health care. This is explained not least by the notion of health care as a hero system. The latter describes how the basic existential condition of mortality is represented in how the psychosocially constituted subject is provided with, or deprived of, social and moral status. This entanglement of the individual with the "worlds", the multiple "referential contexts of significance" in which she/he is "thrown", represents and enhances a sense of apartness, but also inauthenticity and guilt, which is where this discussion is moving next.

Third Concern—Authenticity

In the following paragraphs, I will explore how gaining a voice and giving voice may be explained and related to the research question by existential-psychosocial interpretive means. This implies a further elaboration of Heidegger's conceptual universe and also an application of the psychoanalytic distinction between "true self" and "false self". The ethical dimension inherent in the concern about giving voice to truth, one's own and that of the other, will be elaborated and discussed in the next sub-chapter.

Conspiracies of Silence

Several of the health professionals voiced concern about having privileged knowledge about the impending death of a patient, while the patient was seemingly unaware of his or her situation. The concerns resemble those in Glaser & Strauss' classic grounded theory study from hospitals in the USA, a study which both echoes and complements the findings in this.

The aim of that study resembles those of the present study in that Glaser and Strauss wanted to "help establish surer ground than now exists for understanding the social-psychological dimensions of terminal care". The intention was to explore "whether people can die socially before they die biologically, and what this means for human relationships" (Glaser & Strauss, 1965).

Through extended fieldwork, including observations and interviews, the researchers sought to investigate "contexts of action rather than attitudes toward death" (ibid., viii). "Awareness contexts" is the key concept emerging from their grounded study; it denotes "who, in the dying context, knows what about the probability of death". The authors identify four different "awareness contexts": "closed awareness", "suspected awareness", "mutual pretense awareness", and "open awareness" (ibid., 12).

Glaser & Strauss acknowledge that the problem of telling or not telling a terminally ill patient that she/he has a fatal condition—a problem that also arose across the accounts of the present study—is perhaps the most difficult dilemma regularly facing health professionals, physicians in particular (ibid., 119). Even Herbert, who claimed that he did not want the patient to be inattentive to their own death, was ambivalent about "open awareness". Glaser & Strauss stress that it is a crucial question to settle, as it has an impact on both the patient and those caring for him/her. Their findings suggest though that "quite possibly also physicians, like other Americans, shy away from the embarrassment and brutality of making direct reference to another person about his impending death" (ibid., 31).

More recent studies using audio and video recordings from American (Anderson, Kools, & Lyndon, 2013) and Norwegian (Agledahl, 2011) contexts—the latter discussed in more detail in the final sub-chapter—show a similar response on the part of physicians. The same is evident among nurses, as both the present study and that of Glaser & Strauss show.

Work environments collude in "conspiracies of silence", holding back information or providing wrong information to the patient, in order to sustain "closed awareness". This describes a situation in which "the patient does not recognize his impending death even though the hospital personnel have the information" (Glaser & Strauss, 1965, 29). Structural conditions, which are physically and culturally embedded, facilitate "closed awareness"—as distance and walls, both literal and metaphorical, inhibit the flow of information.

Health professionals are not the only ones inhabiting the contexts of awareness. Echoing interviewees in the present study, Glaser & Strauss speak about patients who do not want to learn about their dire situation and/or relatives that do not want to disclose it to them. A study by Noble et al. describes the detrimental impact on staff when carers act intentionally and unintentionally to prevent the professionals from speaking the truth (Noble, Nelson, & Finlay, 2008).

It is appropriate to label what takes place within the awareness contexts as "dancing around death" (Anderson et al., 2013). One might ask whether the dance originates in the deep-seated resistance to the unbearable truth of man's inherent mortality, outlined above. This sidestepping is evidence of a strong pull toward covering up the fact that death is intrinsic to life. The following offers an existential-psychosocial reading of truth and authenticity and makes the sobering suggestion that inauthenticity is the existential default position and that individual truths are rare and very much socially constituted.

Inauthenticity

On the one hand, gaining a voice and giving voice relate to acquiring the skills needed for what takes place at the bedside of a dying patient—a necessary entangling with "das Man" in order to do one's job, the process of which is reported across the accounts. Illustrative of this was Karla's use of technical medical language and her learning how to be "direct, clear, not vague" when communicating with colleagues, patients, and relatives. The benefit was an experience of shared understandings; the cost, ontologically understood, can be that Dasein "is cut off from the primary and primordially genuine relations of being toward the world, toward Dasein-with, toward being-in itself" (Heidegger, 2010, 164).

The other dimension of gaining a voice and giving voice is that of speaking one's inner truths, voicing the experiences of one's "genuine relations of being toward the world", and allowing the other—patient, relative or colleague—to do the same. This is gaining and giving a voice to that which is not necessarily part of a given and shared repertoire. It is not about mastering a particular professional language, but about being authentically present, truthfully there.

Contemporary culture has a romantic and solipsistic understanding of authenticity as something conditioned solely by the individual (Dreyfus & Wrathall, 2007, 287). In the romantic expressivist idiom, envisioned by philosophers like Rousseau, Hegel, and Dilthey—and to a large degree very much present in popular culture (Taylor, 1992)—the authentic is understood as a kind of essential, unified wholeness or integrity, an achievement, and a conquering of alienation, isolation, fragmentation, and incoherence.

An existential-psychosocial point of view, on the other hand, is far less optimistic with regard to the prospects of authenticity. Heidegger is most cautious concerning promises of authenticity. An authentic (*eigentlich*) mode of existence, according to Heidegger, implies that Dasein stands in a direct first-person relation to itself. The philosopher is hostile toward the concept of subjectivity for the very reason that it may be followed by the assumption that one may be able to grasp the subject as a whole. Such an idea stands in stark contrast to his understanding of Dasein's self-understanding as thrown, evolving, largely implicit and not to be grasped by observational attitudes like perception or intuition (Cerbone, 2008, 288). The subject is "not at hand"—just as death is not at hand.

Heidegger's cautious stance is related not least to his understanding of the individual as always being entangled with the "world". This is part of subject's "essential ontological structure" (Heidegger, 2010, 172) and, as such, not something the individual can opt out of. According to Heidegger, although in principle one is free to be authentic, "the self is initially and for the most part inauthentic" (ibid., 175), which is a way of saying that Dasein, even when speaking in terms of "I", is inauthentically lost in das Man. This suggests that when trying to understand the concern for telling the truth in the narrative accounts, one needs to move beyond "I" statements and claims of truth-telling.

The "We" in the "I"

Let us consider the accounts of Dina and Herbert to shed further light on this point. Both physicians spoke a lot in "I"-language and with what appeared to be a sense of the uniqueness of their respective stories. Nevertheless, despite living their lives in different parts of the world, the stories of the two palliative physicians very much resembled one another.

Both talked about growing up in stoic families in which emotions were not really talked about. Both ended up in marriages that left them feeling estranged. For both, the divorce, followed by therapy and counselling, was an awareness experience in which the world "opened up" to them; part of the enlightening process was an engagement with Eastern beliefs. Both soon found themselves engaged in self-expressive creative activities—Herbert doing carpentry, Dina painting. Finally, both took on "dangerous" hobbies.

Despite these resemblances, there is no doubt that the two biographical narratives are unique, and that the narrators related to their respective "worlds" in idiomatic ways. The point of bringing attention to the similarities is that they reveal not only individual biographical traits, but also significant cultural phenomena with implied discourses, which both inform how the experiences were talked about, as well as how those sharing them felt. Just as the personal trajectories and the reported emotions left by experiencing them resemble one another, it is also true that the very same biographical twist and turns would not have played out, say, thirty years earlier, or perhaps thirty years from now. There is an obvious psychosocial analytic point to be made: namely that the intrapsychic, the felt experience may be informed and limited by a particular culturally given repertoire. Of course this is not to say that the repertoire is not acquired in idiomatic ways.

There are obvious cultural traits implicit in both the narrative accounts: The decline of mainstream Christian churches, and the coming of a secular age in the Western world, and the growing presence of Eastern religion in Western countries are related examples which informed the two interviewees' narratives about life and death. Finally, what is perhaps an even more pressing cultural trait, disguised in romantic notions, is the increased emphasis on autonomy and "authentic" living, facilitated by "the therapeutic turn" of Western societies. These are cultural developments elaborated and discussed by Charles Taylor (Taylor, 1989, 1992, 2007).

This brief consideration of the similarities in the lives and narratives of Herbert and Dina speaks of "entanglement" and "thrownness" as constitutive of human life, and as "the mode of being of a being which always is itself its possibilities in such a way that it understands itself in them and in terms of them [projects itself upon them]" (Heidegger, 2010, 175). Similar to discourse, discussed in a previous chapter, "thrownness" implies a taken-for-grantedness, an in-depth relatedness to "discursive structures". The average everydayness of Dasein can "be determined as entangled-disclosed, thrown-projecting being-in-the-world, which is concerned with its ownmost potentiality in its being together with the world in a being-with with others" (ibid., 175). Dasein thus "maintains itself in the mode of being of the they" (ibid., 161).

In an existential-psychosocial perspective, all genuine understanding, interpreting and communication, rediscovery and new appropriation come about in, out of, and against "worlds of significance". "It is not the case that a Dasein, untouched and unseduced by this way of interpreting, was ever confronted by the free land of a 'world', so that it just looks at what it encounters". This quote may seem at odds with the sense of freedom conveyed by Dina when talking about how she eventually left the "dark valleys" of the southern part of Norway for the culturally open continent. The point is not questioning the subjective experience, but pointing out that one is never confronted by the free land of a "world", but rather "thrown" into a different culturally accepted repertoire of acts and discourses. Even a profound sense of the opposite cannot do away with that.

> Though I may disown my origins, endeavor to start afresh and so on, the ways in which I do so are still pervaded by my (largely unchosen) life until now: that I disown this, that rather than something else, that I start anew in this way, that I find these things worth endorsing and these things worth rejecting, all of this is partly determined, and so revelatory of, my thrownness. (Cerbone, 2008, 96)

The expressed longing for self-expression through speech and creativity, the pursuit of self-development through therapy, traveling the world and pursuing self-realization through kayaking and mountain climbing, present in the narrative accounts of several interviewees, is very much in line with, and can be read as an expression of, embeddedness in a culture encouraging these activities and priorities. It can also very much relate to what may be regarded as a longing for authenticity and self-agency intrinsic to human beings (Taylor, 1992).

Finally and central to this argument is the fact that the enhanced sense of possibility and agency implicit in both Dina and Herbert's narratives do resemble the possible outcomes of being confronted with the prospect of non-being, outlined in previous sub-chapters. In any case, it is anxiety provoking and accompanied by unfamiliarity and uncanniness. I will pursue this train of thought below.

A Call for Authenticity

In the narrative accounts, there were multiple situations and encounters, both inside and outside the clinic, that bore the traits of angst and thus also the promise of authenticity. Encounters with the dying and death of others call for the professional to make a stand, to disentangle self from "how one does it". These are incidents and situations which engender a sense of being accountable to self and the other. Many of them involve a call to speak up and give voice.

Dina reported how part of the breakdown experience she had when leaving her original faith community, and later when getting divorced, involved a sense of not being at home with what used to be her world. It was a realization of entanglement followed by a process of disentanglement. Iris reported a similar profound experience in her twenties, Carl and Herbert when they turned forty. Gail's break with church, but also her current "digging under the fence" to escape an unhealthy work situation, speaks to the same.

When Dasein is individualized and "not-being-at-home" (Heidegger, 2010, 182–183), it is not a pleasant, but an "uncanny" (*unheimlich*) place to be, according to Heidegger. It is possible to identify "uncanny" experiences also among the interviewees' clinical experiences: for example, when Fiona reflected upon a situation way back in which her speaking up could have made a difference to the outcome of the situation. Other experiences go back thirty years, such as Anne not being able to hold the terrified and terrifying gaze of the dying patient; Bente not speaking up when instructed to deliver too much morphine to a seriously ill patient; Karla regretting being too vague too long and feeling responsible for the fact that one of her home-care patients died a not-so-good death at the hospital as a result; Leah witnessing too little being done to relieve the immense pain of a terminally ill patient.

These are stories that "haunt" the professionals (Rashotte, 2005), leaving them with a sense of "uncanniness", perhaps due to a sense of something being revealed that was not supposed to be (Freud & Haughton, 2003). At the same time, these are situations that enhanced a sense of having a say and of the importance of speaking up and thus of being at home with oneself even when among others. They involve the realization that "how one does it" may not be the way to do it. The "world" announces itself and the professional is given an opportunity for authenticity. Yet, individuating situations provoke existential anxiety, as there is a realization of the possibility of one's own non-being, of remaining "fallen prey" to "das Man", staying entangled with the "world". Hence, in these incidents there is a simultaneous actualization of the death of the other and a threat of non-being on the part of the professional.

Caring for the terminally ill and dying can thus have a disentangling effect on the professional. There is a confrontation with freedom, which is accompanied by guilt (May, 1950, 44), which I will address in the next sub-chapter. I left the previous sub-chapter with a promise of coming back to relational qualities that foster a sense of being at home, being a part. It is time to keep the promise.

Homecoming

Jessica Benjamin, Clinical Professor of Psychology and psychoanalyst, proposes that it takes another to be home with oneself. The prototype for this she finds in the mother's holding capacity in relation to the infant, her "ability to maintain internal awareness, to sustain the tension of difference between my needs and yours while still being attuned to you" (Benjamin, 2004, 13). This is simultaneously an ability to maintain identification (empathy) and observation.

Benjamin follows Donald Winnicott, English pediatrician and psychoanalyst, and his discussion on the parent-infant relationship. As part of this, he introduced the distinction between "true self" and "false self", a binary conceptualization resembling that of "dasein" and "das Man", that sits at the center of how Winnicott understood individuation and authentication:

> Let us examine the concept of a central or true self. The central self could be said to be the inherited potential, which is experiencing a continuity of being, and acquiring in its own way and at its own speed a personal psychic reality and a personal body scheme. It seems necessary to allow for the concept of the isolation of this central self as a characteristic of health. (Winnicott, 1960, 6)

The focus is the "primary process" of the individual adjusting to its environment, the entangled relationship with mother, and the early attempts at disentanglement. As in Heidegger's fundamental ontology, anxiety for Winnicott is an interpretive principle when trying to understand just how the infant is adjusting; for him, anxiety relates to the threat of annihilation. The infant is utterly dependent upon the parent to the point that there is no separate existence. Yet, in order to evolve there must be separation:

> I am here supporting the view that the main reason why in infant development the infant usually becomes able to master, and the ego to include, the id, is the fact of the maternal care, the maternal ego implementing the infant ego and so making it powerful and stable. How this takes place will need to be examined, and also how the infant ego eventually becomes free of the mother's ego support, so that the infant achieves mental detachment from the mother, that is, differentiation into a separate personal self. (ibid., 3)

The quality of the process of individuation fundamentally hinges on the capacity of the carer to facilitate a differentiation. In particular, this requires a holding capacity on the part of the parent for the experiencing child. A lack of such holding space implies the isolation of certain experiences, and which engenders the concept of "false self". The point taken and elaborated in the following is that human beings "cannot start to be except under certain conditions" (ibid., 4).

Benjamin calls the required holding capacity "thirdness". "Thirdness" is a notion that designates reciprocal influence (Benjamin, 2004, 20) and is introduced in order to get beyond impasses in communication. The latter are created by breakdowns of recognition due to what Benjamin calls "complementary twoness", "one-way" dynamics marked by reactivity resulting in each person feeling "done to" and the other "doing it to me".

Several of the interviewees' reported experiences of communicative breakdowns, which left the professional with a sense of self being apart and "world" being announced, are illustrative of this "complementary twoness". One such story is that of Bente being instructed by a superior to inject too much morphine which eventually led to a premature death; it left the nurse with a sense of being "done to", to use Benjamin's term. Similar experiences have left many health professionals homeless, with a sense of having lost their personal and professional self, in situations which carried the promise of the opposite—authenticity.

According to Benjamin, "[t]he recovery of subjectivity requires the recognition of our own participation". The "either-or" must be replaced by a "both and" in which there is an acceptance by both parties of each person's contribution to the impasse and thus "surrending our resistance to responsibility" (Benjamin, 2004, 11). This would imply the superior, in Bente's case, taking responsibility for his or her own contribution to the situation. Bente recounted other stories from later in her career which are also illustrative in this respect. These had a similar prospect of feeling "done to" as above, but in contrast to her early experience she acknowledged her responsibility for both speaking up and lending an ear to the other's experience, and thus ensured fewer feelings of being "done to". "Thirdness" offers a conceptualization of the recognition needed by the professional as an experiencing subject, having a legitimate right to authentically express herself, and thus remain a part (cf. discussion in the previous sub-chapter).

Benjamin understands “thirdness” as an “internal mental space” akin to Winnicott’s transitional or potential space. At the same time, Benjamin distances herself from an understanding of thirdness as an observational, interpretive point of reference outside of the dyad. The only usable third is one that is shared. She stresses the importance of not limiting the third to the internal safe haven, the independent observation, the theoretical position, or the interpretation of the analyst, because it leaves the patient feeling “done to”. The third thus must be relational and understood as a mental space to be acquired, an interactive process that creates a dialogical structure, an opportunity to experience mutual recognition (ibid., 23).

There is one story that most poignantly expresses both how unbearable encountering the death of others can be, and how holding capacity is a relevant concept for both patient and professional. This is Anne’s story of being a young nurse not being able to bear holding the gaze of her dying patient. She found an excuse to leave the room, and terminated the communication, potentially leaving both parties feeling “done to”. The unprocessed feelings of shame and guilt haunted the professional for the next thirty years. Was there a similar lack of space for Anne’s unacceptable and unbearable emotions, as there had been for Bente after she emptied the morphine needle into the elderly patient? In contrast, was it this acceptance of the unacceptable and unpleasant, a holding place, that was created when Gail and her colleague Sue could “scream, yell, swear” together?

Benjamin identifies an origin for “thirdness” in the “connections based on affect resonance” that plays out between mother and infant. This is not merely a mirroring of the mother “reducible to a model of action-reaction” (active-passive), but an establishing of a rhythm, resembling that of play and musical improvisation. It is “experienced as a cooperative endeavor… created by both and neither… a nascent or energetic third—as distinct from the one in the mother’s mind—present in the earliest exchange of gestures between mother and child” (ibid., 17, 18). According to Benjamin, thirdness makes a surrender (not submission), an attunement, to the other’s rhythm.

These early pre-symbolic experiences of mutuality, carrying the “intention to recognize and be recognized by the other” (ibid., 19), resembles the intimate sharing of subjective experiences between colleagues referred to, but not always extrapolated, in the narrative accounts: the collegial relationships, which Dina and Bente called friendship, and in which Carl could share "experiences, insecurities and dilemmas". Is thirdness also what occurred in relations between the professional and patients, when Herbert wondered whether he went there "because of me", and Gail said she "loves" being with patients and relatives?

Concluding Remarks

"Did I short-change him" was Herbert's way of describing what was ethically at stake in the concern discussed above. Gaining and giving voice are ultimately a call to authentic living, and to allowing the other the same. Jacob claimed that the most responsible way to deal with knowledge of the other's imminent death was to keep that truth from him and her. This was in stark contrast to Dina, who was censured by relatives for speaking openly about the patient's imminent death. When Jacob denied telling the truth to the patient that he or she was about to die, it was a choice that possibly deprived the other of "an authentic mode of existence". The paradox is that Dina's insistence on telling, was just another expression of a "complementary twoness", which may have had the very same outcome—i.e., the other feeling "done to".

Truth-telling, like the other concerns dealt with above, illustrates the mutual constituency between existential conditions, intrapsychic realities and social context(s). The case has been made that the interviewees' focus on gaining a voice represents a profound quest for authenticity, a basic human existential condition. As explained above, authenticity is very much socially constituted, but one has to move beyond a popular understanding of the term to see just how authenticity is facilitated or suppressed by context(s) of significance, some being conspiracies of silence.

The individual's entanglement with "worlds of significance" has been further explained and the prospects of authentic living proportionally diminished. The case has been made that it requires an accepting holding capacity by another for end-of-life care experiences to be integrated and not "isolated" through shame.

Moving from the singular/isolated to the shared requires more than an internal process, according to Benjamin: "it involves direct or transitionally framed communication about one's own reactivity, mistunement, or misunderstanding" (Benjamin, 2004, 33). She calls it "moral third", because it implies certain values, in particular acceptance, humility, and compassion; values expressed through an honest confrontation with one's own feelings of shame, inadequacy and guilt that enactments and impasses arouse (ibid., 41). Perhaps, this is required in all inter-subjective processes and in all relation-intense work, not least end-of-life care; and its absence may enhance a sense of not being truthfully there.

In what follows, we will further explore the interviewees' entanglement with their "world(s)", and investigate in depth the existential-psychosocial constitution of guilt, the fourth major concern across the narrative accounts.

Fourth Concern—Guilt

Moral Distress and Beyond

What earns guilt a place among the major concerns is what is interpreted as a subtle, but persistent sense conveyed by the narrators, of feeling scrutinized, questioned and held responsible; a sense of having to defend oneself against accusing voices, past and present. This concern is implicit in those already addressed, not least in being apart or a part and in truth-telling. It is a fine thread running across the accounts, making its presence known in various ways, and is most explicit in Dina's narrative, and perhaps most subtle though no less present in Jacob's account of "loose ends".

The "internal court of justice", outlined in the previous chapter, both resembled and exceeded "moral distress". The latter is addressed in the literature as a situation in which "the health care provider feels certain of the ethical course of action but is constrained from taking action" (Piers et al., 2012). Or, it may be related to the contrasting experience of "moral dilemma" when the professional feels "obligated to perform two or more mutually exclusive actions" (Beauchamp & Childress, 2013).

Studies undertaken on moral distress in the context of end-of-life care tend to focus on moral distress related to withholding treatment (Cochrane, 2009; St Ledger et al., 2013; Teixeira, Ribeiro, Fonseca, & Carvalho, 2014) or futile treatment (Muehlbauer, 2014). Quite a few are quantitative, some make use of moral distress scales (Förde & Aasland, 2013; Karanikola et al., 2014; Rice, Rady, Hamrick, Verheijde, & Pendergast, 2008; Whitehead, Herbertson, Hamric, Epstein, & Fisher, 2015), including more open-ended questionnaires (McClendon & Buckner, 2007). There is less research conducted on the subject of moral distress among doctors than nurses (Förde & Aasland, 2013). The growing number of studies addressing the issue bear witness to moral distress as part of being a health care provider, not least in end-of-life care.

The particular interest of the present study is how guilt relates to self-understanding and death. Hence, in what follows we will try to understand the constitution of conscience and guilt within an existential-psychosocial frame. The first part of the discussion will draw heavily upon object relations theory, central to which is the mutual constituency of that which is inside the individual and that which is, or has been, between him/her and significant other(s). The second part of this sub-chapter explores an existential interpretation of guilt, in order to better comprehend guilt not related to particular ideals or wrongdoings, but simply due to being present at the dying and death of others.

Guilt-Inducing Object Representations

Object representation offers a conceptual frame to consider the "internal court of justice" identified in the narrative accounts. The case can be made that what appears across cases—the sense of being accountable, of having to answer to somebody or something—is in fact the elicitation of internalized ideals about how one should be or act. This again relates to what is an integral part of being human, namely "to create nonvisible but meaningful realities capable of containing our potential for imaginative expansion beyond the boundaries of the senses" (Rizzuto, 1979, 47); a fundamental dimension of "being-in-the-world".

The notion of object representation originated with Freud, and is implied in the concept of "super-ego":

> A portion of the external world has, at least partially, been abandoned as an object and has instead, by identification, been taken into the ego and thus become an integral part of the internal world. This new psychical agency continues to carry on the functions which have hitherto been performed by the people (the abandoned objects) in the external world: it observes the ego, gives it orders, judges it and threatens it with punishments, exactly like the parents whose place it has taken. We call this agency the super-ego and are aware of it and its judicial functions as our conscience. (Freud, 1949, 38)

Freud gave the family of origin and in particular the father image, exclusive significance and thus figured that the creation of inner representations is a process that ends in childhood:

> The nature and quality of the human child's relations to people of his own and the opposite sex have already been laid down in the first six years of his life. He may afterwards develop and transform them in certain directions but he can no longer get rid of them. The people to whom he is in this way fixed are his parents and his brother and sisters. All those whom he gets to know later become substitute figures for these first objects of his feelings. (Freud, 1914, cited in Rizzuto, 1979, 5)

Klein, with her concept "inner world", both expanded and challenged Freud's position:

> The phenomenon which was recognized by Freud, broadly speaking, as the voices and the influence of the actual parents established in the ego is, according to my findings, a complex object-world, which is felt by the individual, in deep layers of the unconscious, to be concretely inside himself and for which I and some of my colleagues therefore use the term 'internalized objects' and and 'inner world'. This inner world consists of innumerable objects taken into the ego… . (Klein & Segal, 1998, 362)

Ana-Maria Rizutto (Rizzuto, 1979) undertook a review of the notion of object representation within psychoanalytic literature after Freud. She found the literature:

> … extensive, multifaceted, confusing, and enmeshed in a net of related concepts such as object relations, identification, introjection, ego and superego formation, defenses (projection, splitting, identification with aggressor), the process of individuation and many others, including Winnicott's notion of transitional object. (ibid., 66)

However, across writings and implicit in the various terms listed is a shared acknowledgement that object representations are "immortal" parts of the psychic constitution of humankind, that they "have psychic effects" (ibid., 75) and contribute to console, sustain and organize the world in meaningful ways, but also provoke anxiety, for the individual.

The fact that parents and their respective ideals continued to inform the interviewees, even at the time of the interviews, was made explicit in various ways by the narrators. All of them except Karla explicitly included in various ways the voices of their parents in their accounts. They conveyed (Jacob, Eric, Anne, Carl), praised (Leah, Bente, Herbert) or questioned (Iris, Fiona, Dina, Herbert) their parents' ideals, at times quite vividly through dialogical enactments. Hence, the case can be made that their presence—and possibly also, implicitly, the presence of their grandparents even if they had passed away—remained and possibly informed encounters with the death of others and attendant questions pertaining to responsibility and guilt.

What in particular has been challenged in post-Freudian theorizing on object relations and object representation is the primacy of the father relation (Klein & Segal, 1998; Winnicott, 1960, 267) and, importantly for the present study, the questioning of the family of origin as the sole contributor of significant attachment figures and thus object representations. Klein in particular laid the ground for expanding the notion of who inhabits the "inner world":

> … they also represent all the real people who are continually becoming internalized in a variety of situations provided by the multitude of

> ever-changing external experiences as well as phantasised ones. (Klein & Segal, 1998, 363)

This corresponds well with how all of the interviewees included the ideals of other people in their telling, not least, colleagues whose presence lingered, even though they were no longer in a working relationship. In addition, one might ask whether impersonal normative "voices", such as professional codes, organizational policies and governmental jurisdictions, can also become internalized objects and part of what constitutes "the internal courtroom"; and whether or not the voices of patients and relatives, past and present, expressing themselves in anger or panic, also become part of the internal choir of normative voices informing the professional?

Klein pointed out the complexity of this phenomenon: "In addition, all these objects are in the inner world in an infinitely complex relation both with each other and with the self" (Klein, 1997). Rizzuto echoes this, emphasizing the fact that it is beyond any discipline to provide an exhaustive answer to the nature of object representations, or just how they relate to subjectivity. Even though object representations serve the "remaining", "being" and "becoming" of the self, they are not concrete static entities "with a certain life of [their] own" (Rizzuto, 1979, 78), but rather, "a particular case of more encompassing, processes… representing, fantasizing, interpreting and integrating experiences" (ibid., 75).

Just how object representations inform, relate to other "more encompassing processes" and are appropriated in idiomatic ways, is beyond this (and probably any) endeavor. What is given attention here is the identification of a conflicted sense of guilt in the narrative accounts that bears witness to a dynamic relation to object representations, in that internalized ideals are considered, questioned, opposed, and abandoned.

This corresponds with object relations theory and is echoed in Melanie Klein's discussion of how, from the very beginning of life, dynamics of love and hate for internalized "good" and "bad" objects "combine to produce in the ego a sense of being a prey to contradictory and impossible claims, a condition which is felt as a bad conscience" (Klein & Segal, 1998, 268ff).

Re-negotiations of Object Relations

It is a "rare human experience" to have the freedom "to play with our object representations" (Rizzuto, 1979, 81). This is due to the nature of object representations being "complex thought processes enmeshed in the totality of past, present and anticipated experiences" rather than discrete objects and "entities of the mind capable of exerting actions of their own" (ibid., 83). According to Rizutto "we can only reinterpret our past if these representations can be called back and their component elements in childhood can be re-evaluated" (ibid).

This is in part what is at play in mourning (Freud & Maud, 2005; Klein & Segal, 1998), and seems to be what Dina was doing, namely bringing to attention, exploring, reconsidering and moving toward reconciliation with key objects from her past. Herbert, Eric, Gail, Iris and Carl referred to similar processes in their accounts. Rizzuto talks about this process, which often takes place in relation to a secure other, and implies "an opportunity to re-experience past emotional entanglements with objects and reexamine them by teasing out the component elements of fact, fantasy, wish, fear…" (Rizzuto, 1979, 80). This is worded slightly differently from the way Dina explained her need to "turn every stone", but it seems to resemble the process, which put her in the position to "love or hate, play or fight" with the objects, in particular the God representation.

Rizzuto suggests that this universal process of making "sense of ourselves by finding elaborations that will harmonize our understanding of ourselves and the relevant memories of people who helped to make us who we are" (ibid., 55) is particularly potent when one reaches the age one's parents were when one was growing up, or when encountering one's own death. Both can provide "new encounters with the object of the past". This corresponds with the timing of the negotiations with ideals of the past which were included in the narratives; and perhaps also with the fact that the younger interviewees, Leah and Karla, related critically to a lesser degree to the ideals of their significant others.

The question remains whether encounters with the death of others represent a particular negotiation of object representations. Concerning the dying, Rizzuto states that:

> … approaching death may bring the last occasion for a new encounter with the objects of the past: these cover the entire course of the dying person's life, and give the last occasion for further acceptance or rejection of aspects of the primary objects and others that have remained painfully discordant with the sense of self. (ibid., 78).

What about those who are not dying but who encounter the death of others as part of their everyday work?

In most cases, in encountering the death of others, there is primarily a confirmation of long-established ideals, in many cases explicitly related by the interviewee to the object representations of significant others. Leah and Bente very much related their professional ideals to those of their mothers; Carl to his uncle's, Gail to her parents', and Iris to what she called "wisdom people".

More than encountering the death of others in the clinic, in Dina's case the breakdown situation and the existential angst following her divorce were reported to have aroused object representations in a slumbering state. As outlined in the previous sub-chapter, this seems to resemble the experience of divorce in Herbert's narrative account, illustrating "the power of external events to reactivate the latent content of an object representation" (ibid., 19–20). This is not to say that encounters with terminally ill and dying patients in the clinic did not also contribute to engendering "new encounters with the objects of the past" for the interviewees. Still, the narratives in this study indicated that encounters with the death of others did not trigger actualizations and negotiations of object representations to the same degree as deaths-in-life.

The God Representation

Dina's "turning of every stone" brought attention to one representation carrying particular features, i.e., God. The God representation can be identified, not only in Dina's narrative, but in several of the other accounts. In the others, the God representation was alluded to more, talked about indirectly and thus placed at the borders of the narratives:

in expressions of appreciation of church (Jacob, Iris) or chaplaincy (Karla, Gail) or in claims of non-belief (Bente, Herbert, Leah). The God representation was more explicitly present in the accounts of the chaplains, who also gave more space to addressing re-negotiations of its meaning.

Even if the God representation can be placed on the borders of biographical narratives in "the secular age" (Taylor, 2007), "God" was in fact most central to Freud's discussion of object representation. He was both puzzled and appalled (Freud, 1957; Freud & Strachey, 1962) by "the psychic need to create the representation of a non-experiential being to which so much power is attributed". He regarded it as "the last figure in the series that began with the parents" (Rizzuto, 1979, 44) and intimately related it to "the father complex" and nothing other than an "exalted father".

Rizutto, through her empirical investigation and theoretical consideration of the God representation, finds support for Freud's claim and states that "no child in the western world brought up in ordinary circumstances completes the oedipal cycle without forming at least a rudimentary God representation" (ibid., 200). Following Freud, she claims that:

> There is no such thing as a person without a God representation. Whether the representation lends itself to conscious belief or not depends upon a process of psychic balancing in which other sources may provide what the God representation provides for other people. (ibid., 47)

Rizzuto's appraisal of the God representation, however, differs from that of Freud. Drawing on Winnicott's notion of the "transitional object", she challenges Freud's distinction between "illusion and reality" and claims that instead of it being a childish illusion to be done with, it provides a "potentially available representation for the continued process of psychic integration... at the service of gaining leverage with oneself, with others, and with life itself" (ibid., 180). Rizzuto does not attribute this to God being God, but rather that God, unlike the teddy bear, has:

> ... obtained a good half of his stuffing from the primary object the child has 'found' in his life. The other half of God's stuffing comes from the child's capacity to 'create' a God according to its needs. (ibid., 179)

The God representation thus serves to bestow meaning that transcends individual experiences or individual representations. According to Rizzuto this meaning can be actualized and re-negotiated and serve an integrative function encountering "each epigenetic phenomenon" and "each new life crisis" (ibid., 200) and, with particular relevance for the present study, when encountering death, as explored in regard to terminally ill patients in other studies (van Laarhoven et al., 2010):

> Finally, when death arrives, the question of the existence of God returns. At that point the God representation, which may vary from a long-neglected pre-oedipal figure to a well-known life companion – or to anything in between – will return to the dying person's memory, either to obtain the grace of belief or to be thrown out for the last time. (ibid., 201)

When the interviewees addressed dominant features or major changes in their God representation, they related them partly to experiences in the clinic, and partly to those outside. There are subtle testimonies that encounters and relationships with the dying and their relatives, fostered negotiations, if not alterations, of former ultimate images of God. Anne stated that it was difficult to maintain her former notions of heaven and hell, acquired through her religious upbringing, when working in end-of-life care. Thus, she stated implicitly that her notion of a judging deity had been fundamentally challenged. Carl related his sceptical position in regard to intercessory prayer to multiple encounters with non-improving health conditions despite the sincere practice of prayer by patients and relatives. The chaplain also related his position to having always been a "sceptic". Iris reported that the most important features of her "original" God representation remained unchanged. In contrast, Gail claimed that her God representation had been significantly adjusted, but that this had occurred prior to work with death and dying.

The above merely scratches the surface and does not offer a systematic consideration of the God representation in the narrators' accounts. Anything else, except "under the careful scrutiny of analysis" (ibid., 81), perhaps, would be both impossible and irresponsible. Nonetheless, it identifies a presence of God representations in the material, even though this presence is more often than not left on the boundaries rather than being center-stage. Just how, or to what degree, it works as a "transitional object" that integrates and transcends other representations informing the subject, is more difficult to say. In any case, a close reading of the accounts suggests, as particularly evident in the case of Dina, that it is life outside the clinic rather than encounters with the dying and death of others that primarily actualize or adjust the God representation.

A Guilt-Inducing Territory

In what follows, we will try to come to terms with the paradox that even when the interviewees adhere to the procedural and professional code, doing everything right, it seems as if "the prosecutors" do not leave them alone. It appears as if the narrators' consciences endure a charge against them that goes beyond possible violations of concrete moral and/or legal codes.

The high stakes at play seem to contribute to the professionals' enhanced sense of having a vital part of the dying patient's life in their hands. This enhanced sense of responsibility relates to, and is evoked in, various relations but in particular to dying patients who are still awake. Several of the interviewees shared stories about exchanges of glances that came back to haunt them.

The vulnerability of the dying patient, his/her short time left among the living, the irreversibility of the process, the realization that the professional's words and acts may be the very last experienced by the dying, are the backdrop in all cases and for all the particular clinical incidents recounted. A dimension of the encounters that appeared to be guilt-inducing in and of itself was the notion that "*you get only one chance to do it right*". This implied an ethical demand (Løgstrup, 1997), a relational issue, something that could not be treated medically, but which was a dimension of situations with dying and death that induced a sense of responsibility and guilt in the professionals. It evoked a mood, a *grundstimmung*, that informed the narrators' accounts, and called for a further investigation of guilt as an ontological given.

Guilt as an Ontological Given

In everyday use, conscience and guilt relate to objective legal or moral issues. In conventional understanding, conscience recommends and convicts according to particular ideals and standards. Heidegger proposed a more fundamental understanding when suggesting that conscience and guilt do not relate to specific acts, or to a debt which can be paid off, but rather to a fundamental dimension of Dasein's being, namely that of having to choose and project oneself onto possibilities. Existential guilt, then, is a lasting and inherent basic condition, not something that passes or can be undone. It comes with being and is thus previous to any particular "content", or any particular ideals one can fall short of.

Existential guilt is implicit to "the care structure" (Cerbone, 2008, 56ff; Fløistad, 1968, 258ff; Heidegger, 2010, 186); it is central to Heidegger's fundamental ontology and delineation of being, introduced at the beginning of this chapter. Conscience, according to Heidegger, has a fundamental function resembling that of angst, namely a calling-back from Dasein's lostness in das Man, a summoning to its ownmost potentiality-of-being-a-self, "an attestation in Dasein of its ownmost potentiality-of-being" (Heidegger, 2010, 268).

Thus, an ontological analysis of conscience and guilt:

> … is prior to any psychological description and classification of experiences of conscience, just as it lies outside any biological "explanation", that is, dissolution of this phenomenon. But it is no less distant from a theological exegesis of conscience or any employment of this phenomenon for proofs of God's existence or an 'immediate' consciousness of God. (ibid., 258)

Existential guilt is ontological in that at every point in time Dasein is faced with its ownmost potentiality of being. Thus guilt, as angst, in the Heideggarian universe, serves as a disruption of Dasein's usual routines and makes him and her become aware of their ownmost potentiality of authenticity. As already pointed out, authenticity is not about responding to a given trajectory of actions, particular to each individual, as if relating to him or her own self with the same observational attitude used to understand a second- or third-person relationship. Conscience is a call to self, and according to Heidegger "least of all does it strive to open a 'conversation with itself'" (ibid., 263). Heidegger is thus:

> … replacing the very idea of human existence understood as a unified whole with a concrete phenomenological account of Dasein owning up wholly – that is, wholeheartedly – to itself in its existence. To own up to oneself in one's existence is to exist authentically. (Dreyfus & Wrathall, 2007, 289)

Taylor Carman, Associate Professor of Philosophy, points out how "resoluteness" and "forerunning" link guilt to authenticity in the Heideggerian conceptual universe (ibid., 285ff). The former is "openly facing up to the unique concrete situation in which one finds oneself, in contrast to assimilating it to some preconceived 'general state of affairs'". It implies recognizing oneself as "a locus of accountability". "Forerunning", akin to Kierkegaard's leap of faith, is to "take up my personal commitments as irreducibly mine". I find that the existential interpretation of conscience and guilt as something intrinsic to the human condition helps to consider the kind of guilt identified in the narrative accounts; the guilt that goes beyond a mere transgressing of moral or legal codes.

The case can be made that the narratives include multiple examples of what appears to be the interviewee "openly facing up to the unique concrete situation in which one finds oneself", and a willingness to take up responsibilities as "irreducibly mine". These are situations accompanied by "uncanniness" in which the professionals rise to the occasion, "owning up wholly—that is, wholeheartedly—to itself in its existence", by both "resoluteness" and "forerunning".

Within the same narrative accounts, there are other situations, which leave the professionals with what appears to be the experience of a moral impasse, in which neither resoluteness nor forerunning are possible. There is a summoning and a sense of having to choose, yet there also seems to be a sense of fundamental powerlessness. Illustrative of this was Jacob's claim that his job was "impossible". In his case, it was as if the prosecutors' main accusation pertained to his role as judge over the life and death of patients inherent in his judgments regarding their present or future dignity of life. This aroused conscience and guilt and a demand for resoluteness, but also delivered a sense of "catch 22"—a situation of being caught in unresolvable, larger-than-life dilemmas.

It appears as if end-of-life care implies a call to authenticity, a calling-back from how "one usually does it", yet at the same time leaving the professional with limited ways to respond. Was Jacob's claim of professionalism, discussed in the previous chapter, actually a negotiation of "existential guilt"? Was that perhaps one way of defending self against an "impossible" situation, namely by "assimilating it to some preconceived general state of affairs" evident in passages about how "one"—people like me in situations like this—usually does it?

Despite having done it "right" according to "how one does it", the professionals were still summoned by the (silent) voice of conscience. As in the case of Eric, feeling responsible for that which was beyond his power to control, namely the time of death after the medical equipment was turned off. Similarly, Anne when talking about patients she had treated with the best intentions who had survived, but "possibly shouldn't have". Illustrative of the same kind of dilemma was Karla dedicating most of her account to a time when she did her job faithfully and to the best of her ability, yet when convening a meeting with the family got in the way of a wife being with her husband in the last minutes of his life. The young nurse was not to blame, yet it left her with feelings of guilt. The internal "court of justice" did not bring "positive" content—"information that is actually useful about assured possibilities of 'action' that are avoidable and calculable"; the only "wrongdoing" was having been there.

This sense of guilt related to one's mere presence is perhaps implied in a final point to be made about Heidegger's existential interpretation of guilt, namely that guilt is "being-the-ground of a nullity" (Heidegger, 2010, 272). Carman suggests that "to be the ground of nullity is to be the reason I am not what I am not. This is not to say I am to blame, but simply that it is because of me" (Dreyfus & Wrathall, 2007, 291). The narrators' lingering conflictual sense of responsibility and guilt, impossible to link with any particular ideal, was perhaps partly related to them being the reason that it was not someone else inhabiting the same professional role. It is a fundamental guilt, existential, not exclusive to end-of-life care, but one that "speaks solely and constantly in the mode of silence" (Heidegger, 2010, 262), one which it takes an existential reading of guilt and conscience to identify.

Illustrative of this is Karla lingering with the story about the bereaved wife who didn't get to say good-bye to her husband.

Concluding Remarks

An existential-psychosocial argument has been outlined above, in order to theoretically come to terms with what I have identified across the cases as an "internal court of justice". Lines of thoughts have been established that account for object-relational dynamics of conscience and guilt, how the introjection of significant others contributes to the internal choir of voices. The case is made that the hierarchy of attachment figures, the "cast" on the inner stage, is negotiated throughout life. Thus, working in end-of-life care may inform the "inner world" of the professionals. This seems evident in that ideals related to both living and dying seem to be adjusted not only to encounters with the terminally ill and dying, but also with mentors, "wise people" and colleagues.

In order to account for what is identified as guilt that is not easily related to particular ideals, an existential interpretation of guilt has been introduced. This reading suggests that the mere participation, the just being-there, in the dying and death of others may evoke a latent fundamental guilt; an existential guilt not exclusive to end-of-life care professionals. Yet, the irreversibility of death and thus the high stakes involved, and the sense of having a limited repertoire of responses, may facilitate an enhanced and lingering feeling of unresolved guilt.

Different from other hearings and other courtrooms, these "trials" do not seem to have an end, as there are always new clinical cases and unsettled older ones that are brought to the table. There are limits to how long a trial may go on, even for the most brutal of criminals. The prospect for the end-of-life care professionals though, is a continued conflicted sense of responsibility, even for that which is beyond what anyone can be held responsible for, namely when the last breath of the other is to be drawn and what existential state of mind the patient, or relative, might be in when death comes.

Fifth Concern—The Good Object

The discussion so far has very much been an extrapolation of the relationship, or lack thereof, between the personal and the professional in the narrative accounts. The simultaneous thinking of the different concerns and the research question have been a consideration of the personal in the professional. Discussion of the first four major concerns has elicited how the personal, the individual and the existential are represented, and how in end-of-life care there is something personal at stake for the professional. In the following, I will undertake a fundamental ontological and psychosocial investigation of the dotted lines separating the personal and the professional that run through all the accounts.

A Matter of the Existential Situation?

Following the lines of thought in this discussion, intrinsic to an existential-psychosocial interpretation, is the constant entanglement of the personal and the professional. Any distinction between the two should be regarded as primarily rhetorical. This is not to say that separating the two, as with the psychic and the social, in everyday conventional use, carries no meaning.

Hence, it both makes sense and calls for explanation when the interviewees, in various ways and at crucial points in their accounts, seem to operate with a line between the two, as if the personal may not be part of the professional. This is so despite the fact that several of them explicitly adhered to a discourse that supports the consideration of the personal in the professional. This is illustrated by Iris's claim that considering the personal in the professional is fundamental to relational work. Yet, what appeared as obvious possibilities for relating the two in her own narrative, were left unaccounted for by the narrator.

The conflictual relation between the personal and the professional is not merely a distinction between different spheres of life inside and outside the clinic. It is, rather, the identified hesitation by the professionals to consider self in the context of the professional. This emerged particularly in the accounts of emotionally-charged critical clinical incidents in which the reader would have expected a consideration of the narrator's own emotional experience. It also came through as a lack, on the part the narrators, of attention to paradoxes and contradictions in their own narratives.

Intrinsic to an existential-psychosocial perspective, as made evident in the previous sub-chapters, is that self is never "at hand" as the individual can never have a self-understanding that grasps it all. In a first-, second- or third-person perspective, or a synoptic reading of the three, the self evades full identification. How this relates to its psychosocial constitution and constant entanglement with its "world" has been established. Hence, a "complicating" factor, perhaps explaining "dots" in the line between the personal and the professional, is that intrinsic to the everydayness of the individual is a being "fallen prey" to the discursive structures in which s/he is thrown. Thus, the lack of linking the personal in the professional may align with how the individual for the most part makes his or her own being an issue by navigating "mindlessly" in the "referential totality", the "discursive structure", that comprises one's "thrownness". This way of relating to self is evident across the accounts, even though the variety of social contexts makes for very different narratives.

An existential reading of death complicates the matter further. The possibility of non-being is accompanied by angst and leaves the individual in an "uncanny" situation, a place in which one does not want to linger, and thus a condition against which one defends oneself. Karla pointed out how ICU professionals would not last in their jobs if they were to "take in" everything they experienced. It is a defensive stand, but also a realistic one. Perhaps, it is even a necessary stand, if we consider the "experiential burden" outlined above, which human beings deal with by taking necessary defensive measures. Is it perhaps such a defensive stand that emerged in Dina's and Iris' non-inclusion of almost any experiences from the clinic in their narratives, in Eric's tendency toward one-sided positive talk about death, and in Karla's "deflecting" when coming close to her own emotions?

An existential-psychosocial reading of the subject relativizes the notion of "the personal" and should make us cautious about using it diagnostically. Illustrative of this perhaps was the fact that Gail, in contrast to Jacob, did not apologize for bringing in her world. Was this the expression of a more "personal" account than Jacob's, or rather the expression of already "being-at-home" within another discourse, another part of her referential totality? Whether the interviewees, or anyone else, speak in terms of using "I" or "one" cannot be used as a diagnostic tool.

The interviewees' manner of telling resembles how the individual relates to self and death as outlined in "the care structure"; but it is also in line with the defensive and conflicted subject of psychoanalytic theory. What appears to be a demarcation line between the personal and the professional, it can be argued, relates, in part at least, to the narrators' existential situation. What is metaphorically identified as a dotted line between the personal and the professional in the narrative accounts may thus in part be an explication of limitations intrinsic to life itself.

A Matter of Care for Self and Others

The narrative accounts include the playing-out of a drama with high stakes: representations of being as a moral and social person; in the silent summoning of guilt and angst, a call for authenticity. The conflicted relation between the personal and the professional may be linked to a conflict intrinsic to being, namely that between "existing" or "complying" with the social contexts into which one is thrown (Levine, 2013, 19).

Heidegger does not make "the care structure", nor the different modes ("forgetful" or "mindful") of being an ethical issue, but only part of his delineation of being. He understands "care" to be constitutional for what it means to be a human being as opposed to other beings. Dasein's care for its own being—its ability to make own being an issue for itself—is fundamental to its very being, but also constitutional for "care" for other human beings or other things. Levine, on the other hand, makes a value statement when he claims that:

> Our capacity to connect with others in a way that expresses and affirms psychic existence is the starting point for ethical conduct. (Levine, 2013, x)

Levine thus relates the care of self to the care of others. This is to be understood not as "the capacity to make doing express being per se, but the capacity to exist as a center of initiative in relations" (ibid., 19). Care is not merely a matter of "care for" through specific concrete tasks, but "care about", which is more of a relating to self and others (Hollway, 2006, 4).

Authentic and inauthentic modes of existence, being "mindful" or "forgetful", in the Heideggarian discourse resemble that of "false self" and "true self" in psychoanalytic theory. Considering the binary concepts ethically as denoting capacity for care, Levine suggests that "moral conduct" is an expression of the former, as "false self" implies compliance with established rules. "Ethical conduct", by contrast, implies being "a separate and autonomous center of initiative" (Levine, 2013, 33), a "true self".

In this, there is a resemblance of Heidegger's relation between *Sorge, Besorge* and *Fürsorge* (Cerbone, 2008, 57): "even if only in private, care is always taking care and concern" (ibid., 187). Thus, implicit in making own being an issue (care) is a relation to the other(s) (care). Therefore, within a relation-intense professional context, it is a developmental task to "integrate their personal self into a coherent professional self", which "finds its expression when the practitioner is able to be coherent and genuine when relating to clients" (Rønnestad & Skovholt, 2013, 99).

A recent empirical study from a Norwegian hospital undertaken by Kari Agledahl (Agledahl, Førde, & Wifstad, 2011), who is herself a physician, is illustrative of how such a "humanistic medical ideal" is not always easy to attain in the everyday care of professionals. The study shows how seventy-one medical doctors in conversations with patients focused primarily on the medical aspect of the patient's condition and did not pick up on personal or existential clues from either the patients or their relatives. This was the case even in encounters with patients receiving palliative care: "The doctors actively directed the focus away from their patients' existential concerns onto medical facts and rarely addressed the personal aspect of a patient's condition, treating them in a biomechanical manner" (ibid., 650). Thus, they were exclusively practicing "care for" and not including "care about".

In so doing they disregarded the patient's personal account, missing out on information that was clinically important. More important still, according to Agledahl, this was a "moral offense against the patient" (ibid.). "When it comes to professional caring, the study reveals the importance of distinguishing between doctors' existential care, which they mostly lack, and their courteousness, which they clearly display" (ibid., 653). What the author perhaps found most troubling was the seeming lack of awareness on the part of these physicians that patients were reduced to "medical objects", and that they were missing what was happening for the patient. The authors conclude that the "'offence' appears to be intrinsically bound to modern medical practice" (ibid., 650) thus introducing a psychosocial point, which I will pick up on below when looking at who cares for the carer.

A Matter of Care for "The Good Object"

In the following, I will elaborate on how the professional is situated in a context in which what is "true good" is contested, and thus the personal, as "psychic reality", is not always given legitimacy.

Taking object-relational thinking as the point of departure, following Winnicott's conceptual universe, Levine identifies gaining a voice for the "true self" as the "true good". As outlined above, Winnicott took as his point of departure the original object relation, namely the mother-infant relation, and showed this to be the primary context out of which the discrepancy between the baby's "inner reality" (Levine, 2013, 193) and expressive self emerges.

The "false self" is the infant's way of dealing with the fact that the mother, according to Winnicott, doesn't always give good enough space for the weak ego that needs her support for its omnipotent expressions. "False self" is thus an adjustment to the demands of the environment, a complacency and introjection of the expectations of significant others (becoming just like them), a way of defending one's self from the spontaneous, with the cost of being left isolated.

Truth-telling, a major concern across the cases, is one way the individual disentangles self from das Man. Yet the ideal of truth-telling may also be illustrative of "the complex relation between virtuous intentions and the capacity for ethical conduct" (ibid., 101). A conflicted relation to truth-telling is conveyed in the narrative accounts in response to the question about whether it is necessarily a caring act to share one's privileged knowledge about the patient's imminent death. There is a more subtle dimension to the relation between knowledge and care though. In the question of truth-telling, there is more at stake for the professional than the mere delivery of medical information. This relates in part to truth-telling reflecting the fact that "knowledge" and "care" may in fact be mutually exclusive.

In health care, the "good object" is promoting health, defeating sickness, robbing death of casualties, saving lives. It is this prospect that attracts many professionals in the first place, because the ideal of the organization corresponds with one of her or his internalized good objects. The "shared fantasy" (ibid.) is that through medical means one can make a difference between life and death. This contains a certain amount of truth. A competing truth, elaborated above, is that death wins in the end anyway; we are all going to die. Too much knowledge about the good object can alter one's perception of it, and this threatens one's willingness or ability to care for it. Hence, one will take measures to defend oneself from such knowledge in order to keep the object good. It is a shared "responsibility" for the employing organization and the individual professional to protect the good object of health care. The measures taken to achieve this may explain yet another part of the dotted line between the personal and the professional in the narrative accounts.

The fact that an increasing amount of money invested in health care goes toward treatment for the very end of life may also speak to such defensive measures. The hierarchy of medical disciplines, in which the medical fields at the very top are those with the highest rate of saving life, may speak to the same. Both Herbert and Jacob talked about colleagues at the threshold of death refusing to acknowledge its presence and continuing to treat the patient as if s/he were going to survive. Both expressed indignation at such a "triumph of fantasy over reality" (ibid., 94), at the implied limitless grandiosity and prolonging of suffering it entailed. Yet, at the same time, they acknowledged being locked into the same dynamics, continuously encountering the expectations and demands of employers, patients and relatives, to protect the good object of health care.

A Matter of Negative Capability

The case is made throughout this chapter that there is something personal at stake for the professional end-of-life care worker. I have argued how allowing space for the psychic reality of the professional, a care for self, is at the heart of care for others since authenticity, "true self", is a prerequisite for ethical conduct (Levine, 2013; Taylor, 1992).

Amin Maalouf, a French-Lebanese writer, in his book *On identity* (Maalouf, 2012) dismantles the notion of self and identity as "one", as a "pure pole". He shows both how common and how "murderous" (metaphorically and literally) such a way of thinking of self and identity can be:

> … the notion that reduces identity to one single affiliation – encourages people to adopt an attitude that is partial, sectarian, intolerant, domineering, sometimes suicidal, and frequently changes them into killers or supporters of killers. (ibid., 26)

Maalouf argues that it is cruel to demand of the other to be only "one", monophonic, uncomplicated, totally integrated and committed subject. It is not hard to recognize the cruelty of such a demand when voiced by terrorists, which is Maalouf's particular interest. It is harder to identify both these demands and their implications in well-intentioned philanthropic organizations, in helping professions within the modern welfare state, or in research that is supposed to promote understanding. Yet, the values and principles at stake are the same here, when we demand that the other be one pure pole of professionalism.

The point taken from Maalouf is the potentially oppressive effect of relating to the other "as if" he or she were not a center of psychic reality. According to Levine, and thus echoing what has been argued throughout this chapter, there are significant forces that seek to control experience rather than give it legitimacy: internalized norms and "self-ideals", but also the application of certain management models. The religious environment of Dina's upbringing is perhaps easier to recognize as having had a potentially oppressive role than more culturally-recognized benevolent health contexts. I will make the claim that in contexts working for the unambiguously "good", with professionals for whom "nothing is impossible", it may be equally hard for an ambiguous and contradictory self to express itself. The case can be made that these contexts can be just as threatening to the subtle and "silent call" to authenticity as those of ecstatic religiosity. Agledahl's study showed how problematic it may be when the individual psychic reality of patients is not validated by health professionals. Invalidations of the professional as an experiencing subject may have similar detrimental effects.

When there is a lack of "transitional space" for the evolution of the "potential self", Levine speaks of "an assault on self". Dina's traumatic experience when "committing the unforgivable sin" is illustrative of how the "discursive structure" may "assault" the individual. This may also be the case in other normative contexts, like health care. In Dina, it invoked both shame, but also a strong and lasting desire to speak her mind. This resembles experiences in the clinic, shared by the interviewees, of the lack of recognition that implies "assault on the self as a center of emotional experience". When successful, "it replaces connection with disconnection, self-regard with self-contempt" (Levine, 2013, 15), underscoring what is existentially at stake for the professional in end-of-life care.

"Negative capability" is the alternative position to an "assault on self". It denotes giving legitimacy and providing space for psychic reality, countering pressures toward conformity. Negative capability represents a possible bulwark against reducing the other to one pole, as it indicates the ability to create inner space in which "normless" and "deliberate" thinking that "doesn't already know what will [be] produce[d]" can take place (Levine, 2013, 35). It is neither compliant with the already-known, nor acting on impulse. Negative capability is rather "the capacity to *have* the experience" (ibid.), not avoid it. It is "transformative thinking" which replaces repetition and fosters novelty and originality. Hence, as pointed out by Levine, it is intrinsic to ethical conduct and care for others. Relating negative capability to Heidegger's terminology, then, implies making one's being an issue by not remaining in das Man, not totally subjecting oneself to the "discursive structure", but rather challenging that which is taken for granted.

Negative capability implies validation of the individual's psychic reality, "everything in the psyche that takes on the force of reality for the subject" (ibid., 49) and thus "respect for the unique presence of being" (ibid., 55). Negative capability is related to "thirdness", introduced in the previous sub-chapter. Both arise in the infant–parent relation, but may be part of the communication of emotions in other important relationships in life, for example between the professional and the patient, or between the professional and his/her colleagues, as discussed above.

Intrinsic to both negative capability and thirdness is curiosity. A malfunctioning capacity to link is marked by a limited or damaged "capacity for curiosity" (Bion, 1962, 314). Professional development is a "continuous and focused search for a more comprehensive, nuanced, and in-depth understanding of oneself and others, and of the processes and phenomena that the practitioner meets in his or her work" (Rønnestad & Skovholt, 2013, 149), implied in which is curiosity. In a dotted demarcation line between the personal and the professional one may identify a thwarting of curiosity, perhaps both by the context and the individual. If so, following the outlined argument, it may impact not only the professional's care for self, but also his/her care of others.

Concluding Remarks

The final part of this chapter has underscored the entanglement between the personal and the professional, and the fact that the former is at the heart of the latter, not least in relation-intense professions. It may be important to separate the two for both professional and personal purposes. Still, the Heideggerian "care structure", object-relational thinking and the application of both perspectives in the present study, testify to their intimate inter-relatedness.

I have undertaken an existential-psychosocial investigation of some of the concerns that make up the dotted line between the personal and the professional in the narrative accounts. One concern is related to the existential situation of the health professional: the fact that it is not for anyone to apply a first-, second- or third-person perspective on self; the self always evades full identification. This is part of the human condition, and no one can opt out.

The next concern is related and as embedded in the human condition, namely that the default existential situation of humankind is that of being "fallen prey" to the social environment(s) into which one is thrown at any particular time. It is not easy to disentangle oneself from this state of fallen-ness; particularly not if part of the entanglement relates, as it often does, to the "the good object", which was the third concern explored above.

In end-of-life care, two good objects might at times be at odds with one another. One is the "true self"—the starting point of ethical conduct; the inner psychic reality of the professional and a prerequisite for curiosity and creativity, fundamental or ethical conduct and care for others. The other is "defeating sickness", understood as robbing death of casualties. At times, and also in the narrative accounts, the former is subdued by the latter. This may lead to futile treatment and leave the professional in line with professional expectations, but at odds with his or her own ethical convictions.

The final concern, which is also related to the former three, is that the demarcation line identified between the personal and the professional is related to a lack of negative capability. The case is made, that in order to ensure quality in patient care and the health of the professional, efforts must be made to make space for, and give legitimacy to, experiences and feelings of professionals at odds with the official norm, the agreed-upon "good object". This calls for negative capability and care for the carer.

References

Agledahl, K. M., Førde, R., & Wifstad, Å. (2011). Courteous but not curious: How doctors' politeness masks their existential neglect. A qualitative study of video-recorded patient consultations. *Journal of Medical Ethics, 2011*(37), 650–654.

Anderson, G. M., Kools, S., & Lyndon, A. (2013). Dancing around death: Hospitalist–patient communication about serious illness. *Qualitative Health Research, 23*(1), 3–13. https://doi.org/10.1177/1049732312461728.

Antonovsky, A. (1987). *Unraveling the mystery of health: How people manage stress and stay well.* San Francisco: Jossey-Bass.

Ariès, P. (1976). *Western attitudes toward death: From the middle ages to the present.* London: Marion Boyars.

Auchincloss, E. L., & Samberg, E. (2012). *Psychoanalytic terms and concepts.* New Haven, CT: Yale University Press.

Bassett, J. F. (2007). Psychological defenses against death anxiety: Integrating terror management theory and firestone's separation theory. *Death Studies, 31*(8), 727–750.

Baumeister, R. F. (1986). *Public self and private self.* New York: Springer.

Beauchamp, T. L., & Childress, J. F. (2013). *Principles of biomedical ethics* (7th ed.). New York: Oxford University Press.

Becker, E. (1973). *The denial of death.* New York: Free Press.

Benjamin, J. (2004, January). Beyond doer and done to: An intersubjective view of thirdness. *The Psychoanalytic Quarterly*, LXXIII(1), 5–46

Benktson, B. E. (1976). *Varat och tiden: introduktion till Martin Heideggers tänkande* [Being and time: An introduction to Martin Heidegger's philosophy] (Ny utg. ed.). Lund: LiberLäromedel.

Benner, P. (1984). *From novice to expert: Excellence and power in clinical nursing practice.* New Jersey: Prentice Hall.

Bion, W. R. (1962). *Learning from experience* (3rd ed.). Oxford: Rowman & Littlefield.

Bion, W. R. (1984). *Transformations.* London: Karnac Books.

Black, K. (2007). Health care professionals' death attitudes, experiences, and advance directive communication behavior. *Death Studies, 31*(6), 563–572. https://doi.org/10.1080/07481180701356993.

Braun, M., Gordon, D., & Uziely, B. (2010). Associations between oncology nurses' attitudes toward death and caring for dying patients. *Oncology*

Nursing Forum, 37(1), E43–E49, 41p. https://doi.org/10.1188/10.onf.e43-e49.
Candrian, C. (2014). Taming death and the consequences of discourse. *Human Relations, 67*(1), 53–69, 17p. https://doi.org/10.1177/0018726713485472.
Cerbone, D. R. (2008). *Heidegger: A guide for the perplexed.* Guides for the perplexed. London: Continuum International Publishing Group.
Clarke, S., Hahn, H., & Hoggett, P. (2008). *Object relations and social relations: The implications of the relational turn in psychoanalysis.* London: Karnac.
Cochrane, T. I. (2009). Unnecessary time pressure in refusal of life-sustaining therapies: Fear of missing the opportunity to die. *American Journal of Bioethics, 9*(4), 47–54. https://doi.org/10.1080/15265160902718857.
Dahlstrom, D. O. (2013). *The Heidegger dictionary, Bloomsbury philosophy dictionaries.* London: Bloomsbury.
Douglas, P. M., & Douglas, M. (2013). *Purity and danger: An analysis of concepts of pollution and taboo.* Hoboken: Taylor and Francis.
Dreyfus, H. L., & Wrathall, M. A. (2007). *A companion to Heidegger.* Malden, MA: Blackwell.
Dunne, S., Gallagher, P., & Matthews, A. (2015). Existential threat or dissociative response? Examining defensive avoidance of point-of-care testing devices through a terror management theory framework. *Death Studies, 39*(1), 30–38, 39p. https://doi.org/10.1080/07481187.2014.885469.
Edo-Gual, M., Monforte-Royo, C., Aradilla-Herrero, A., & Tomás-Sábado, J. (2015). Death attitudes and positive coping in Spanish nursing undergraduates: A cross-sectional and correlational study. *Journal of Clinical Nursing, 24*(17/18), 2429–2438. https://doi.org/10.1111/jocn.12813.
Fløistad, G. (1968). *Heidegger: En innføring i hans filosofi ved Guttorm Fløistad* (2nd ed.) [Heidegger: An introduction to his philosophy by Guttorm Fløistad]. Oslo: Pax forlag AS.
Frank, A. W. (2013). *The wounded storyteller: Body, illness, and ethics* (2nd ed.). Chicago: University of Chicago Press.
Freud, S. (1949). *An outline of psychoanalysis.* New York: Norton.
Freud, S. (1957). *The future of an illusion.* New York: Doubleday Anchor Books.
Freud, S., & Haughton, H. (2003). *The uncanny.* New York: Penguin Books.
Freud, S., & Maud, E. (2005). *On murder, mourning and melancholia.* London: Penguin.

Freud, S., & Strachey, J. (1962). *Civilization and its discontents*. New York: Norton.

Froggett, L. (2002). *Love, hate and welfare—Psycho-social approaches to policy and practice*. Great Britain: The Policy Press.

Froggett, L., Manley, J., & Roy, A. (2015). The visual matrix method: Imagery and affect in a group-based research setting. *Forum: Qualitative Social Research, 16*(3), 1–31.

Frommelt, K. H. M. (2003). Attitudes toward care of the terminally ill: An educational intervention. *American Journal of Hospice & Palliative Care, 20*(1), 13–11p, 12p.

Förde, R., & Aasland, O. G. (2013). *Moralsk stress og faglig ytringsfrihet blant leger* [Moral distress and professional freedom of speech among doctors]. *The Journal of the Norwegian Medical Association, 133*(12–13).

Gama, G., Barbosa, F., & Vieira, M. (2012). Factors influencing nurses' attitudes toward death. *International Journal of Palliative Nursing, 18*(6), 267–273, 267p.

Gifford, S. (1969). Some psychoanalytic theories about death: A selective historical review. *Annals of the New York Academy of Sciences, 164*(3), 638–668.

Glaser, B. G., & Strauss, A. L. (1965). *Awareness of dying*. New York: Aldine.

Goffman, E. (1968). *Stigma: Notes on the management of spoiled identity*. Harmondsworth: Penguin.

Heidegger, M. (2002). *On time and being*. Chicago: University of Chicago Press.

Heidegger, M. (2010). *On time and being*. Albany: State University of New York Press.

Hinshelwood, R. D. (1991). *A dictionary of Kleinian thought* (2nd ed.). London: Free Association Books.

Hochschild, A. R. (2003). *The managed heart: Commercialization of human feeling* (Twentieth Anniversary Edition, with a new afterword). Berkeley, Los Angeles and London: University of California Press.

Hollway, W. (2006). *The capacity to care: Gender and ethical subjectivity*. London: Routledge.

Honneth, A. (1995). *The struggle for recognition: The moral grammar of social conflicts*. Cambridge: Polity Press.

Honneth, A., & Margalit, A. (2001). Recognition. *Proceedings of the Aristotelian Society, Supplementary Volumes, 75*, 111–139.

Hood, C. (1991). A public management for all seasons? *Public Administration, 69*(1), 3–19. https://doi.org/10.1111/j.1467-9299.1991.tb00779.x.

Hui, C. H., Chan, S. W. Y., Lau, E. Y. Y., Cheung, S.-F., & Mok, D. S. Y. (2014). The role of religion in moderating the impact of life events on material life goals: Some evidence in support of terror management theory. *Mental Health, Religion & Culture, 17*(1), 52–61, 10p. https://doi.org/10.1080/13674676.2012.745494.

Iranmanesh, S., Ghazanfari, Z., Sävenstedt, S., & Häggström, T. (2011). Professional development: Iranian and Swedish nurses' experiences of caring for dying people. *Journal of Palliative Care, 27*(3), 202–209, 208p.

Kalicińska, M., Chylińska, J., & Wilczek-Różyczka, E. (2012). Professional burnout and social support in the workplace among hospice nurses and midwives in Poland. *International Journal of Nursing Practice, 18*(6), 595–603, 599p. https://doi.org/10.1111/ijn.12003.

Karanikola, M. N. K., Albarran, J. W., Drigo, E., Giannakopoulou, M., Kalafati, M., Mpouzika, M., et al. (2014). Moral distress, autonomy and nurse-physician collaboration among intensive care unit nurses in Italy. *Journal of Nursing Management, 22*(4), 472–484. https://doi.org/10.1111/jonm.12046.

Kessler, I., Heron, P., & Dopson, S. (2012). Opening the window: Managing death in the workplace. *Human Relations, 65*(3), 291–312, 222p. https://doi.org/10.1177/0018726711430002.

Kiser, B. (2015). The worm at the core: On the role of death in life. *Nature, 522*(7544), 33.

Klein, M. (1959). *The psycho-analysis of children*. London: Hogarth Press.

Klein, M. (1997). *Envy and gratitude and other works 1946–1963*. London: Vintage.

Klein, M., & Segal, H. (1998). *Love, guilt and reparation and other works 1921–1945*. London: Vintage.

Lasch, C. (1991). *The culture of narcissism: American life in an age of diminishing expectations*. New York: Norton.

Lester, D., & Abdel-Khalek, A. (2003). The Collett-Lester fear of death scale: A correction. *Death Studies, 27*(1), 81–85, 85p.

Levine, D. P. (2013). *The capacity for ethical conduct: On psychic existence and the way we relate to others*. London and New York: Routledge.

Lewis, A. M. (2014). Terror management theory applied clinically: Implications for existential-integrative psychotherapy. *Death Studies, 38*(6), 412–417, 416p. https://doi.org/10.1080/07481187.2012.753557.

Løgstrup, K. E. (1997). *The ethical demand*. Notre Dame, IL: University of Notre Dame Press.

Maalouf, A. (2012). *In the name of identity: Violence and the need to belong*. New York: Arcade Publishing.

Mastroianni, C., Piredda, M., Taboga, C., Mirabella, F., Marfoli, E., Casale, G., et al. (2015). Frommelt attitudes toward care of the dying scale form B: Psychometric testing of the Italian version for students. *Omega: Journal of Death & Dying, 70*(3), 227–250. https://doi.org/10.1177/0030222815568944.

Matsui, M., & Braun, K. (2010). Nurses' and care workers' attitudes toward death and caring for dying older adults in Japan. *International Journal of Palliative Nursing, 16*(12), 593–598, 596p.

May, R. (1950). *The meaning of anxiety*. New York: Ronald Press Company.

McClendon, H., & Buckner, E. B. (2007). Distressing situations in the intensive care unit. *Dimensions of Critical Care Nursing, 26*(5), 199–206.

McMullen, L. (2007). Oncology nursing and compassion fatigue: Caring until it hurts. Who is caring for the caregiver? *Oncology Nursing Forum, 34*(2), 491–492.

Michal, B., Dalya, G., & Beatrice, U. (2010). Associations between oncology nurses' attitudes toward death and caring for dying patients. *Oncology Nursing Forum, 37*(1), E43–E49. https://doi.org/10.1188/10.onf.e43-e49.

Muehlbauer, P. (2014). Sort through ethical dilemmas in medically futile care. *ONS Connect, 29*(2), 42–42.

Neimeyer, R. A. (1994). *Death anxiety handbook: Research, instrumentation, and application*. London and New York: Taylor & Francis.

Noble, S. I. R., Nelson, A., & Finlay, I. G. (2008). Challenges faced by palliative care physicians when caring for doctors with advanced cancer. *Palliative Medicine, 22*(1), 71–76.

Peters, L., Cant, R., Payne, S., O'Connor, M., McDermott, F., Hood, K., et al. (2013). Emergency and palliative care nurses' levels of anxiety about death and coping with death: A questionnaire survey. *Australasian Emergency Nursing Journal, 16*(4), 152–159. http://dx.doi.org/10.1016/j.aenj.2013.08.001.

Piers, R. D., Van den Eynde, M., Steeman, E., Vlerick, P., Benoit, D. D., & Van Den Noortgate, N. J. (2012). End-of-life care of the geriatric patient and nurses' moral distress. *Journal of the American Medical Directors Association, 13*(1), 80. e87–e80, e13. https://doi.org/10.1016/j.jamda.2010.12.014.

Powell, I. (2013). Can you see me? Experiences of nurses working night shift in Australian regional hospitals: A qualitative case study. *Journal of Advanced Nursing, 69*(10), 2172–2184, 2113p. https://doi.org/10.1111/jan.12079.

Rank, O. (1932). *The myth of the birth of the hero and other writings*. New York: Random House.

Rashotte, J. (2005). Dwelling with stories that haunt us: Building a meaningful nursing practice. *Nursing Inquiry, 12*(1), 34–42. https://doi.org/10.1111/j.1440-1800.2005.00248.x.

Rice, E. M., Rady, M. Y., Hamrick, A., Verheijde, J. L., & Pendergast, D. K. (2008). Determinants of moral distress in medical and surgical nurses at an adult acute tertiary care hospital. *Journal of Nursing Management, 16*(3), 360–373. https://doi.org/10.1111/j.1365-2834.2007.00798.x.

Rizzuto, A.-M. (1979). *The birth of the living god: A psychoanalytic study*. Chicago: University of Chicago Press.

Rønnestad, M. H., & Skovholt, T. M. (2013). *The developing practitioner: Growth and stagnation of therapists and counselors*. New York: Routledge.

Skovholt, T. M., & Trotter-Mathison, M. J. (2011). *The resilient practitioner: Burnout prevention and self-care strategies for counselors, therapists, teachers, and health professionals*. New York: Routledge.

Snyder, C. R., & Forsyth, D. R. (1991). *Handbook of social and clinical psychology: The health perspective* (Vol. 162). New York: Pergamon Press.

St Ledger, U., Begley, A., Reid, J., Prior, L., McAuley, D., & Blackwood, B. (2013). Moral distress in end-of-life care in the intensive care unit. *Journal of Advanced Nursing, 69*(8), 1869–1880. https://doi.org/10.1111/jan.12053.

Stevens, E. (2009). Extending knowledge of terror management theory to improve palliative nursing care. *International Journal of Palliative Nursing, 15*(8), 368–370.

Strachey, J. (1957). *The standard edition of the complete psychological works of Sigmund Freud* (Vol. xiv). London: The Hogarth Press.

Taylor, C. (1989). *Sources of the self: The making of the modern identity*. Cambridge: Cambridge University Press.

Taylor, C. (1992). *The ethics of authenticity*. Cambridge, MA: Harvard University Press.

Taylor, C. (2007). *A secular age*. Cambridge, MA: Belknap Press of Harvard University Press.

Taylor, L. D. (2012). Death and television: Terror management theory and themes of law and justice on television. *Death Studies, 36*(4), 340–359, 320p. https://doi.org/10.1080/07481187.2011.553343.

Teixeira, C., Ribeiro, O., Fonseca, A. M., & Carvalho, A. S. (2014). Ethical decision making in intensive care units: A burnout risk factor? Results from a multicentre study conducted with physicians and nurses. *Journal of Medical Ethics, 40*(2), 97–103. https://doi.org/10.1136/medethics-2012-100619.

Thiemann, P., Quince, T., Benson, J., Wood, D., & Barclay, S. (2015). Medical students' death anxiety: Severity and association with psychological health and attitudes toward palliative care. *Journal of Pain and Symptom Management, 50*(3), 335–342, e332. http://dx.doi.org/10.1016/j.jpainsymman.2015.03.014.

Tillich, P. (2000). *The courage to be* (2nd ed.). Yale: Yale University Press.

van Laarhoven, H. W. M., Schilderman, J., Vissers, K. C., Verhagen, C. A. H. H. V. M., & Prins, J. (2010). Images of god in relation to coping strategies of palliative cancer patients. *Journal of Pain and Symptom Management, 40*(4), 495–501. https://doi.org/10.1016/j.jpainsymman.2010.02.021.

Wengraf, T. (2001). *Qualititative research interviewing: Biographic narrative and semi structured methods*. London: Sage.

Whitehead, P. B., Herbertson, R. K., Hamric, A. B., Epstein, E. G., & Fisher, J. M. (2015). Moral distress among healthcare professionals: Report of an institution-wide survey. *Journal of Nursing Scholarship, 47*(2), 117–125. https://doi.org/10.1111/jnu.12115.

Winnicott, D. W. (1960). The theory of the parent-infant relationship. *International Journal of Psycho-Analysis, 41*, 585–595.

Yalom, I. D. (1998). *The Yalom reader: Selections from the work of a master therapist and storyteller*. New York: Basic Books.

Yalom, I. D. (2008). *Staring at the sun: Overcoming the terror of death*. San Francisco: Jossey-Bass.

Zhang, B., Wright, A. A., Huskanip, H. A., Nilsson, M. E., Maciejewski, M. L., Earle, C. C., et al. (2009). Health care costs in the last week of life. *Archives of Internal Medicine, 169*(5), 480–488.

Zyga, S., Malliarou, M., Lavdaniti, M., Athanasopoulou, M., & Sarafis, P. (2011). Greek renal nurses' attitudes towards death. *Journal of Renal Care, 37*(2), 101–107, 107p. 10.1111/j.1755-6686.2011.00210.x.

10

Implications for Research and Future Practice

Stop a moment, cease your work, look around you, consider what you are...
Leo Tolstoy

In *Hamlet*, the most famous play by Shakespeare, the question "to be or not to be" is the "hub in the wheel", around which the whole drama evolves. Still, death, as termination of physical life, is not the only threat, and perhaps not even the most significant, that Hamlet faces in the dramatic hours through which the drama unfolds. Death wears many faces and the question to be or not to be, for Hamlet, encompasses both the possibility of a termination of life and non-being in a social and moral sense.

In a similar vein, there is something existentially at play for the professional due to encounters with the death of others: not only, or primarily, in regard to the termination of one's life, but also threats to one's own moral and social being. So what? The following is a brief outline of possible implications of the findings, identified and discussed above. Implications for those who in specific ways tend to the carer: educational institutions and employing organizations, but also researchers and policy-makers.

K. Moen, *Death at Work*, Studies in the Psychosocial,
https://doi.org/10.1007/978-3-319-90326-2_10

A Call to Recognize the Existentially Concerned Professional

The case is increasingly made that responsible health care encompasses and takes seriously the existential suffering that no medicine can deal with adequately–the pain that comes with existence (Hutchinson & Hutchinson, 2011; Kearney, 2000; Svenaeus, 2017). There is a growing expectation that health professionals are willing and able to provide existential care to terminally ill and dying patients. This position rests on a model of care that is not merely able to address physical pain, but also existential suffering. Implied is a recognition of Cicely Saunders's concept of "total pain" (Saunders, 1960) and understanding of a suffering that also relates to the human being as spirit (Kearney, 2000).

The present study demonstrates that existential care is intrinsic to health care also because the health professional is existentially engaged and informed by encounters with the dying. The suffering that comes with humankind as spirit pertains not only to the dying patient, but also to the end-of-life care professional. Hence, any effort toward whole-person care must start with a recognition and consideration of the humanity of those providing it.

The present study elucidates how the existential, psychic, and social intersect and inform the self-understanding and practice of end-of-life care professionals. A case is thus made for an existential–psychosocial understanding and against the notion of the health professional being solely an autonomous, free, and rational human being intentionally moving upon his/her world. The health professional is informed by the "experiential burden" and moved upon and defending self against the mandatory basic conditions, as well as past and present systems of meaning in which he/she is embedded and which relate to the social contexts in which he/she is situated. Hence, any attempt to understand the health professional, or any other human being, as independent of his/her social context(s) and existential conditions, is fundamentally off the mark.

These insights gained in the present study, and echoed in others, have several implications for research, education, and professional practice.

First, there is a need for future hermeneutic phenomenological narrative research to supplement and expand the understanding of end-of-life care professionals. The findings of the present study suggest further systematic investigations of how the general situation (ontological) of entanglement manifests in individual and idiomatic (ontic) expressions.

Second, any institution offering education in end-of-life care, or any other relation-intense profession for that matter, needs to take account of the students as living and dying human beings. An increasing focus on the acquisition of knowledge, exams, grades, and marks must be balanced by an interest in the student as an evolving subject or spirit. This resonates with old educational ideals (*Geisteswissenschaft*) outlined in Chapter 3, but also current efforts to ensure that education is not reduced to an activity that leaves out the self, but rather helps the student to relate actively to his/her own being—ongoing discussions about whether and how to make space for humankind as spirit, and thus for the formative dimension of higher education (Ognjenovic & Hagtvet, 2011). The present study is affiliated with this tradition and contributes to its argument: It explains how self-understanding is intrinsic to being, and how being as self-understanding is realized in encounters taking place within professional contexts.

Third, any organization offering employment in relation-intense professions needs to be not only "communicating and encouraging" with its employees, but also facilitating "containment for the containers" (Kearney, 2000, 266). It is the responsibility of the individual professional to have an active relation to self, but it is a communal and political responsibility to foster "resilience" not merely as a character trait of health professionals, but as a communal quality, a mark of educational institutions and employing organizations. There is a call for reflective spaces, in the contexts of education and work, in which the student and the health professional may digest experience, think the unthought (Bion, 1962), and "make own being an issue" (Heidegger, 2010).

Giving space and legitimacy to the existential concerns of the professionals is important for several reasons, not least because whether or not one does has an impact on the longevity of the health professional, the capacity for ethical conduct and for the quality of patient care provided.

This may take countercultural measures, particularly so in contexts in which death has moved out of the home and is placed at the margins (the unspoken yet present) of society, but also where New Public Management (NPM) (Hood, 1991) is making its mark on educational institutions and employing welfare organizations.

A Need for Habitable Professional "Worlds"

This study offers a philosophical anthropology that underscores the inter-subjectivity of the professional subject—how it always resides within, and is fundamentally informed by past and present social contexts, at both the meso- and macro-levels. The study suggests how professional encounters at the border between life and death actualize all three levels—micro, meso, macro—simultaneously. The main concern, as the personal and subjective are constitutive for professionalism in this field, is whether the meso and macro allow for the professional as a unique experiencing subject. Hence, attention should be given to links and tensions between the professional subject, his or her professional affiliations, and discursive structures.

The professions, the meso-level of end-of-life care, have different tasks and different responsibilities toward the patients and their relatives; their respective paths to learning mirror and enhance these differences. Hence, it is fair to suggest that the various professions represented at the bedside of the terminally ill and dying patient may represent different "worlds", cultures and languages, and hence different "houses of being".

What has been just as evident in the narrative accounts of this study is how the interviewees' immediate collegial clinical community, also part of the meso in our equation, becomes their "world". This study shows how social contexts work to make their inhabitants conform to certain beliefs and actions. Such conformity is intrinsic to social life (das Man) and makes itself evident also in health professions and in end-of-life care. The interpretation of the narrative accounts in the present study elucidates the struggle between conformity and authenticity and how engaging in end-of-life care is accompanied both by the gift of meaning and becoming and by the threat of extinction for the professional.

Thus, the collegial community has great importance and takes on characteristics resembling those of home and family. In different ways, all the narrators explicitly state, and give significance to, their present professional context, or parts of it, providing them with acceptance, recognition, and a sense of "we-ness"—and thus with a habitable world and a strong reason to stay in the field. Professionals who have had to leave end-of-life care due to different forms of stress may, of course, tell a different story.

Polyphony Rather Than Monologism

The previous chapters have also explored the macro-level of end-of-life care and how it may relate to the micro and meso. In his book *Western Attitudes toward Death*, the French historian Philippe Ariès (1976) undertakes a brief, yet compelling, historical survey of death's position in Western societies during the last millennium. In regard to our own time in history, he calls it the time of "forbidden death":

> Death, so omnipresent in the past that it was familiar, would be effaced, would disappear. It would become shameful and forbidden... one no longer died at home, in the bosom of one's family, but in the hospital, alone. (Ariès, 1976, 85)

Ariès shows how despite its undeniable presence, its fundamental impact on our lives, death has been removed from everyday life. In modern times, we entertain more separate lives—and deaths. Dying has become "a technical phenomenon", which has "erased the great dramatic act of death", according to Ariès. Hence, modern end-of-life care is no longer situated in a world with a shared set of beliefs about what dying and death require of society, or of the individual encountering death. Such a shared notion—the *ars moriendi*, the art of dying, more present in the Middle Ages—faded as societies became less homogenous, more individualistic, and diverse.

Implicitly and explicitly, the interviewees in my study echoed this discursive development when they expressed a sense of feeling estranged from people outside their clinical field due to their own attained "familiarity" and "natural relation to" death. At the same time, there is, from several of the interviewees, a voicing of a concern of the felt impact of NPM , in which there is, in Gail's terms, an implied "mathematical reason" that does not have the means to take account of matters of the heart. NPM and its potential impact on health professionals is discussed in the previous chapter.

Still, it is appropriate to once again voice the question whether NPM is about to fill the void after what used to be a culturally shared *ars moriendi and* monologize the discourse in end-of-life care? Mikhail Bakhtin distinguishes between monological and dialogical novels (Mørch, 2003). The dialogical author allows a polyphony of voices in which he treats his literary persons as equals and is thus able to relinquish control over his own work as he develops it as a dialogue with his characters. The monological author, on the other hand, tries to monopolize discourse, dominate voices, and force them to speak his language, hence limiting the options for the thoughts that could be expressed. The novel may have the outward shape of a dialogue, but you won't find in it voices in the plural.

Turning welfare organizations into clusters of productivity units risks a potential monopolization of important discourses. This may limit the amount of thinking that could be expressed about the reality and experience of life and death within the health context. In a "world" in which efficiency, productivity, and accountability are ultimate concerns, there is potentially little space for what does not add up, such as death, or for the professional as a unique center of subjective experience. There is a concern that NPM applies a measuring stick to complex social realities that are difficult to account for on an Excel spreadsheet; this way of measuring may reduce health professionals to accountants and leave them with a subordination of professional concerns to managerial imperatives.

Is NPM monopolizing the discourse in end-of-life care totally? Has it become its "house of being"? I would be hesitant to conclude in the affirmative. Still, if relating Bakhtin's perspective to health care, one may make the point that even though NPM is not the only discursive structure, it is a system of significance. It includes a set of rewards related to a certain kind of loyalty to particular standards. As monological literary works tend to become monolithic unities that are closed, ended, perfect, and static, NPM can be monopolizing, in danger of undermining the dialogism and the polyphony of voices required to ensure whole-person care as well as care for the carer.

In an article entitled "Retrieving the ars moriendi tradition", Carlo Leget makes the case that palliative care is about to take on a form that resembles that of an ars moriendi in that it entails certain values and practices that are shared across countries and continents, not dependent upon or related to, any particular religion (Leget, 2007). Still, the philosophy of palliative care seems too unequally distributed in the clinic to be regarded a shared horizon. In its emergence though, one may hear a reclaiming of the professions and the need of health professions to rediscover their historical value base, founded on the unique encounter between the health worker and the patient.

Humanization Through Narration

What marks monologism—whether it is religious, political, or more subtly present through reductionist images of the helper in the welfare system—is the lack of curiosity and the willingness to extinguish individual narratives. In professional contexts marked by rapid change, technological development, demands of efficiency, and profitability, it is critical to make space for personal testimonies. Allowing for narratives is one way of re-humanizing, and thus, it is an essential, ethical, and ontological imperative to counter de-personalizing tendencies. Narration allows for the psychic reality of the individual, "the given uniqueness of every voice". Without narration, nothing would remain either of the individual or of the communal life (Cavarero, 2005).

Applying the term "hero" to health professionals may be appropriate at times, but, as pointed out in the previous chapter, it may also be a limiting and unfair categorization, which inhibits narration. It can serve to dehumanize, as it tends to disallow the complex psychic reality, the vulnerability, and thus the humanity of the professional. The result can be an under-communicating of difficult "un-heroic" experiences, thus depriving both the individual and the organization of opportunities to learn from experience. What is called for instead—in research, education, and professional practice—is a thinking of, and relating to, end-of-life workers in ways that challenge stereotypical images, foster curiosity, invite narration, and allow for the humanity of the professional encountering death at work.

References

Ariès, P. (1976). *Western attitudes toward death: From the middle ages to the present.* London: Marion Boyars.

Bion, W. R. (1962). *Learning from experience* (3rd ed.). Oxford: Rowman & Littlefield.

Cavarero, A. (2005). *For more than one voice: Toward a philosophy of vocal expression.* Stanford: Stanford University Press.

Heidegger, M. (2010). *On time and being.* Albany: State University of New York Press.

Hood, C. (1991). A public management for all seasons? *Public Administration, 69*(1), 3–19. https://doi.org/10.1111/j.1467-9299.1991.tb00779.x.

Hutchinson, T. A., & Hutchinson, T. A. (2011). *Whole person care.* New York: Springer.

Kearney, M. (2000). *A place of healing: Working with suffering in living and dying.* Oxford: Oxford University Press.

Leget, C. (2007). Retrieving the ars moriendi tradition. *Medicine, Health Care and Philosophy, 10*(313). https://doi.org/10.1007/s11019-006-9045-z

Moore, C. D. (2006). *Leo Tolstoy: Spiritual writings.* Maryknoll, NY: Orbis Books.

Mørch, A. J. (2003). *Mikhail Bakhtin, latter og dialog, utvalgte* Skrifter. [Mikhail Bakhtin, laughter and dialogue, selected writings]. Oslo: Cappelen akademiske.

Ognjenovic, G., & Hagtvet, B. (2011). *Dannelse: Tenkning, modning, refleksjon: Nordiske perspektiver på allmenndannelsens nødvendighet i høyere utdanning og forskning.* [Formation: Thinking, maturing, reflection: Nordic

perspectives on the necessity of formation in higher education and in research]. Oslo: Dreyers forl.
Saunders, C. (1960). *Care of the dying: Euthanasia, control of pain in terminal cancer, and mental distress in the dying*. London: Macmillan.
Svenaeus, F. (2017). *Phenomenological bioethics: Medical technologies, human suffering and the meaning of being alive*. New York: Routledge.

Bibliography

Agledahl, K. M., Førde, R., and Wifstad Å. (2011). Courteous but not curious: How doctors' politeness masks their existential neglect. A qualitative study of video-recorded patient consultations. *Journal of Medical Ethics, 37, 650–654.*

Album, D., & Westin, S. (2008). Do diseases have a prestige hierarchy? A survey among physicians and medical students. *Social Science & Medicine, 66*(1), 182–188. https://doi.org/10.1016/j.socscimed.2007.07.003.

Anderson, H. (1997). *Conversation, language, and possibilities: A postmodern approach to therapy.* New York: Basic Books.

Anderson, H. (2003). *Samtale, sprog og terapi: Et postmoderne perspektiv* [Conversation, language, and possibilities: A postmodern approach to therapy]. København: Hans Reitzels Forlag.

Anderson, G. M., Kools, S., & Lyndon, A. (2013). Dancing around death: Hospitalist—Patient communication about serious illness. *Qualitative Health Research, 23*(1), 3–13. https://doi.org/10.1177/1049732312461728.

Antonovsky, A. (1987). *Unraveling the mystery of health: How people manage stress and stay well.* San Francisco: Jossey-Bass.

Ariès, P. (1976). *Western attitudes toward death: From the Middle Ages to the present.* London: Marion Boyars.

Auchincloss, E. L., & Samberg, E. (2012). *Psychoanalytic terms and concepts.* New Haven, CT: Yale University Press.

K. Moen, *Death at Work*, Studies in the Psychosocial,
https://doi.org/10.1007/978-3-319-90326-2

Bang, S. (2003). *Rørt, rammet og rystet: faglig vekst gjennom veiledning* [Professional growth through supervision]. Oslo: Gyldendal akademisk.

Bassett, J. F. (2007). Psychological defenses against death anxiety: Integrating terror management theory and Firestone's separation theory. *Death Studies, 31*(8), 727–750.

Bateson, G. (1972). *Steps to an ecology of mind.* Chicago and London: The University of Chicago Press.

Baumeister, R. F. (1986). *Public self and private self.* New York: Springer.

Beauchamp, T. L., & Childress, J. F. (2013). *Principles of biomedical ethics* (7th ed.). New York: Oxford University Press.

Becker, E. (1973). *The denial of death.* New York: Free Press.

Benjamin, J. (2004, January). Beyond doer and done to: An intersubjective view of thirdness. *The Psychoanalytic Quarterly, LXXIII*(1), 5–46.

Benktson, B. E. (1976). *Varat och tiden: introduktion till Martin Heideggers tänkande* [Being and Time: An introduction to Martin Heidegger's philosophy] (Ny utg. ed.). Lund: LiberLäromedel.

Benner, P. (1984). *From novice to expert: Excellence and power in clinical nursing practice.* Upper Saddle River, NJ: Prentice Hall.

Benner, P. (1994). *Interpretive phenomenology: Embodiment, caring, and ethics in health and illness.* Thousand Oaks, CA: Sage.

Benner, P. (2011). Formation in professional education: An examination of the relationship between theories of meaning and theories of the self. *Journal of Medicine & Philosophy, 36*(4), 342–353.

Benner, P., & Sutphen, M. (2007). Learning across the professions: The clergy, a case in point. *Journal of Nursing Education, 46*(3), 103–108.

Bion, W. R. (1962). *Learning from experience* (3rd ed.). Oxford: Rowman & Littlefield.

Bion, W. R. (1984). *Transformations.* London: Karnac Books.

Black, K. (2007). Health care professionals' death attitudes, experiences, and advance directive communication behavior. *Death Studies, 31*(6), 563–572. https://doi.org/10.1080/07481180701356993.

Bollas, C. (1989). *Forces of destiny: Psychoanalysis and human idiom.* London: Free Association Books.

Bollas, C. (1992). *Being a character: Psychoanalysis and self experience.* New York: Hill and Wang.

Booth, A., Carroll, C., Ilott, I., Low, L. L., & Cooper, K. (2013). Desperately seeking dissonance: Identifying the disconfirming case in qualitative evidence synthesis. *Qualitative Health Research, 23*(1), 126–141. https://doi.org/10.1177/1049732312466295.

Bourdieu, P. (1977). *Outline of a theory of practice*. Cambridge: Cambridge University Press.

Bowlby, J. (1997). *Attachment and loss*. London: Pimlico.

Braun, M., Gordon, D., & Uziely, B. (2010). Associations between oncology nurses' attitudes toward death and caring for dying patients. *Oncology Nursing Forum, 37*(1), E43–E49, 41p. https://doi.org/10.1188/10.onf.e43-e49.

Braun, V., & Clarke, V. (2013). *Successful qualitative research: A practical guide for beginners*. Los Angeles, CA: Sage.

Brewin, C. R. (2003). *Posttraumatic stress disorder: Malady or myth?* New Haven, CT: Yale University Press.

Candrian, C. (2014). Taming death and the consequences of discourse. *Human Relations, 67*(1), 53–69, 17p. https://doi.org/10.1177/0018726713485472.

Casey, B., Proudfoot, D., & Corbally, M. (2016). Narrative in nursing research: An overview of three approaches. *Journal of Advanced Nursing*. https://doi.org/10.1111/jan.12887.

Cavarero, A. (2005). *For more than one voice: Toward a philosophy of vocal expression*. Stanford: Stanford University Press.

Cerbone, D. R. (2008). *Heidegger: A guide for the perplexed*. Guides for the perplexed. London: Continuum International Publishing Group.

Chamberlayne, P., Bornat, J., & Wengraf, T. (2002). *The turn to biographical methods in social science: Comparative issues and examples*. London and New York: Routledge, Taylor & Francis.

Charmaz, K. (2006). *Constructing grounded theory: A practical guide through qualitative analysis*. London: Sage.

Clark, A. (2006). Anonymising research data. *ESRC National Centre for Research Methods, Real Life Methods Working Paper Series*. Retrieved from http://eprints.ncrm.ac.uk/480/1/0706_anonymising_research_data.pdf.

Clarke, S., Hahn, H., & Hoggett, P. (2008). *Object relations and social relations: The implications of the relational turn in psychoanalysis*. London: Karnac.

Cochrane, T. I. (2009). Unnecessary time pressure in refusal of life-sustaining therapies: Fear of missing the opportunity to die. *American Journal of Bioethics, 9*(4), 47–54. https://doi.org/10.1080/15265160902718857.

Cummings, C. L. (2011). What factors affect nursing retention in the acute care setting. *Journal of Research in Nursing, 16*(6), 489–500.

Dahlberg, K., Dahlberg, H., & Nyström, M. (2008). *Reflective lifeworld research* (2nd ed.). Lund: Studentlitteratur.

Dahlstrom, D. O. (2013). *The Heidegger dictionary, Bloomsbury Philosophy Dictionaries*. London: Bloomsbury.

Dennett, D. (1992). The self as a center of narrative gravity. In F. Kessel, P. Cole, & D. Johnson (Eds.), *Self and consciousness: Multiple perspectives*. Hillsdale, NJ: Erlbaum.

Douglas, P. M., & Douglas, M. (2013). *Purity and danger: An analysis of concepts of pollution and taboo*. Hoboken: Taylor & Francis.

Draucker, C. B. (1999). The critique of Heideggerian hermeneutical nursing research. *Journal of Advanced Nursing, 30*(2), 360–373. https://doi.org/10.1046/j.1365-2648.1999.01091.x.

Dreyfus, H. L., & Wrathall, M. A. (2007). *A companion to Heidegger*. Malden, MA: Blackwell.

Dunne, S., Gallagher, P., & Matthews, A. (2015). Existential threat or dissociative response? Examining defensive avoidance of point-of-care testing devices through a terror management theory framework. *Death Studies, 39*(1), 30–38, 39p. https://doi.org/10.1080/07481187.2014.885469.

Edo-Gual, M., Monforte-Royo, C., Aradilla-Herrero, A., & Tomás-Sábado, J. (2015). Death attitudes and positive coping in Spanish nursing undergraduates: A cross-sectional and correlational study. *Journal of Clinical Nursing, 24*(17/18), 2429–2438. https://doi.org/10.1111/jocn.12813.

Emerson, R. W. (2000). *The essential writings of Ralph Waldo Emerson* (B. Atkinson ed.). New York: Classic Books International.

Engeland, A., Bjørge, T., & Brunborg, G. (2015, April 9). Kreft i Norge - Folkehelserapporten 2014 [Cancer in Norway—The public health report 2014]. Retrieved from http://www.fhi.no/eway/default.aspx?pid=239&trg=Content_7242&Main_6157=7239:0:25,8904&MainContent_7239=7242:0:25,8906&Content_7242=7244:110413::0:7243:3:::0:0#eHandbook1104133.

Fay, B. (1996). *Contemporary philosophy of social science: A multicultural approach*. Oxford: Blackwell.

Fløistad, G. (1968). *Heidegger: En innføring i hans filosofi ved Guttorm Fløistad* (2nd ed.) [Heidegger: An introduction to his philosophy by Guttorm Fløistad]. Oslo: Pax forlag AS.

Fotaki, M., Long, S., & Schwartz, H. S. (2012). What can psychoanalysis offer organization studies today? Taking stock of current developments and thinking about future directions. *Organization Studies, 33*(9), 1105–1120. https://doi.org/10.1177/0170840612448152.

Frank, A. W. (2013). *The wounded storyteller: Body, illness, and ethics* (2nd ed.). Chicago: University of Chicago Press.

Frankl, V. E. (1964). *Man's search for meaning: An introduction to logotherapy*. London: Hodder & Stoughton.

Freud, S. (1949). *An outline of psychoanalysis*. New York: Norton.
Freud, S. (1957). *The future of an illusion*. New York: Doubleday Anchor Books.
Freud, S., & Haughton, H. (2003). *The uncanny*. New York: Penguin Books.
Freud, S., & Maud, E. (2005). *On murder, mourning and melancholia*. London: Penguin.
Freud, S., & Strachey, J. (1962). *Civilization and its discontents*. New York: Norton.
Froggett, L. (2002). *Love, hate and welfare—Psycho-social approaches to policy and practice*. Great Britain: The Policy Press.
Froggett, L., Manley, J., & Roy, A. (2015). The visual matrix method: Imagery and affect in a group-based research setting. *Forum: Qualitative Social Research, 16*(3), 1–31.
Froggett, L., Ramvi, E., & Davies, L. (2014). Thinking from experience in psycho-social practice: Reclaiming and teaching 'Use of Self'. *Journal of Social Work Practice*. https://doi.org/10.1080/02650533.2014.923389.
Frommelt, K. H. M. (2003). Attitudes toward care of the terminally ill: An educational intervention. *American Journal of Hospice & Palliative Care, 20*(1), 13–11, 12p.
Frosh, S. (2010). *Psychoanalysis outside the clinic: Interventions in psycho-social studies*. Basingstoke: Palgrave Macmillan.
Frosh, S., Phoenix, A., & Pattman, R. (2003). Taking a stand: Using psychoanalysis to explore the positioning of subjects in discourse. *British Journal of Social Psychology, 42*(1), 39–53. https://doi.org/10.1348/014466603763276117.
Förde, R., & Aasland, O. G. (2013). *Moralsk stress og faglig ytringsfrihet blant leger* [Moral distress and professional freedom of speech among doctors]. *The Journal of the Norwegian Medical Association, 133*(12–13).
Gadamer, H.-G. (1989). *Truth and method* (2nd, rev. ed. translation revised by J. Weinsheimer and D. G. Marshall). London: Sheed & Ward.
Gadamer, H.-G., & Holm-Hansen, L. (2010). *Sannhet og metode: grunntrekk i en filosofisk hermeneutikk* [Truth and method: The fundamentals of a philosophical hermeneutic]. Oslo: Pax Forlag AS.
Gallagher, S., & Zahavi, D. (2008). *The phenomenological mind: An introduction to philosophy of mind and cognitive science*. London and New York: Routledge.
Gama, G., Barbosa, F., & Vieira, M. (2012). Factors influencing nurses' attitudes toward death. *International Journal of Palliative Nursing, 18*(6), 267–273, 267p.
Geertz, C. (1973). *The interpretation of culture*. London: Fontana Press.

Gifford, S. (1969). Some psychoanalytic theories about death: A selective historical review. *Annals of the New York Academy of Sciences, 164*(3), 638–668.
Giordano, J., O'Reilly, M., Taylor, H., & Dogra, N. (2007). Confidentiality and autonomy: The challenge(s) of offering research participants a choice of disclosing their identity. *Qualitative Health Research, 17*(2), 264–275.
Glaser, B. G., & Strauss, A. L. (1965). *Awareness of dying*. New York: Aldine.
Goffman, E. (1968). *Stigma: Notes on the management of spoiled identity*. Harmondsworth: Penguin.
Grinyer, A. (2002). The anonymity of research participants: Assumptions, ethics and practicalities. *Social Research Update*. Retrieved from http://sru.soc.surrey.ac.uk/SRU36.html.
Haugsgjerd, S. (1990). *Lidelsens karakter i ny psykiatri* [The character of suffering in psychiatry]. Oslo: Pax forlag.
Hayes, J., Schimel, J., Arndt, J., & Faucher, E. H. (2010). A theoretical and empirical review of the death-thought accessibility concept in terror management research. *Psychological Bulletin, 136*(5), 699–739. https://doi.org/10.1037/a0020524.
Heidegger, M. (2002). *On time and being*. Chicago: University of Chicago Press.
Heidegger, M. (2010). *On time and being*. Albany: State University of New York Press.
Hinshelwood, R. D. (1991). *A dictionary of Kleinian thought* (2nd ed.). London: Free Association Books.
Hochschild, A. R. (2003). *The managed heart: Commercialization of human feeling* (Twentieth Anniversary Edition, with a new afterword). Berkeley, Los Angeles, and London: University of California Press.
Holloway, M. (2006). Death the great leveller? Towards a transcultural spirituality of dying and bereavement. *Journal of Clinical Nursing, 15*(7), 833–839. https://doi.org/10.1111/j.1365-2702.2006.01662.x.
Hollway, W. (2006). *The capacity to care: Gender and ethical subjectivity*. London: Routledge.
Hollway, W., & Froggett, L. (2013). Researching in-between subjective experience and reality. *Historical Social Research, 38*(2), 140–157.
Hollway, W., & Jefferson, T. (2000). *Doing qualitative research differently: Free association, narrative and the interview method*. London: Sage.
Holm, U. (2005). *Empati* [Empathy]. Oslo: Gyldendal Norsk Forlag AS.
Honneth, A. (1995). *The struggle for recognition: The moral grammar of social conflicts*. Cambridge: Polity Press.

Honneth, A., & Margalit, A. (2001). Recognition. *Proceedings of the Aristotelian Society, Supplementary Volumes, 75*, 111–139.

Hood, C. (1991). A public management for all seasons? *Public Administration, 69*(1), 3–19. https://doi.org/10.1111/j.1467-9299.1991.tb00779.x.

Hood, C., & Dixon, R. (2015). What we have to show for 30 years of new public management: Higher costs, more complaints. *Governance, 28*(3), 265–267. https://doi.org/10.1111/gove.12150.

Hui, C. H., Chan, S. W. Y., Lau, E. Y. Y., Cheung, S.-F., & Mok, D. S. Y. (2014). The role of religion in moderating the impact of life events on material life goals: Some evidence in support of terror management theory. *Mental Health, Religion & Culture, 17*(1), 52–61, 10p. https://doi.org/10.1080/13674676.2012.745494.

Hutchinson, T. A., & Hutchinson, T. A. (2011). *Whole person care*. New York: Springer.

Iranmanesh, S., Ghazanfari, Z., Sävenstedt, S., & Häggström, T. (2011). Professional development: Iranian and Swedish nurses' experiences of caring for dying people. *Journal of Palliative Care, 27*(3), 202–209, 208p.

Jennings, L., & Skovholt, T. M. (1999). The cognitive, emotional, and relational characteristics of master therapists. *Journal of Counseling Psychology, 46*(1), 3–11. https://doi.org/10.1037/0022-0167.46.1.3.

Kaasa, S. (2008). *Palliasjon: Nordisk lærebok* [Palliation: Nordic textbook]. Oslo: Gyldendal akademisk.

Kalicińska, M., Chylińska, J., & Wilczek-Różyczka, E. (2012). Professional burnout and social support in the workplace among hospice nurses and midwives in Poland. *International Journal of Nursing Practice, 18*(6), 595–603, 599p. https://doi.org/10.1111/ijn.12003.

Karanikola, M. N. K., Albarran, J. W., Drigo, E., Giannakopoulou, M., Kalafati, M., Mpouzika, M., et al. (2014). Moral distress, autonomy and nurse-physician collaboration among intensive care unit nurses in Italy. *Journal of Nursing Management, 22*(4), 472–484. https://doi.org/10.1111/jonm.12046.

Kearney, M. (2000). *A place of healing: Working with suffering in living and dying*. Oxford: Oxford University Press.

Kessler, I., Heron, P., & Dopson, S. (2012). Opening the window: Managing death in the workplace. *Human Relations, 65*(3), 291–312, 222p. https://doi.org/10.1177/0018726711430002.

Kiser, B. (2015). The worm at the core: On the role of death in life. *Nature, 522*(7544), 33.

Klein, M. (1959). *The psycho-analysis of children*. London: Hogarth Press.

Klein, M. (1997). *Envy and gratitude and other works 1946–1963*. London: Vintage.
Klein, M., & Segal, H. (1998). *Love, guilt and reparation and other works 1921–1945*. London: Vintage.
Kubler-Ross, E. (1973). *On death and dying*. Hoboken: Taylor & Francis.
Lasch, C. (1991). *The culture of narcissism: American life in an age of diminishing expectations*. New York: W. W. Norton & Company.
Lave, J., & Wenger, E. (1991). *Situated learning: Legitimate peripheral participation*. Cambridge: Cambridge University Press.
Leget, C. (2007). Retrieving the ars moriendi tradition. *Medicine Health Care and Philosophy, 10*, 313. https://doi.org/10.1007/s11019-006-9045-z.
Lerner, R. M. (1983). *Developmental psychology: Historical and philosophical perspectives*. Mahwah, NJ: L. Erlbaum Associates.
Lester, D., & Abdel-Khalek, A. (2003). The Collett-Lester fear of death scale: A correction. *Death Studies, 27*(1), 81–85, 85p.
Levine, D. P. (2013). *The capacity for ethical conduct: On psychic existence and the way we relate to others*. London and New York: Routledge.
Lewis, A. M. (2014). Terror management theory applied clinically: Implications for existential-integrative psychotherapy. *Death Studies, 38*(6), 412–417, 416p. https://doi.org/10.1080/07481187.2012.753557.
Lindseth, A., & Norberg, A. (2004). A phenomenological hermeneutical method for researching lived experience. *Scandinavian Journal of Caring Sciences, 18*(2), 145–153. https://doi.org/10.1111/j.1471-6712.2004.00258.x.
Løgstrup, K. E. (1997). *The ethical demand*. Notre Dame, IL: University of Notre Dame Press.
Maalouf, A. (2012). *In the name of identity: Violence and the need to belong*. New York: Arcade Publishing.
Martins Pereira, S., Fonseca, A. M., & Sofia Carvalho, A. (2011). Burnout in palliative care: A systematic review. *Nursing Ethics, 18*(3), 317–326. https://doi.org/10.1177/0969733011398092.
Mastroianni, C., Piredda, M., Taboga, C., Mirabella, F., Marfoli, E., Casale, G., De Marinis, M. G. (2015). Frommelt attitudes toward care of the dying scale form B: Psychometric testing of the Italian version for students. *Omega: Journal of Death & Dying, 70*(3), 227–250. https://doi.org/10.1177/0030222815568944.
Matsui, M., & Braun, K. (2010). Nurses' and care workers' attitudes toward death and caring for dying older adults in Japan. *International Journal of Palliative Nursing, 16*(12), 593–598, 596p.
May, R. (1950). *The meaning of anxiety*. New York: Ronald Press Company.

McClendon, H., & Buckner, E. B. (2007). Distressing situations in the intensive care unit. *Dimensions of Critical Care Nursing, 26*(5), 199–206.

McMullen, L. (2007). Oncology nursing and compassion fatigue: Caring until it hurts. Who is caring for the caregiver? *Oncology Nursing Forum, 34*(2), 491–492.

Menzies-Lyth, I. ([1959] 1988). The function of social systems as a defence against anxiety in selected essays: Containing anxiety in institutions (Vol. 1, pp. 43–48). London: Free Association Books. (The function of social systems as a defence against anxiety: A report on a study of the nursing service of a general hospital, first published in*Human Relations* (1959) *13*, 95–121).

Michal, B., Dalya, G., & Beatrice, U. (2010). Associations between oncology nurses' attitudes toward death and caring for dying patients. *Oncology Nursing Forum, 37*(1), E43–E49. https://doi.org/10.1188/10.onf.e43-e49.

Mishler, E. G. (1986). *Research interviewing: Context and narrative*. Cambridge and London: Harvard University Press.

Moore, C. D. (2006). *Leo Tolstoy: Spiritual writings*. Maryknoll, NY: Orbis Books.

Moore, N. (2012). The politics & ethics of naming: Questioning anonymisation in (archival) research. *International Journal of Social Research Methodology, 15*(4), 331–340. https://doi.org/10.1080/13645579.2012.688330.

Mørch, A. J. (2003). *Mikhail Bakhtin, Latter og Dialog, Utvalgte Skrifter* [Mikhail Bakhtin, laughter and dialogue, selected writings]. Oslo: Cappelen akademiske.

Muehlbauer, P. (2014). Sort through ethical dilemmas in medically futile care. *ONS Connect, 29*(2), 42.

Murty, S. A., Sanders, S., & Stensland, M. (2015). End-of-life care as a field of practice in the social work curriculum. *Journal of Social Work in End-of-Life and Palliative Care, 11*(1), 11–26. https://doi.org/10.1080/15524256.2015.1021071.

Nasjonalt handlingsprogram for pallliasjon i kreftomsorgen. (2015). *National program for pallation in cancer care*. Retrieved from https://helsedirektoratet.no/retningslinjer/nasjonalt-handlingsprogram-med-retningslinjer-for-palliasjon-i-kreftomsorgen.

Neimeyer, R. A. (1994). *Death anxiety handbook: Research, instrumentation, and application*. London and New York: Taylor & Francis.

Nicholson, C. (2013, September). Holding it together: A psycho-social exploration of living with frailty in old age. *International Journal of Nursing Studies, 50*(9), 1172–1179. https://doi.org/10.1016/j.ijnurstu.2012.01.006. Epub 2012 February 4.

Noble, S. I. R., Nelson, A., & Finlay, I. G. (2008). Challenges faced by palliative care physicians when caring for doctors with advanced cancer. *Palliative Medicine, 22*(1), 71–76.

Noyes, R., Jr. (1980). Attitude change following near-death experiences. *Psychiatry, 43*(3), 234–242.

Nyeng, F., & Taylor, C. (2000). *Det autentiske menneske: med Charles Taylors blikk på menneskevitenskap og moral* [The authentic human being: With Charles Taylor's perspective on human sciences and morality]. Bergen: Fagbokforl.

Ognjenovic, G., & Hagtvet, B. (2011). *Dannelse: tenkning, modning, refleksjon: nordiske perspektiver på allmenndannelsens nødvendighet i høyere utdanning og forskning* [Formation: thinking, maturing, reflection: Nordic perspectives on the necessity of formation in higher education and in research]. Oslo: Dreyers forl.

Olesen, H. S. (2013). The societal nature of subjectivity: An interdisciplinary methodological challenge. *Historical Social Research, 38*(2), 7–25.

Pearlman, L. A., & Saakvitne, K. W. (1995). *Trauma and the therapist: Countertransference and vicarious traumatization in psychotherapy with incest survivors*. New York: Norton.

Peters, L., Cant, R., Payne, S., O'Connor, M., McDermott, F., Hood, K., et al. (2013). Emergency and palliative care nurses' levels of anxiety about death and coping with death: A questionnaire survey. *Australasian Emergency Nursing Journal, 16*(4), 152–159. https://doi.org/10.1016/j.aenj.2013.08.001.

Petrovskaya, O. (2014). Is there nursing phenomenology after Paley? Essay on rigorous reading. *Nursing Philosophy, 15*(1), 60–71. https://doi.org/10.1111/nup.12045.

Piers, R. D., Van den Eynde, M., Steeman, E., Vlerick, P., Benoit, D. D., & Van Den Noortgate, N. J.s (2012). End-of-life care of the geriatric patient and nurses' moral distress. *Journal of the American Medical Directors Association, 13*(1), 80.e87–80.e13. https://doi.org/10.1016/j.jamda.2010.12.014.

Pizzi, M. A. (2014). Promoting health, wellness, and quality of life at the end-of-life. *Journal of Allied Health, 43*(4), 212–220, 219p.

Powell, I. (2013). Can you see me? Experiences of nurses working night shift in Australian regional hospitals: A qualitative case study. *Journal of Advanced Nursing, 69*(10), 2172–2184, 2113p. https://doi.org/10.1111/jan.12079.

Ramvi, E. (2007). *Læring av erfaring? et psykoanalytisk blikk på læreres læring*. Forskerskolen i livslang læring [Learning from experience? A psychoanalytic perspective on teachers' learning]. Roskilde: Roskilde universitetscenter.

Rank, O. (1932). *The myth of the birth of the hero and other writings*. New York: Random House.

Rank, O. (1973). *The trauma of birth*. New York: Harper Torchbooks.

Rashotte, J. (2005). Dwelling with stories that haunt us: Building a meaningful nursing practice. *Nursing Inquiry, 12*(1), 34–42. https://doi.org/10.1111/j.1440-1800.2005.00248.x.

Rendtorff, J. D. (2000). *Paul Ricoeurs filosofi* [The philosophy of Paul Ricoeur]. København: Hans Reitzels Forlag.

Rice, E. M., Rady, M. Y., Hamrick, A., Verheijde, J. L., & Pendergast, D. K. (2008). Determinants of moral distress in medical and surgical nurses at an adult acute tertiary care hospital. *Journal of Nursing Management, 16*(3), 360–373. https://doi.org/10.1111/j.1365-2834.2007.00798.x.

Ricoeur, P. (1988). *Time and narrative* (Vol. 3). Chicago: University of Chicago Press.

Ricoeur, P. (1992). *Oneself as another*. Chicago: University of Chicago Press.

Rittel, H., & Webber, M. (1973). Dilemmas in a general theory of planning. *Integrating Knowledge and Practice to Advance Human Dignity, 4*(2), 155–169. https://doi.org/10.1007/BF01405730.

Rizzuto, A.-M. (1979). *The birth of the living God: A psychoanalytic study*. Chicago: University of Chicago Press.

Rogers, C. R. (1965). *Client-centered therapy*. Boston, MA: Houghton Mifflin Company.

Roseneil, S. (2009). Haunting in an age of individualization: Subjectivity, relationality and the traces of the lives of others. *European Societies, 11*(3), 411–430. https://doi.org/10.1080/14616690902764823.

Rønnestad, M. H., & Skovholt, T. M. (2013). *The developing practitioner: Growth and stagnation of therapists and counselors*. New York: Routledge.

Sabin-Farrell, R., & Turpin, G. (2003). Vicarious traumatization: Implications for the mental health of health workers? *Clinical Psychology Review, 23*(3), 449–480. https://doi.org/10.1016/S0272-7358(03)00030-8.

Saunders, B., Kitzinger, J., & Kitzinger, C. (2015). Anonymising interview data: Challenges and compromise in practice. *Qualitative Research, 15*(5), 616–632. https://doi.org/10.1177/1468794114550439.

Saunders, C. (1960). *Care of the dying: Euthanasia, control of pain in terminal cancer, and mental distress in the dying*. London: Macmillan.

Schön, D. A. (1991). *The reflective practitioner: How professionals think in action*. Aldershot: Avebury.

Sedgwick, E. K., & Frank, A. (2003). *Touching feeling: Affect, pedagogy, performativity*. Durham, NC: Duke University Press.

Sinclair, H. A. H., & Hamill, C. (2007). Does vicarious traumatisation affect oncology nurses? A literature review. *European Journal of Oncology Nursing, 11*(4), 348–356. https://doi.org/10.1016/j.ejon.2007.02.007.

Skjervheim, H. (1974). Objectivism and the study of man. *Inquiry: An Interdisciplinary Journal of Philosophy, 17*, 213–239, 265–302.

Skovholt, T. M. (2012). *Becoming a therapist: On the path to mastery*. Hoboken, NJ: Wiley.

Skovholt, T. M., & Trotter-Mathison, M. J. (2011). *The resilient practitioner: Burnout prevention and self-care strategies for counselors, therapists, teachers, and health professionals*. New York: Routledge.

Skovholt, T. S., Hage, S. M., Kachgal, M. M., & Gama, E. P. (2007). An interview with Sunny Hansen: Pioneer and innovator in counseling and career development. *Journal of Counseling & Development, 85*(2), 216–226.

Snyder, C. R., & Forsyth, D. R. (1991). *Handbook of social and clinical psychology: The health perspective* (Vol. 162). New York: Pergamon Press.

St Ledger, U., Begley, A., Reid, J., Prior, L., McAuley, D., & Blackwood, B. (2013). Moral distress in end-of-life care in the intensive care unit. *Journal of Advanced Nursing, 69*(8), 1869–1880. https://doi.org/10.1111/jan.12053.

Stevens, E. (2009). Extending knowledge of terror management theory to improve palliative nursing care. *International Journal of Palliative Nursing, 15*(8), 368–370.

Stokkeland, J. M. (2011). *Å gi og å ta imot: Donald Meltzers psykoanalytiske tenkning i tradisjonen fra Melanie Klein og Wilfred Bion* [To give and to receive: Donald Meltzer's psychoanalytic thinking in the tradition of Melanie Klein and Wilfred Bion]. Tromsø: Universitetet i Tromsø, Fakultet for humaniora, samfunnsvitenskap og lærerutdanning, Institutt for lærerutdanning og pedagogikk.

Stolorow, R. D. (2011). *World, affectivity, trauma: Heidegger and post-Cartesian psychoanalysis*. New York: Routledge.

Stolorow, R. D., & Atwood, G. E. (1992). *Contexts of being: The intersubjective foundations of psychological life*. Hillsdale, NJ: Analytic Press.

Stolorow, R. D., Atwood, G. E., & Brandchaft, B. (1994). *The intersubjective perspective*. Northvale, NJ: J. Aronson.

Strachey, J. (1957). *The standard edition of the complete psychological works of Sigmund Freud* (Vol. xiv). London: The Hogarth Press.

Stubblefield, C., & Murray, R. L. (2002). A phenomenological framework for psychiatric nursing research. *Archives of Psychiatric Nursing, 16*, 149–155.

Svenaeus, F. (2017). *Phenomenological bioethics: Medical technologies, human suffering and the meaning of being alive*. New York: Routledge.

Taylor, C. (1989). *Sources of the self: The making of the modern identity*. Cambridge: Cambridge University Press.

Taylor, C. (1992). *The ethics of authenticity*. Cambridge, MA: Harvard University Press.

Taylor, C. (2007). *A secular age*. Cambridge, MA: Belknap Press of Harvard University Press.

Taylor, L. D. (2012). Death and television: Terror management theory and themes of law and justice on television. *Death Studies, 36*(4), 340–359, 320p. https://doi.org/10.1080/07481187.2011.553343.

Teixeira, C., Ribeiro, O., Fonseca, A. M., & Carvalho, A. S. (2014). Ethical decision making in intensive care units: A burnout risk factor? Results from a multicentre study conducted with physicians and nurses. *Journal of Medical Ethics, 40*(2), 97–103. https://doi.org/10.1136/medethics-2012-100619.

Thagaard, T. (2013). *Systematikk og innlevelse. En innføring i kvalitativ metode* (4rd ed.) [An introduction to qualitative method]. Bergen: Fagbokforlaget.

Thiemann, P., Quince, T., Benson, J., Wood, D., & Barclay, S. (2015). Medical students' death anxiety: Severity and association with psychological health and attitudes toward palliative care. *Journal of Pain and Symptom Management, 50*(3), 335–342, 332p. https://doi.org/10.1016/j.jpainsymman.2015.03.014.

Tillich, P. (1951). *Systematic theology* (Vol. 1). Chicago: The University of Chicago Press.

Tillich, P. (2000). *The courage to be* (2nd ed.). Yale: Yale University Press.

Tolstoy, L. (1989). *The death of Ivan Ilych*. London: Penguin Books.

Trotter-Mathison, M., Koch, J. M., Sanger, S., & Skovholt, T. M. (2010). *Voices from the field: Defining moments in counselor and therapist development*. New York and London: Taylor & Francis.

Van Laarhoven, H. W. M., Schilderman, J., Vissers, K. C., Verhagen, C. A. H. H. V. M., & Prins, J. (2010). Images of god in relation to coping strategies of palliative cancer patients. *Journal of Pain & Symptom Management, 40*(4), 495–501. https://doi.org/10.1016/j.jpainsymman.2010.02.021.

Van Mol, M. M. C., Kompanje, E. J. O., Benoit, D. D., Bakker, J., & Nijkamp, M. D. (2015). The prevalence of compassion fatigue and burnout among healthcare professionals in intensive care units: A systematic review. *PLoS One, 10*(8), e0136955–e0136955. https://doi.org/10.1371/journal.pone.0136955.

Vetlesen, A. J., & Stänicke, E. (1999). *Fra hermeneutikk til psykoanalyse: muligheter og grenser i filosofiens møte med psykoanalysen* [From hermeneutics to psychoanalysis: Possibilities and limitations in the encounter between philosophy and psychoanalysis]. Oslo: Ad notam Gyldendal.

Von Gennep, A. (1960). *Rites of passage*. London: Routledge & Kegan Paul Ltd.

Walkerdine, V. (2008). Contextualizing debates about psycho-social studies. *Psychoanalysis, Culture and Society, 13*, 341–345.

Webster (1989). *Webster'sencyclopedic unabridged dictionary of the English language*. New York: Gramercy Books.

Wengraf, T. (2001). *Qualititative research interviewing: Biographic narrative and semi structured methods*. London: Sage.

Wengraf, T. (2011). *BNIM short guide bound with the BNIM detailed manual.* Interviewing for life-histories, lived periods and situations, and ongoing personal experiencing using the Biographic-Narrative Interpretive Method (BNIM).

Whitehead, P. B., Herbertson, R. K., Hamric, A. B., Epstein, E. G., & Fisher, J. M. (2015). Moral distress among healthcare professionals: Report of an institution-wide survey. *Journal of Nursing Scholarship, 47*(2), 117–125. https://doi.org/10.1111/jnu.12115.

Whittemore, R., Chase, S. K., & Mandle, C. L. (2001). Validity in qualitative research. *Qualitative Health Research, 11*(4), 522.

WHO. (2011, 2016). http://www.who.int/cancer/palliative/definition/en/.

Winnicott, D. W. (1960). The theory of the parent-infant relationship. *International Journal of Psycho-Analysis, 41*, 585–595.

Yalom, I. D. (1998). *The Yalom reader: Selections from the work of a master therapist and storyteller*. New York: Basic Books.

Yalom, I. D. (2008). *Staring at the sun: Overcoming the terror of death*. San Francisco: Jossey-Bass.

Zhang, B., Wright, A. A., Huskanip, H. A., Nilsson, M. E., Maciejewski, M. L., Earle, C. C., et al. (2009). Health care costs in the last week of life. *Archives of Internal Medicine, 169*(5), 480–488.

Zyga, S., Malliarou, M., Lavdaniti, M., Athanasopoulou, M., & Sarafis, P. (2011). Greek renal nurses' attitudes towards death. *Journal of Renal Care*, 37(2), 101–107, 107p. https://doi.org/10.1111/j.1755-6686.2011.00210.x.

Index

K. Moen, *Death at Work*, Studies in the Psychosocial,
https://doi.org/10.1007/978-3-319-90326-2

FSC
www.fsc.org
MIX
Papier | Fördert
gute Waldnutzung
FSC® C083411

Kolibri 360 GmbH
Ferdinand-Jühlke-Straße 7
99095 Erfurt, Deutschland
produktsicherheit@kolibri360.de